the *everyday* supermodel

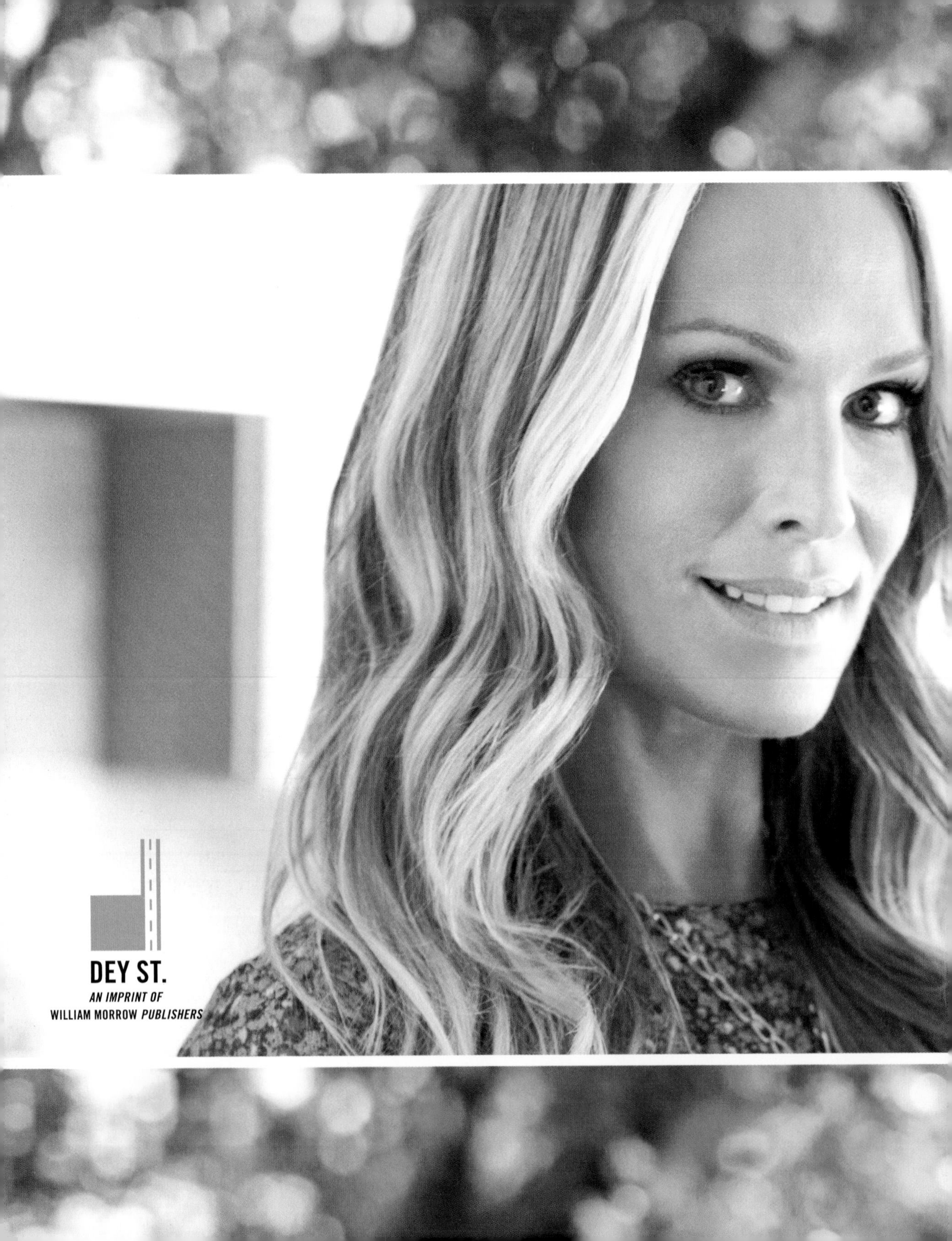
DEY ST.
AN IMPRINT OF
WILLIAM MORROW PUBLISHERS

MOLLY SIMS

with TRACY O'CONNOR

the *everyday* supermodel

MY BEAUTY, FASHION, and WELLNESS SECRETS MADE *simple*

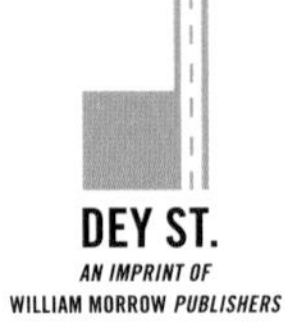

Page 328 constitutes a continuation of the copyright page.

FIRST EDITION

BOOK DESIGN BY SHUBHANI SARKAR

Library of Congress Cataloging-in-Publication Data has been applied for.

ISBN 978-0-06-227415-1

15 16 17 18 19 OV/RRD 10 9 8 7 6 5 4 3 2

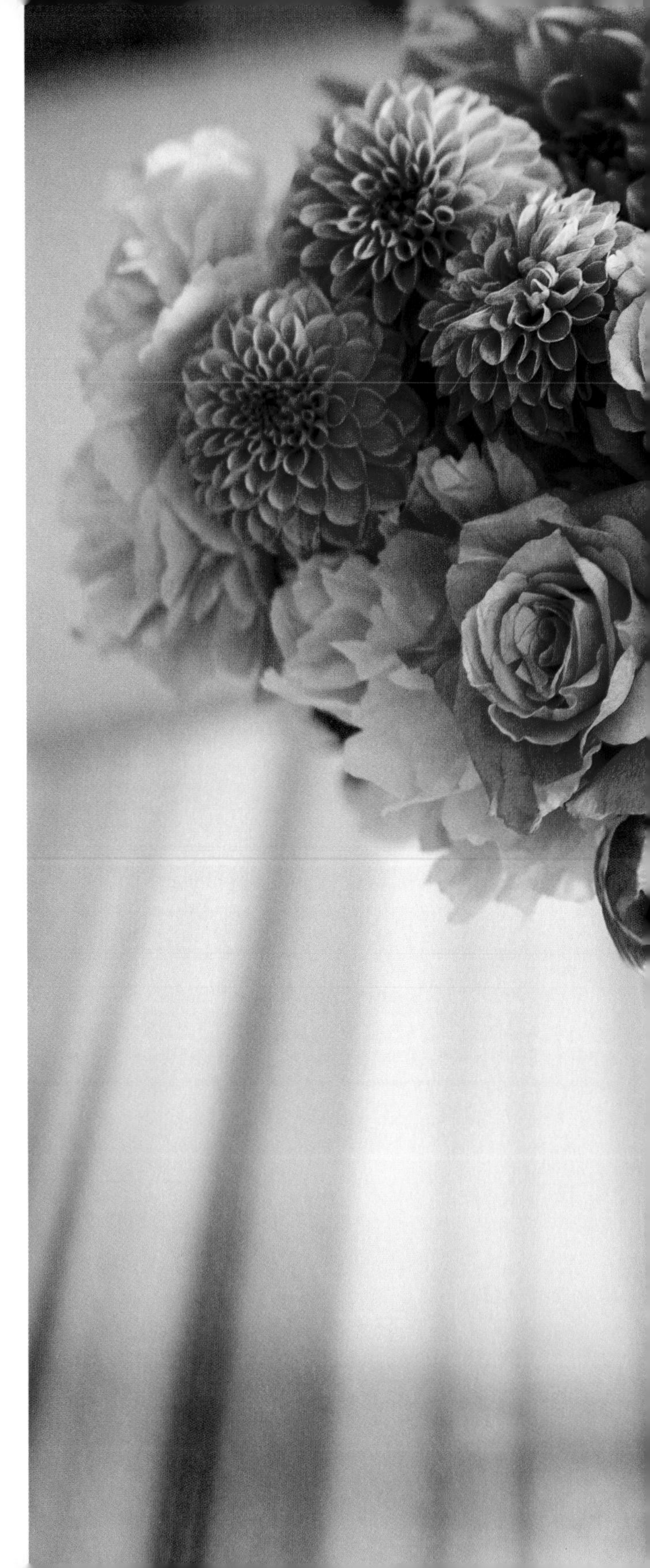

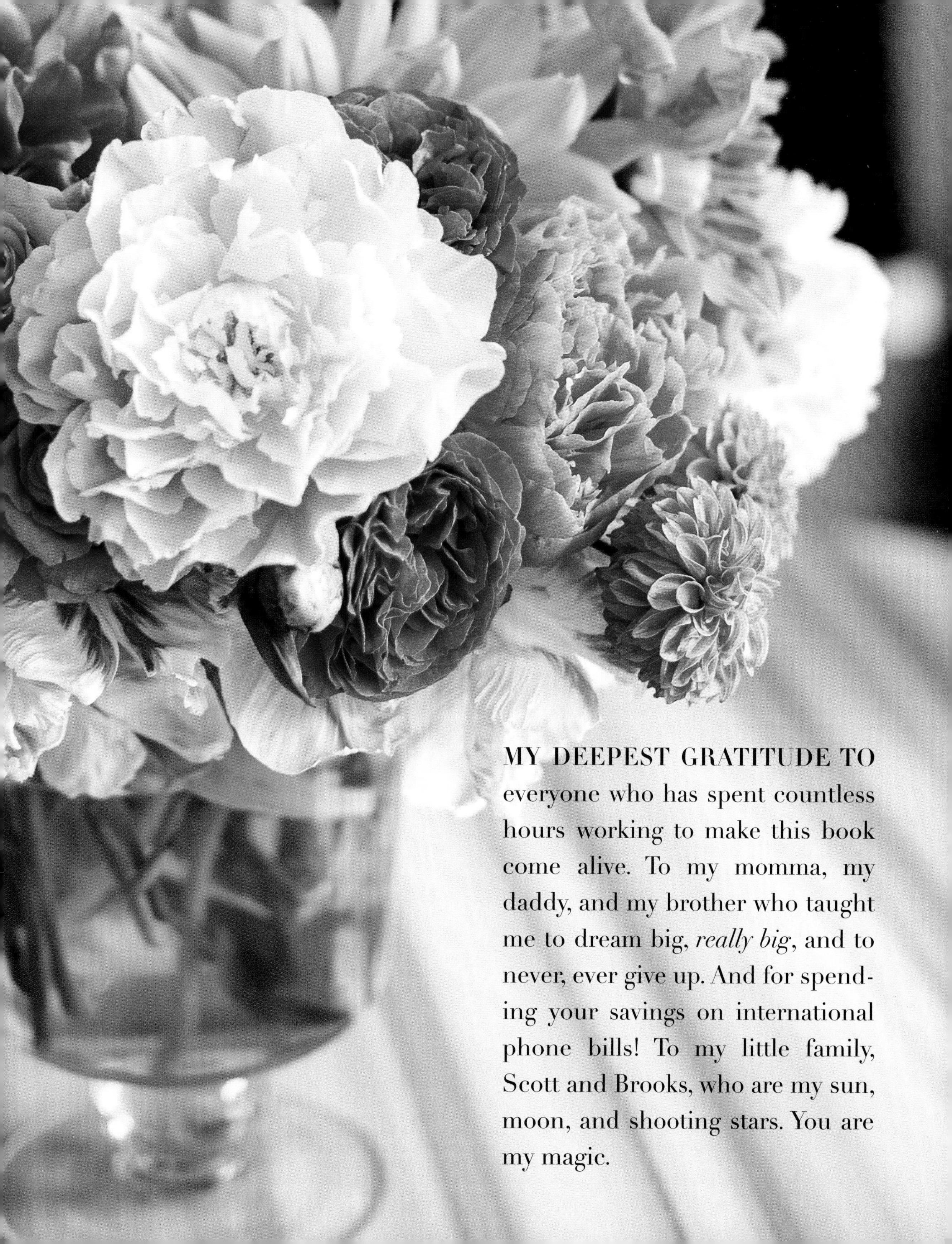

MY DEEPEST GRATITUDE TO everyone who has spent countless hours working to make this book come alive. To my momma, my daddy, and my brother who taught me to dream big, *really big*, and to never, ever give up. And for spending your savings on international phone bills! To my little family, Scott and Brooks, who are my sun, moon, and shooting stars. You are my magic.

CONTENTS

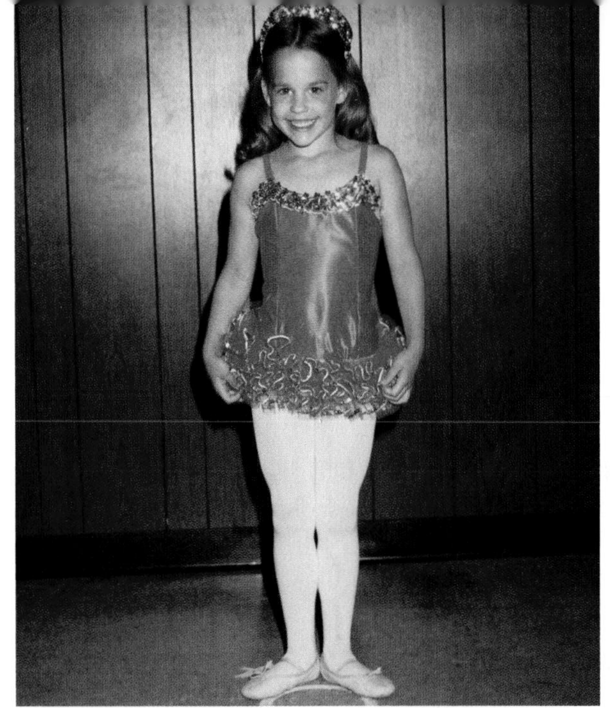

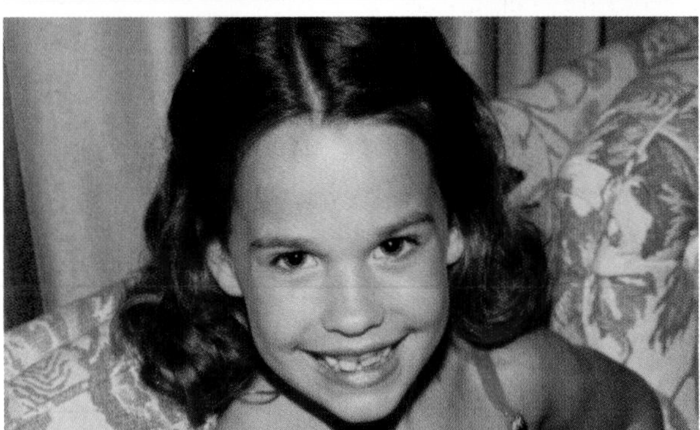

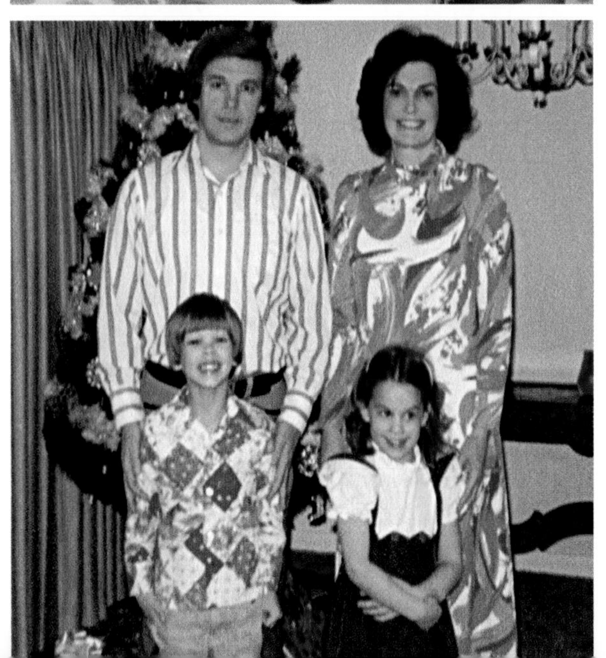

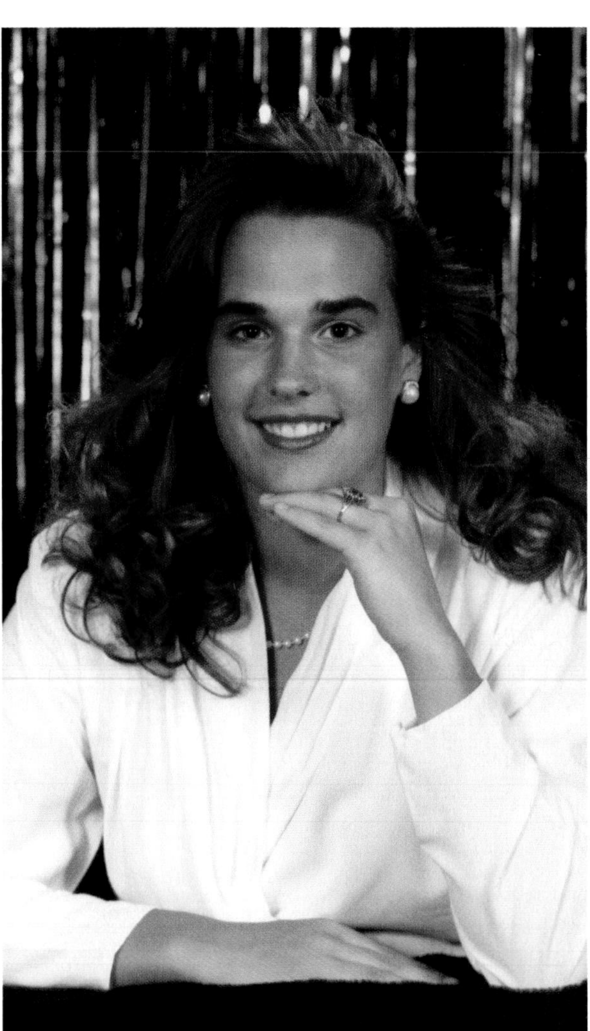

I have the top trainers, hair colorists, nutritionists, and acupuncturists on speed dial. Consider this book a three-way call between you, me, and all of them!

introduction

SOUTHERN GIRL TURNED SUPERMODEL

I'm going to let you in on a little secret, right now, right here: I wasn't born this way. I wasn't born a supermodel. My early teen years could be described in one word: awkward. I had a unibrow. I had acne. I had braces with fluorescent rubber bands, and even better, headgear. I wore flats to the prom. And surprise, my natural body weight isn't how you see me in magazines and on TV. (That's me because of six-days-a-week, balls-to-the-wall exercising, and watching what I eat like Homeland Security watches airports and borders.) It's been a long road from headgear to high heels. I've worked my ass off to get to supermodel status. Literally.

You might be thinking: bullsh*t. *But I mean it.* When it comes to looking good and feeling great—I have tried it all. The supermodel has literally been yanked out of me. I have Weight-Watched, Atkinsed, and Zoned. I've yogaed, spinned, danced, and boxed. I've been dressed up in every kind of outfit imaginable. And when it comes to beauty? I've been potioned, lotioned, plucked and prodded, bleached, bronzed, waxed and makeuped, extensioned, curled, blow-dried and straightened . . . into an entirely new human form.

The truth is, I have stealthily studied and applied my way into supermodeldom. What I didn't get in the genetic lottery, I sure as heck went after. I am the ultimate guinea pig and I know what works because of years of trial and error. I didn't just google this stuff on the Internet. I've lived it. Every piece of advice in this book is road tested and *regular girl turned supermodel* approved. And I want to share it with you. Thinking about a new diet or hair product? I've probably tried them. And if I haven't—I know ten people who have. In my circle of friends, I am the go-to girl for all the goods. If your hair is brassy, I will tell you. Why? Because you need to know that it doesn't have to be. Don't settle! Especially if it can be gorgeous and golden instead.

As difficult and judgmental as modeling can be, it gives me access to the best of the best in beauty, fashion, health, and wellness. I have the top trainers, hair colorists, nutritionists, and acupuncturists on speed dial. Consider this book a three-way call

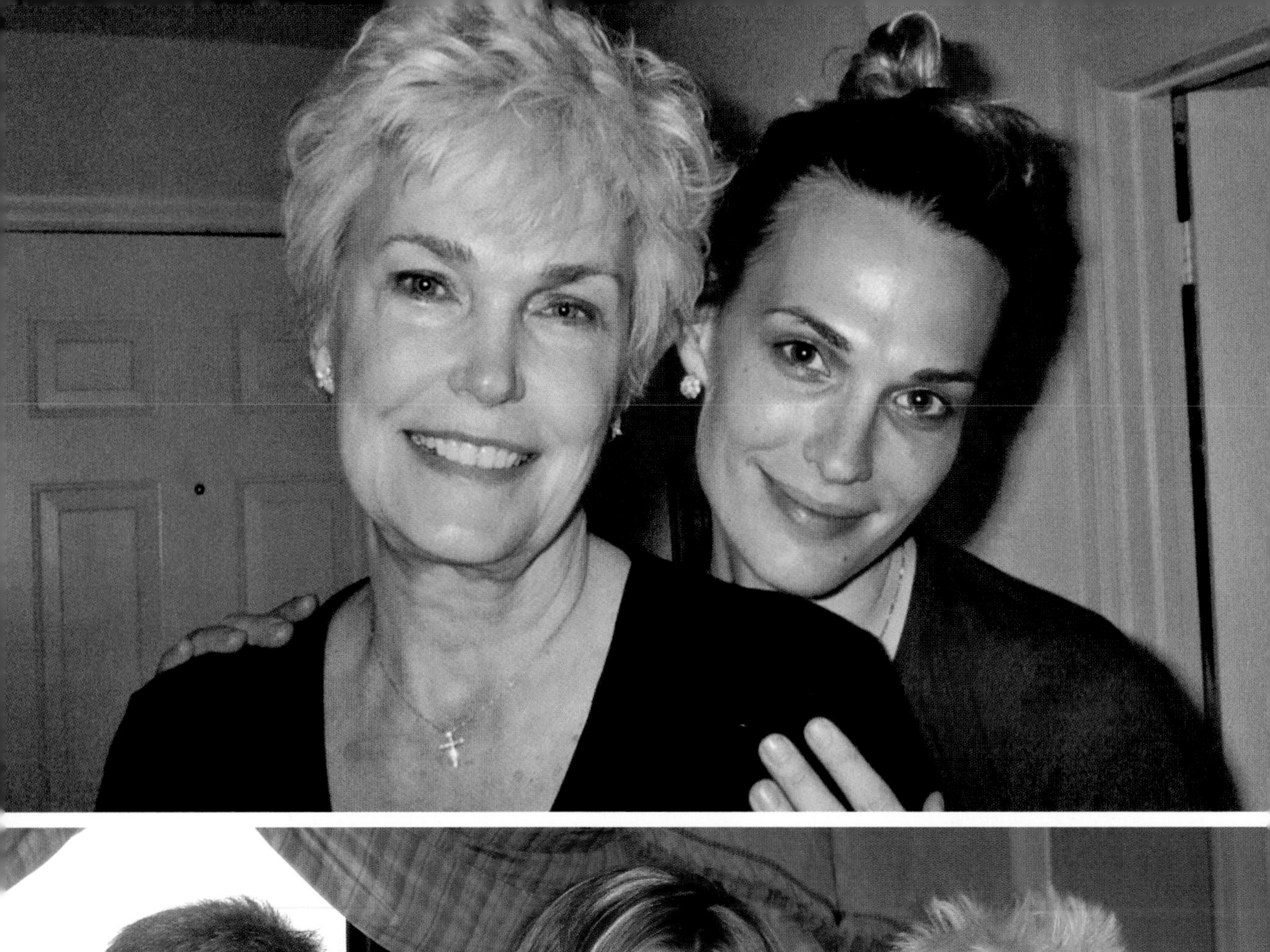
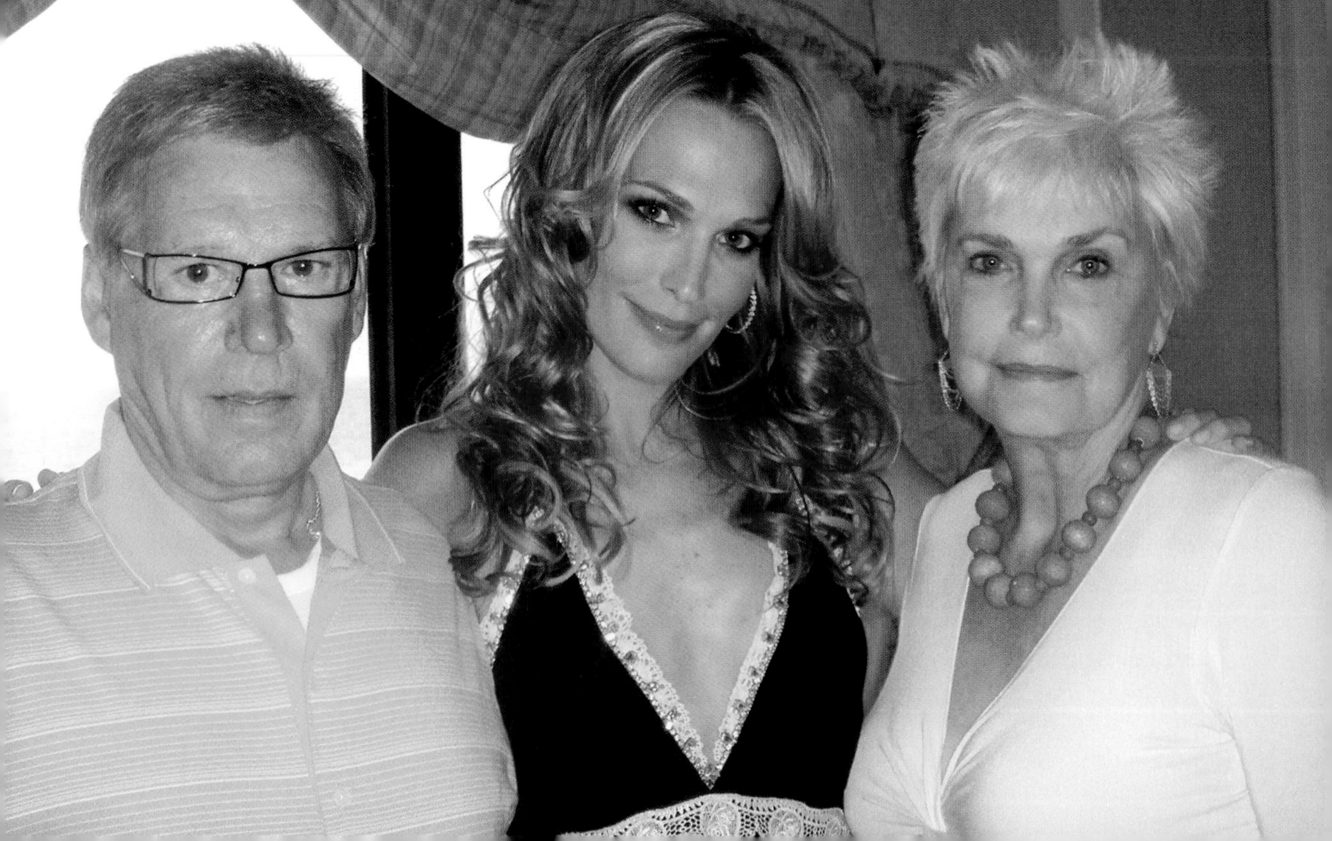

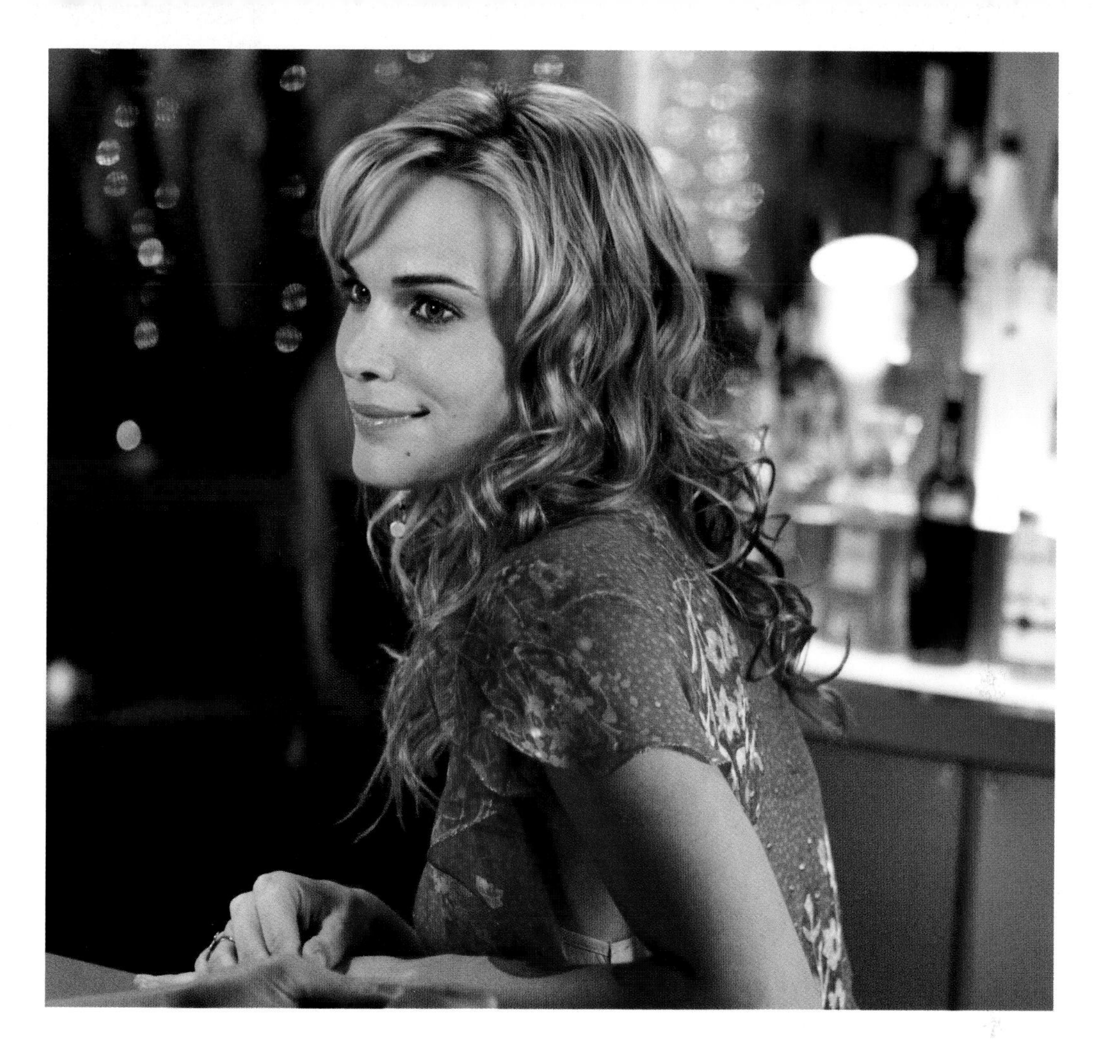

between you, me, and all of them! I want you to look and feel great too. I want to share my supermodel secrets because I 100 percent believe that when you feel good about yourself and the way you look, it shows.

Like anyone else, I've struggled with body issues. I've wanted to get hired for a job and didn't. I've stressed out about my next paycheck, or whether or not I could have children. I may not have all the answers, but one thing I do know for sure—you gotta go big or go home. At every turn we can always choose to be the best versions of ourselves. You want to get married? Lose fifteen pounds? You want glowing skin? To be noticed in a room? You want a better job, a raise, or to feel sexy in bed with your partner? Then let's do this. Let's go big together in this book and make sh*t happen for you!

In these pages, you will find enough fashion, beauty, fitness, and health advice to transform yourself into the very best version of you. And while I might have extra resources to spend on expensive treatments and clothes, the truth is—I'm always looking for the best deal because that's how I was raised. My parents raised me to believe I could do anything, and I believe that together we can do this. I'm from a small town in Kentucky and what I learned growing up there is that it's all about focus, perseverance, and fortitude—a little southern grit never hurt anyone. There is an everyday supermodel in each one of us. There was in me. And there is one in you. Let's go get her!

---

the *everyday* supermodel

The *everyday supermodel* is happy, healthy, and hot! What does that mean? She feels fabulous, looks fabulous, and loves herself head to toe, inside and out. Why? She respects herself, challenges herself, and doesn't give up. Who is she? The *everyday supermodel* is YOU—she is the very best version of each one of us.

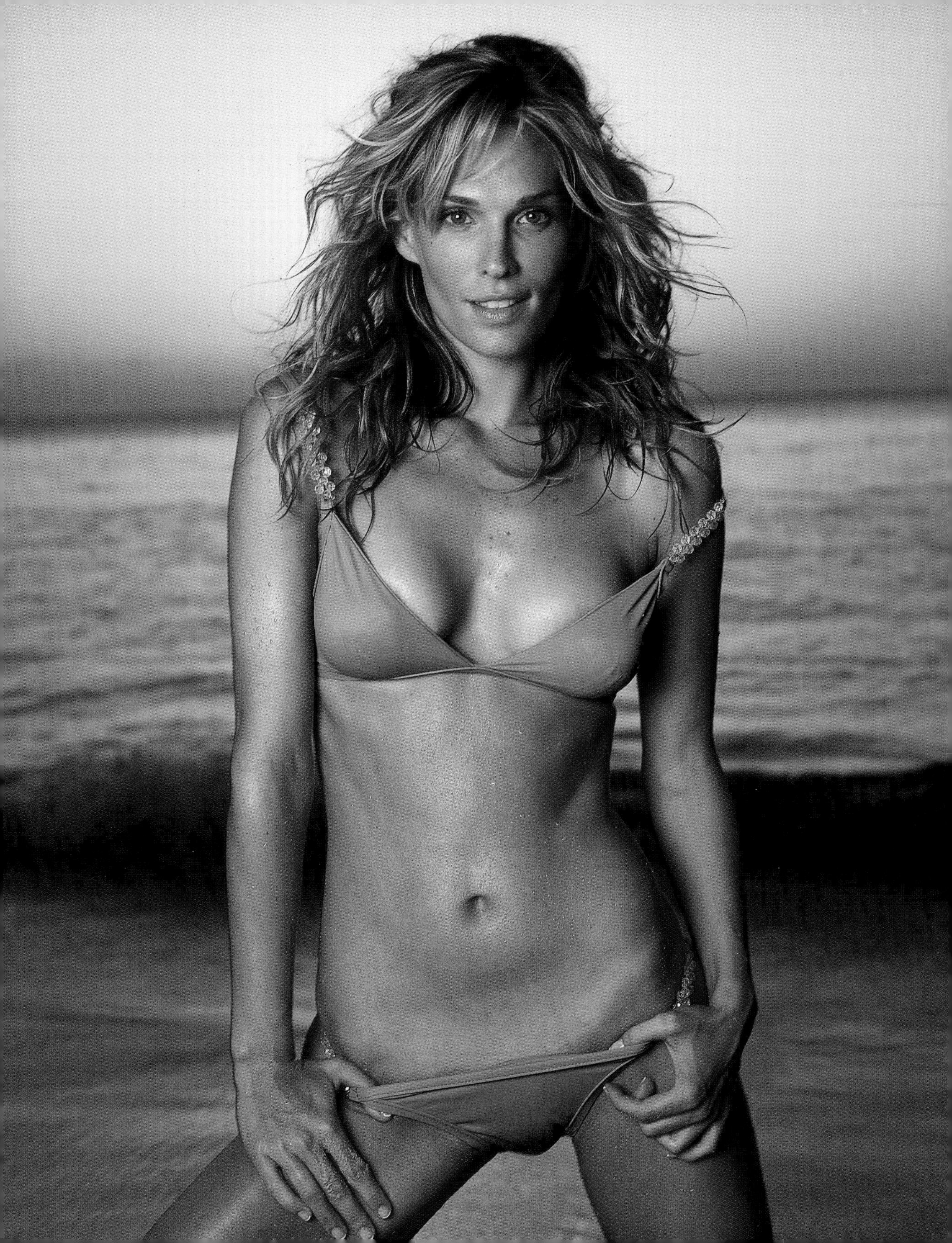

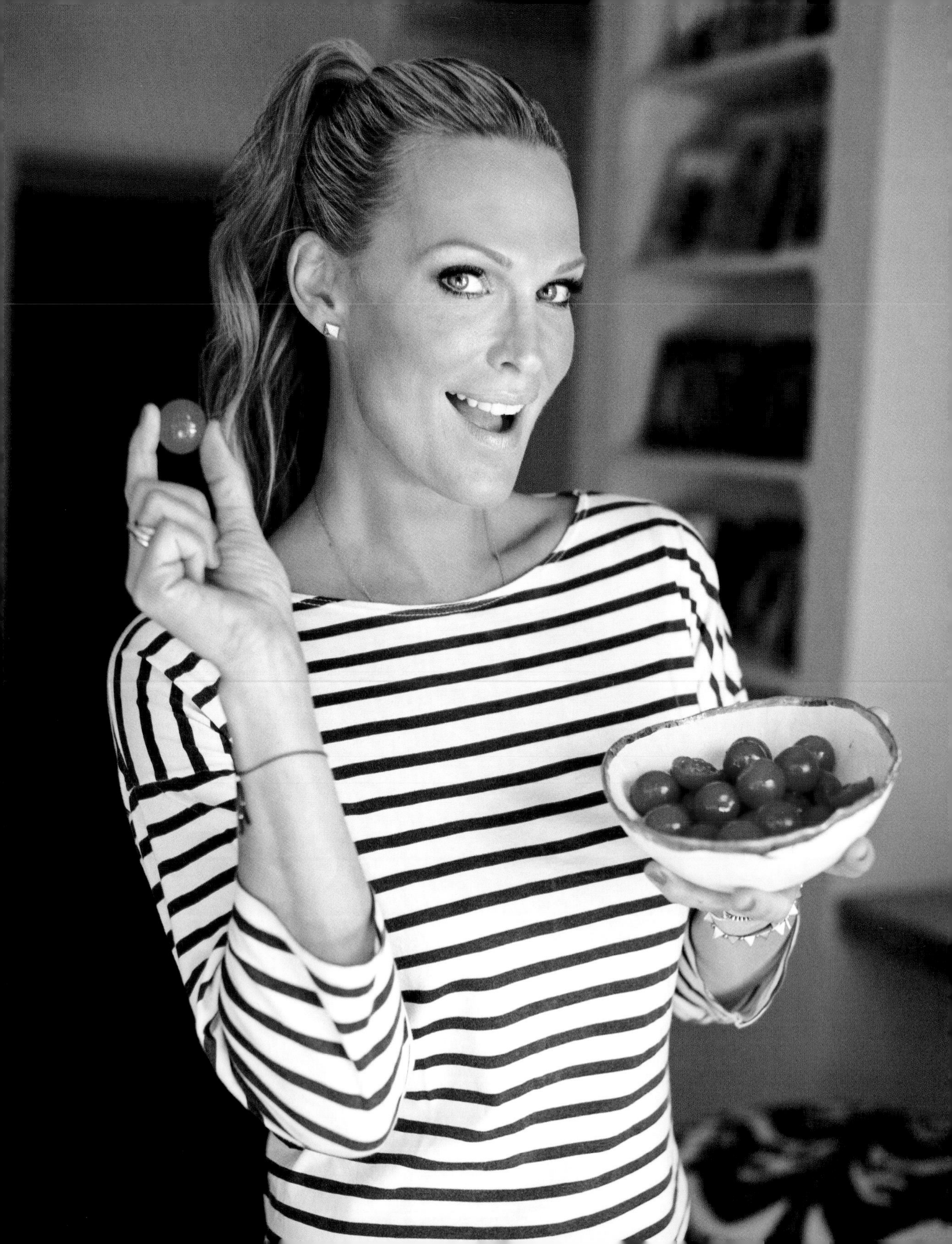

ch/1

food is not the frenemy

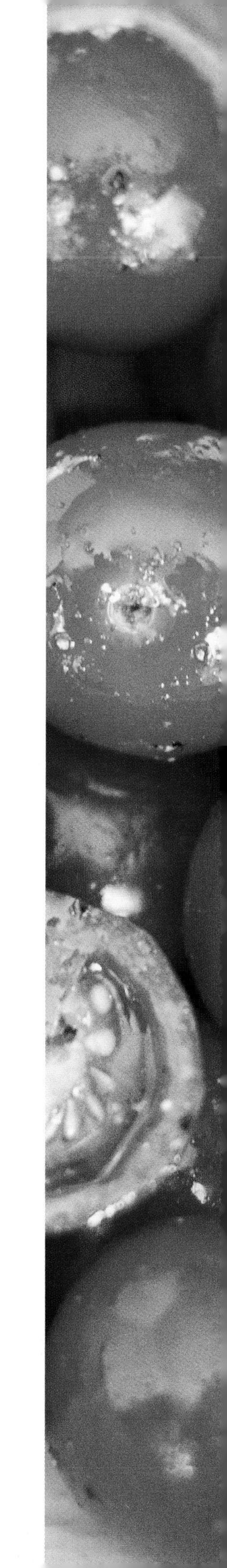

Dear food: Can't we just get along? The answer is yes. *Finally.*

Forget starving yourself. Or going from one fad diet to the next. I've been there, done that. Let's stop this love/hate relationship and end the food fight. Food is good, it gives us energy, it brings us together, and it is deeply linked to our physical and emotional well-being. Once you find the right balance, your relationship with food is one that will give back to you in so many ways. It wasn't until I was in my thirties that I finally gave up the yo-yoing and decided to commit to eating. And eating healthy. The way we eat should be a lifestyle—not a *lifestruggle*.

I did not inherit the "skinny genes." My mom and brother can eat three jars of peanut butter and lose weight. I walk past one and gain it. You name the diet—Atkins, Weight Watchers, South Beach, Macrobiotic—I've done it. So, woman to woman, I know what most of you are going through. You won't see a ton of pictures of me in a "fat stage" because, as a working model, I have never been allowed to go through one. My livelihood depends on my weight. *No pressure there.*

But I promise you—inside me is a chubbier person just waiting for me to get lazy on healthy eating and exercise. I am NOT one of those girls who can eat whatever she wants. So many celebs say, "I'm just naturally skinny. I eat burgers and french fries all day." *Bullsh*t.* Most can't eat like that, and neither can I. Since I was twenty my body has been plastered in magazine spreads, on billboards, and now high-def television. What you see is the result of intense dedication and an eating strategy/ workout regimen that keeps me fit—not some kind of special supermodel gene.

Like so many of us women, I've spent way too much mental energy on food in my lifetime. So now my plan is simple—I do what I can to be healthy and get over what I can't control. Here's a fun fact! I gained seventy-two pounds during my first pregnancy. It took me a year to get it off, and I still struggle with a few pounds. I am not lying to you when I say—I didn't recognize myself or my body in the mirror. And there were days I thought I'd never lose the weight. But I didn't give up.

I was dedicated and made weight loss *and myself* a priority. I was not happy where I was—so I wasn't going to settle for it.

I won't ever be stick thin, but I don't want to be. I've learned to love my body. It's strong. And I've learned by trial and error to make healthy choices instead of unhealthy ones (i.e., at age twenty-one, eating celery sticks, rice cakes, sucking down Dieter's Tea, and calling it a day!). I've been educated by the best of the best and I now know what's healthy and what works.

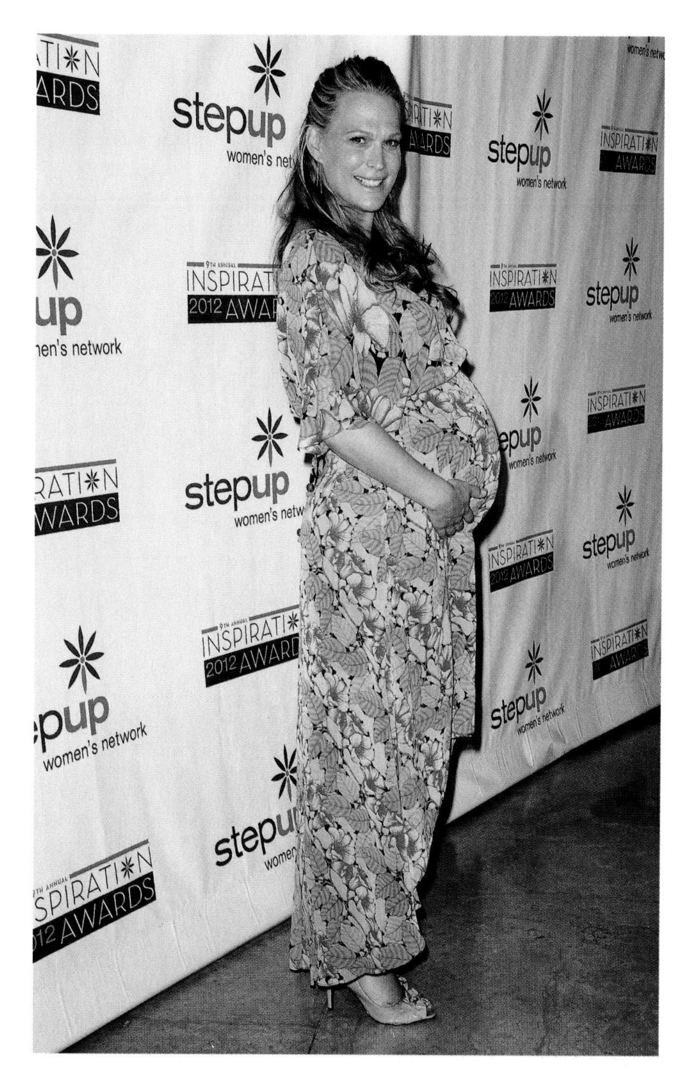

Very pregnant!

In this chapter, I focus on eating styles, strategies, and tips that have worked for me. I talk about practical, day-to-day stuff that anyone can integrate into their lifestyle. Start by making a commitment to yourself. Get organized. And get your friends, your mother, your sister, your dog, and your man on board to help you. Chubby, tall, skinny, short, mature in age, or younger in years—you can do this. Everything might not work for you in this chapter. But a lot will. And, I promise, the pieces of advice that do hit home will change your life and make a big difference in the way you look and feel every day.

Many of us are addicted to food in the same way some people are addicted to alcohol, cigarettes, and drugs. Bad food habits can be just as destructive and as challenging to kick. I want you to enjoy making better choices for yourself, because that means you are putting yourself first. I want to help you establish a healthy relationship with food. These plans and strategies aren't a diet; rather, they are tools for creating a new, healthier lifestyle. I want you to feel good about who you are and where you are. And if you don't, I want you to know *that you can do something about it.*

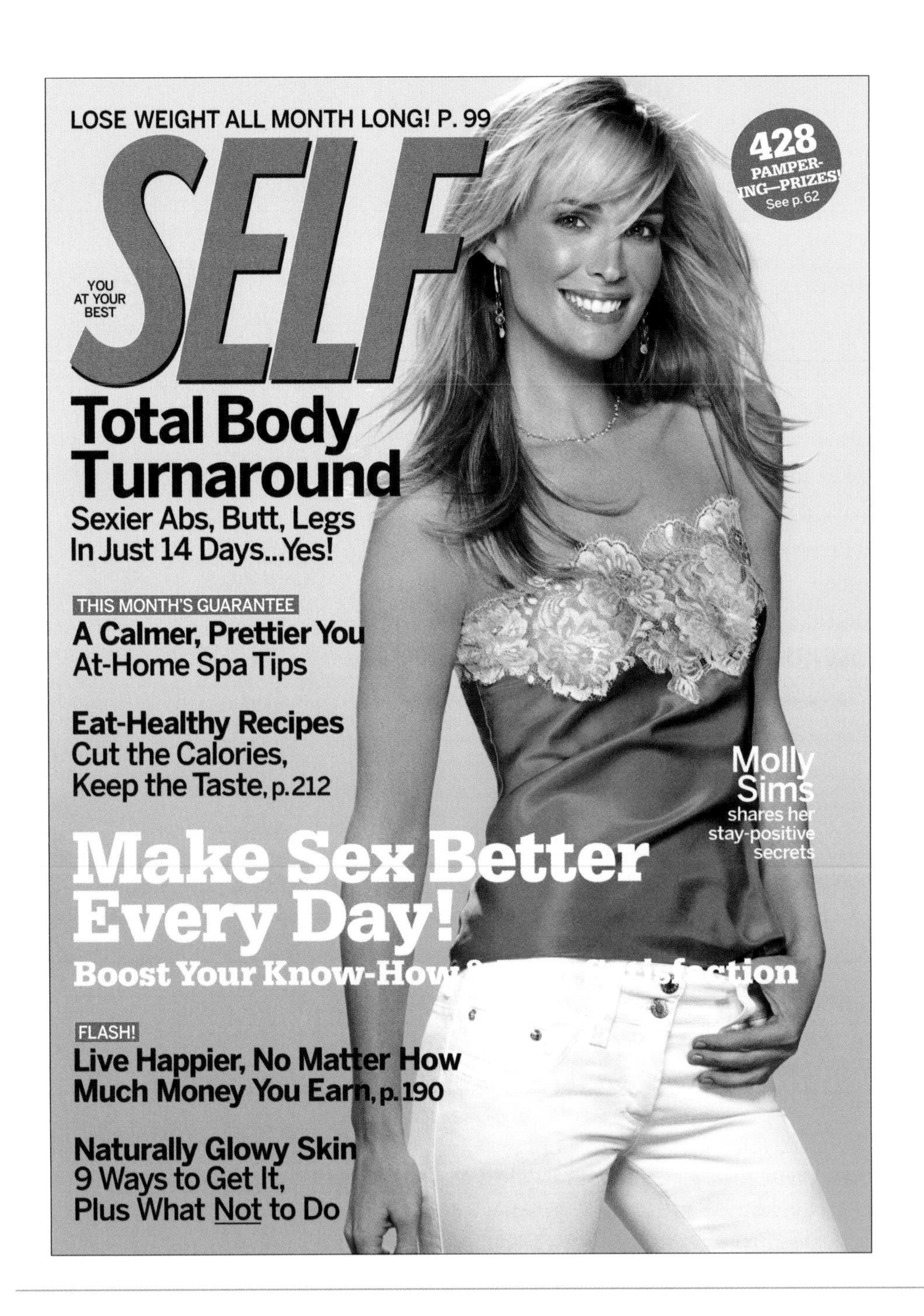

molly's motto: *If you look good, you feel good—and when you feel good, you look good. So you might as well feel f***ing fabulous!*

Before trying any specific diet or wellness strategy—you should always consult a doctor. Every program isn't for everyone. For example, my momma is on heart medicine, so she can't have all the green juices, smoothies, and spinach salads that I am always recommending. Check in with your team first. Make sure any strategy or supplement you are considering is safe for you personally—and then go for it!

My *health heroes* and *food fantastics*

- **REBECCA BAER, BAER NUTRITION**—Rebecca is a registered dietician and my partner in fat-fighting crime. She walks the walk, talks the talk, and has personally coached me to trim—before my wedding and after my first pregnancy (baby weight . . . banished!).
- **LORI BREGMAN**—I owe my sanity during pregnancy to this woman! Intuitive healer, inspirational life coach, doula, and transformational body worker—you name it, Lori does it. She educated and guided me through every stage. Food and mind wise, she kept me on track.
- **CHEF GAVAN MURPHY**—a.k.a. the Healthy Irishman. Gavan has been a private chef to many a supermodel, including Cindy Crawford, and he currently works with me and my husband. Trained in the Ballymaloe Cookery School, he is highly adept at transforming traditional meals into healthier, more vibrant versions.

---

supermodel *secret*

The modeling business can be brutal. At the age of twenty-one, I was a size six and told I was *too fat* to be a model. I was just a kid and was traumatized by this piece of news. So what did I do? I starved myself. I took laxatives to lose weight. I drank Dieter's Tea all the time. I did coffee enemas. I started smoking to speed up my metabolism. I really didn't eat. And if I did—it wasn't until 4:00 P.M. and consisted of pretzels and celery. Eating disorders are prevalent in the industry because of the pressure to be stick-thin. That pressure rules every aspect of your life. You wake up thinking about it (because you are hungry) and go to bed the same way. I was at least fifteen to twenty pounds more than all the other girls when I started modeling, so I felt added pressure. I became anemic, had dark circles under my eyes at all times—it wasn't good. As I approached my late twenties, I began to stop the madness and started to eat better. But I had to retrain my brain. I had to learn there are such things as healthy fats and that all carbs aren't the devil. Whether we overeat, or undereat, we have to unwind our mind. The decision to be fitter and healthier always begins there.

Today, the foundation of my healthy eating program involves the following:

1. A fiber-focused eating plan. It incorporates lots of veggies, healthy carbs, lean proteins, and of course plenty of water and exercise.
2. Juicing daily and doing a liquid cleanse or juice fast one to two times per year.
3. Incorporating the occasional plant-based or vegan meal into my eating plan a few meals a week.
4. Taking the phrase "on a DIET" out of my vocabulary. I highly recommend you do it. Swap it with "getting healthy" or "making food choices that are about loving myself."

let's break it all down!

1. GETTING FIBER FOCUSED

How I lost fifteen pounds before my wedding and sixty-five and counting after my first pregnancy. And . . . how I keep it off.

When I first met Molly, she was eating about a box a day of Soy Crisps and Nut-Thins, thinking that these were healthy snack foods. Her diet consisted mainly of fats and proteins—with barely any whole grains, fruits, or vegetables. Molly was relying on caffeine from coffee and diet soda to help her go to the bathroom. And like many women who have spent years doing different diets, she no longer had much of a grasp on what she should be eating.

—REBECCA BAER, dietician, Baer Nutrition

I met Rebecca Baer, a New York–based nutritionist, a few months before my wedding. I had been eating a lot of dinners out with Scott, my fiancé, and let's face it, I was heavier (and happier!) than I'd been in a long time. But! I was fifteen pounds from where I wanted to be on my wedding day. So I decided to have a consultation with Rebecca and get on her program. I wanted help getting my rear *aisle-ready*—and I wanted to do it in a healthy way. Rebecca's program not only did that, but it also helped me to mend my mercurial relationship with food.

According to Rebecca, the majority of women are eating and dieting the wrong way. She says that there isn't a soul who steps into her office who eats enough fiber or vegetables. Yours truly included. What I love about a fiber-focused plan is that it's sustainable day to day. It doesn't require me to buy a bunch of special foods (although there are a few I now enjoy) or be puritanical in my eating habits. And I can pretty much stay committed to the eating suggestions anywhere/anytime. I can be on a television set, out with the baby, racing around in my car, or with my friends who eat rubbish, and I can stick to the diet and feel good about it.

And I didn't have to quit drinking! Rebecca taught me to drink responsibly. In other words, to choose the least-caloric alcoholic beverages in addition to drinking less (more alcohol = lower inhibitions = stuffing face late night with fatty foods and Fritos). Upping my fiber, eating the right amount of protein, and following the rest of the plan worked for me. It waged war on my extra weight and currently helps to keep it off. Although there are plenty of "diets" that help you lose weight in the short term, the real key is finding something that is sustainable for the long term and that you will stick with.

I love working with people to help them achieve their goals and become the healthiest and happiest they can be. With commitment, focus, and a belief in yourself, anything is possible. And when it's all said and done, there is a huge transformation in body and mind. I watch people gain back the confidence they had lost; they become better mothers, wives, daughters, and friends all because they feel great both inside and out.

—REBECCA BAER, dietician, Baer Nutrition

WHAT IS *fiber* AND WHY SHOULD WE "ROUGH" IT?

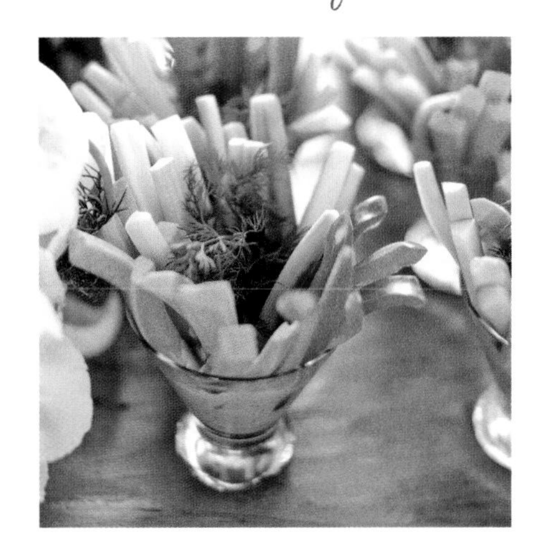

By adding fiber to your diet, "roughing" it can actually help you reduce that number on the scale. The basic building block of a regular carbohydrate is *a sugar molecule.* Our digestive system converts ALL carbs we eat into sugar. Those sugar molecules are then converted into the glucose that fuels our activity and gives us energy for shopping, sex, swimming, and whatnot. But what if you don't burn up all that glucose? Your body will hold on to it in glycogen stores. The body will only store so much before it eventually turns the excess glycogen stores *into fat. Muffin tops. Pooches. Teacher arms, and the like.*

But high-fiber carbs are different. *They are special.* Why? Fiber cannot be broken down into sugar so it moves through the body undigested and never gets stored. So it will never turn to fat. Rebecca explained to me that carbs are not the enemy. We need them—they are an essential macronutrient, but it's important to choose wisely. Choose carbs that are high in fiber so we don't end up with excess saddle-baggage.

benefits of a High-Fiber Diet

* A study published in the journal *Nutrition* concluded that people who add more fiber to their diets lose more weight than those who don't.
* A high-fiber eating plan is generally lower in calories than a low-fiber diet. Insoluble fiber essentially contains zero calories.
* Fiber expands in the belly and makes us feel fuller faster and longer.
* Fiber requires more chewing, slows down eating, and gives our body more time to send signals that say "Stop! I'm full!," which keeps you from overeating.
* Insoluble fiber (like in veggie juices) helps push food through the intestinal tract, keeping you regular.
* Other health benefits? Studies show fiber helps lower cholesterol, prevents constipation, helps with hemorrhoids (even more reason to eat a lot of fiber when preggers), keeps blood pressure in check, and may reduce the risk of colon and breast cancer.

Rebecca's Fiber-Focused Plan: *six mantras* for Success!

1. **THREE AND THREE:** Enjoy three meals and three snacks a day. Eating regularly and spreading out meals consistently keeps your metabolism in high gear and you burn calories more efficiently throughout the day. Get in a combo of high-fiber carbs (see page 20) and a healthy dose of lean protein (see page 19) for lasting energy.

2. **EAT. MORE. FIBER. PERIOD:** Focus on getting more fiber into your diet, any way you can! As noted earlier, fiber is generally lower in calories, you will feel fuller and will naturally begin to eliminate bad foods on your own. You do NOT have to stop eating carbs. But you DO have to choose the "good" ones. We list good carbs, bad carbs, and good sources of fiber later.

   GENERAL GOAL:

   - **FIBER INTAKE:** 30–40 grams a day
   - **NET CARBS:** 35 grams per day

3. **KEEP A DIET DIARY:** Why? Journaling keeps you honest, keeps you accountable, and helps you stay on track with calorie count, fat count, carb count, and fiber count. As Rebecca says, "Calories do count. If more calories go in than out . . . that's when we gain weight." A detailed diary can expose unhealthy patterns that you can then correct (mine showed I was eating most of my calories after 4 P.M.!—not good). For the tech savvy, there are helpful apps that assist with food journaling. (Check out Loseit! and My Fitness Pal).

4. **EAT LEAN, MEAN . . . PROTEIN!:** Choose lean, healthy proteins. Adequate protein intake is important for building muscle and losing weight. Lean proteins are generally low in calories and contain essential amino acids and nutrients necessary for an *everyday supermodel* bod.

5. **WATER IS YOUR WEIGHT WARRIOR:** Okay, simple enough. The more fiber you eat, the more water you need to drink. Fiber needs liquid in order to move through the body and get its sweep on. Also, oftentimes sugar and fat cravings are actually the result of dehydration, water cravings displaced. So drink up!

6. **SWEAT IT OUT:** A regular fitness program is essential to a fit frame. Rebecca suggests working out five days a week, for at least thirty to forty-five minutes a day. I did more, but everybody is different. Weight doesn't just slide off me. It tends to drag its heels. The key, Rebecca says, is to combine both cardio and resistance training—you need both!

supermodel *secret*

My whole life, I've never drunk enough water. Perhaps you can relate. So I make it *irresistible* by dressing it up a little. How? By squeezing fresh lemon or adding a sprig of mint to flat or sparkling water. Also, it might sound simple, but drinking with a straw helps me down more in a day.

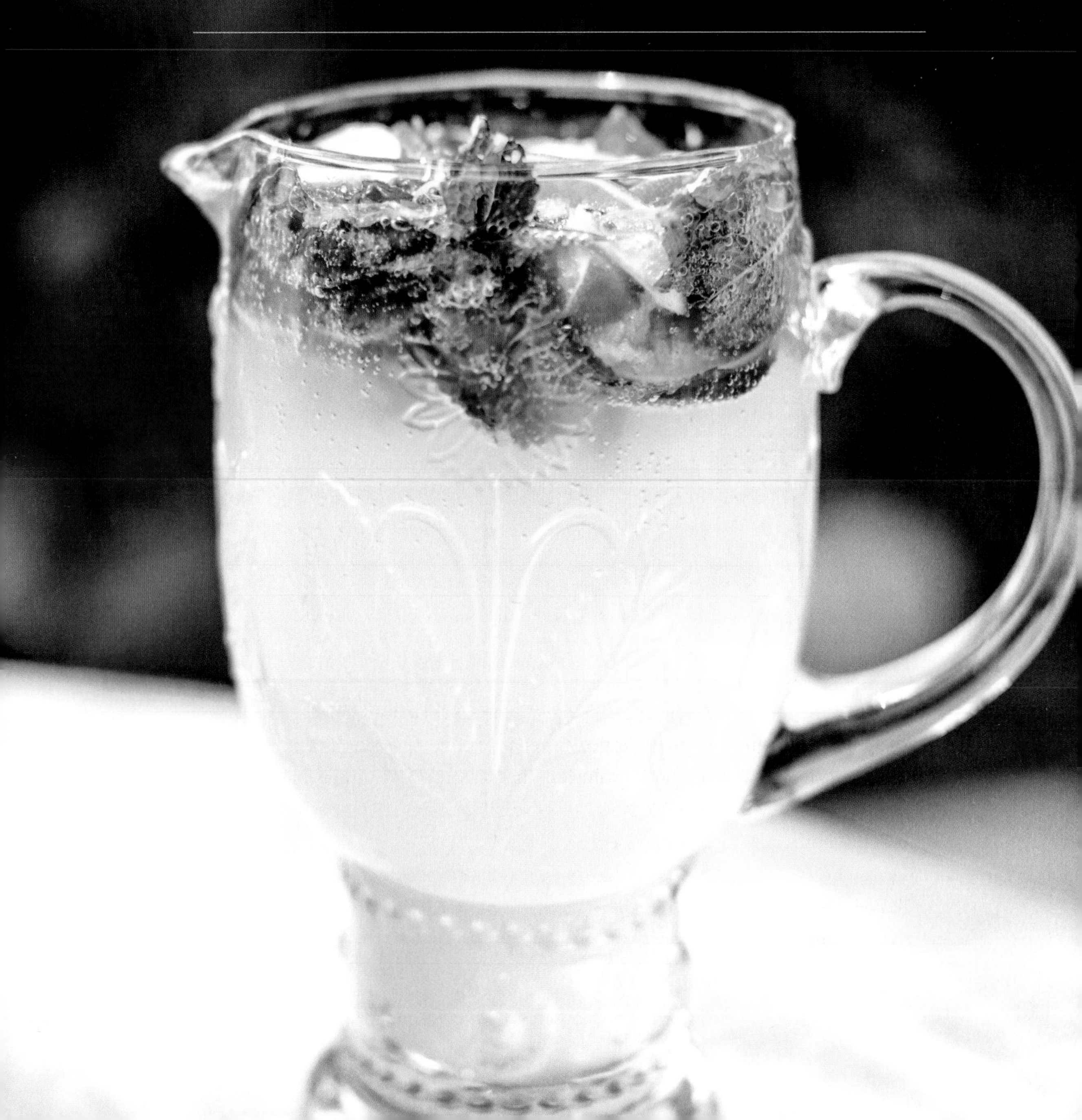

I would recommend writing EVERYTHING you consume down for a week and then have a look at areas you can improve. I did this and saw that I was consuming a lot more sugar than I imagined.

—ELETTRA WIEDEMANN, model

Rebecca's program was designed to help me lose two to six pounds a week. Below are goals and guidelines Rebecca set for me based on my specific stats. I outline my exact program and discuss ways to tailor it to your goals and your body type.

General *dietary goals* for Weight Loss and Maintenance

- **GOAL WEIGHT:** For me, 130–135 pounds. (I was about 15 pounds over this before my wedding). How can you get the number right for you? By doing the Ideal Body Weight (IBW) Equation. It's easy, you can do it for yourself!
    - **IBW EQUATION:** 100 lb. + 5 lb. for each inch you are over five feet (and then plus or minus 10% for your frame size)
    - **EXAMPLE:** Me = Height 5'10". I am medium to smaller frame, so I subtract (rather than add) 10%.
    - 100 + 50 lb. for the 10 inches over 5 feet = 150 lb. I then subtract 10% of 150 for my small/medium frame and get my goal weight of 135 lb.
- **GOAL CALORIC INTAKE:** For me, 1,400 calories per day for weight-loss mode. 1,600–2,000 for maintenance. To find out your own calorie goal, plug in your own stats at www.choosemyplate.gov.
- **GOAL FAT INTAKE:** Should be 20–30% of your total calories per day for both the weight-loss phase and maintenance. Twenty percent of a 1,400 calorie diet is 280 total fat calories. That's about 31–46 grams of fat. (For easy reference 1 tablespoon of olive oil contains 15 grams of fat.) No more than 10% of total calories should be saturated fat.
- **GOAL FIBER INTAKE:** 30–40 grams of fiber per day. The 2010 Dietary Guidelines recommend at least 28 grams of fiber a day for women, and there is no upper limit.

- **GOAL NET CARB INTAKE:** 20–50 net carbs per day. What are net carbs? Basically, the carbs leftover (that turn to sugar!) after you subtract the carbs assigned to fiber.
- **GOAL PROTEIN INTAKE:** Our goal for me was between 8 and 10 ounces of protein per day. Eight to ten ounces is a generally good rule of thumb for most women, but to get your exact recommended intake, look for a protein intake calculator online. Based on this goal, I ate about 3 ounces of protein for breakfast, 3 for lunch, 3 for dinner, and 1 ounce of protein as a snack. For reference: 3 ounces of protein is approximately the size of the palm of your hand and thickness of a deck of cards; 1 ounce of protein looks like a 1-inch cube or slice of cheese.
- **GOAL SLEEP HOURS:** 7–8 hours a night. Good sleep is important for a healthy metabolism.
- **GOAL EXERCISE:** 30–60 minutes a day, 5x a week—combine cardio with at least two days of strength training.
- **GOAL WATER INTAKE:** 9–12 cups per day.

REBECCA'S *go-to* HEALTH AND NUTRITION SOURCES

- Academy of Nutrition and Dietetics: www.eatright.org
- Centers for Disease Control and Prevention: www.cdc.gov
- USDA Choose My Plate: www.choosemyplate.gov
- National Institute for Health: www.nhlbi.nih.gov

so . . . what *can* you eat?!?

A GUIDE TO LEAN PROTEINS AND HIGH-FIBER FOODS

Lean Protein *choices*

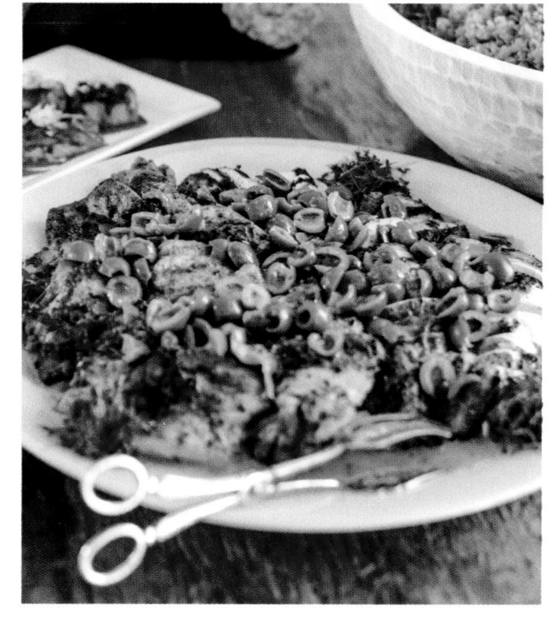

- Beef: flank, filet, sirloin, tenderloin, and lean ground chuck
- Lamb, pork, poultry (turkey, chicken, duck)
- Low-cholesterol seafood, including: salmon, tuna, sardines, etc.
- Egg whites and reduced-fat dairy (1% cottage cheese, low-fat cheese, and Greek yogurt)
- Tofu and meat substitutes, including: tofu, soy crumbles, Boca Burgers, edamame, and seitan.
- Quinoa and beans, including black and navy beans. (Technically these contain both proteins and high-fiber carbs, bonus!)

  FYI: I also ate a very limited amount of nut and seed butters, including peanut, almond, and sunflower seed. These aren't necessarily "lean," but they contain good fats essential to radiant health. But I kept them to a minimum!)

THE PROTEIN PLEDGE: Keep it *clean and lean*. Nothing fried, breaded, battered, or overly processed. Choose lean cuts of meat—not the fatty ones. Avoid certain shellfish, like lobster and shrimp, as they tend to be high in cholesterol. Always be aware of invisible oils, especially when it comes to fish in restaurants. You may think you are making a good choice, but you never really know what's happening back in the kitchen. Your fish could be creamed, buttered, or soaked in oil. Quiz your server about the preparation! Ask for steamed or poached whenever possible.

I do find that I feel better and have more energy when I include a small portion and healthy source of lean protein in every meal, especially breakfast. That sustains me so I'm not tempted to snack idly on foods I don't need throughout the day.

—JESSICA ALBA, actress

How Lean Proteins *whittle* the Middle

- Lean proteins take longer to digest than simple carbohydrates and, like fiber, they can help us feel fuller for longer periods. Hallelujah! That helps us curb sneaky snacking and contributes to reduced calorie intake.
- Eating lean protein also builds lean muscle mass in our bodies, and muscle, *everyday supermodels*, burns more calories than fat! The more muscle you have, the more fat you lose.
- Get this: Per gram, protein contains only four calories, while fats can contain up to nine. So, in contrast to fat, lean meats are a relatively low-calorie food.

High-Fiber Food *choices*

Here are the good carbs, not the bad ones. There are so many to choose from—never fear food boredom.

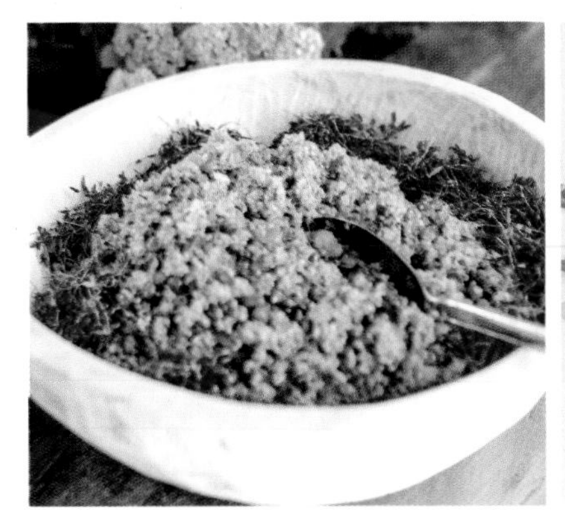

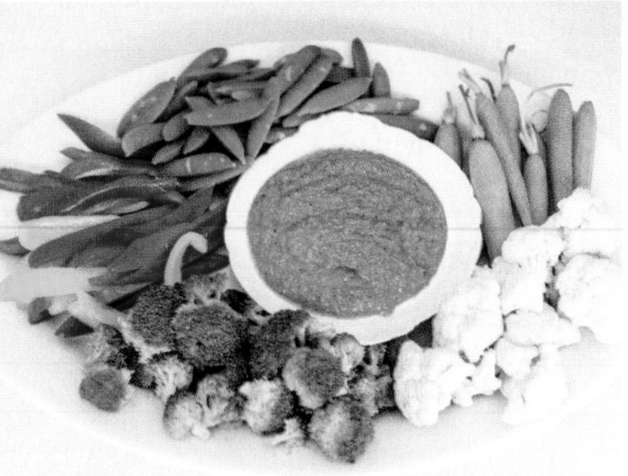

- **VEGGIES:** artichoke hearts, green beans, sugar snap peas, beets, broccoli, Brussels sprouts, cabbage, carrots, cauliflower, celery, cucumber, daikon radish, eggplant, greens (collard, kale, mustard, turnip, Swiss chard), salad greens (iceberg, endive, arugula), hearts of palm, jicama, mushrooms, okra, onion, garlic, sprouts, spinach, squash, tomato, turnips, water chestnuts.
- **FRUITS:** apples, pears, berries, and other fruits. Whenever possible, choose the fruits that are lower in natural sugars, rather than those higher in natural sugar, such as very ripe bananas.

- **WHOLE GRAINS:** brown rice, quinoa, millet, spelt, or whole wheat pasta.
- **BEANS AND LEGUMES:** white beans, pinto, adzuki beans, black, navy, and lentils.

Basically, these high-fiber foods are awesome. They have the antioxidants, vitamins, and minerals your body needs to help you lose weight, look younger, have better skin, hair and nails, and be the *everyday supermodel* you deserve to be. These are your new superfoods. Yes, they contain carbs, but they contain fewer carbs and calories because they are HIGH IN FIBER. So your net carbs are always lower when consuming these over empty, starchy carbs. Speaking of those foods, that brings us to . . . WHAT NOT TO EAT!

FOODS TO AVOID WHILE BEING FIBER FOCUSED: These are your high-carbohydrate/low-fiber foods. They are considered simple carbohydrates versus complex carbohydrates. These foods will increase your net carb intake. They will turn to sugar—and then to FAT. Most of them are calorie dense, but not nutrient or fiber dense. They will cause your blood sugar to spike and fall, giving you dramatic highs and lows. We all know about the crash! They pretty much suck nutritionally.

- Bleached grains, so anything with white flour, such as breads, pastas, and white rice, as well as most commercially baked breads and pastries.
- Starchy veggies, like potatoes, squash, corn, and peas. Did you know that eating common white potatoes is basically the equivalent of spooning down table sugar?
- Dried fruit (as opposed to fresh or frozen). Dried fruits are sky-high in sugars and calories, and the water content is low, reducing the volume and the serving size. Ten juicy grapes or two meager tablespoons of raisins? You decide.
- White sugars, including foods and drinks with high fructose corn syrup and other sneaky names for sugar—read your labels. Sugar is a high-calorie food and it's hidden in a lot more foods than you think. Some sneaky names for sugar that *sound healthy* include: fruit juice concentrate, corn sweetener, dehydrated cane juice, and fructose. Be a sugar sleuth.
- Certain processed and packaged foods, crackers, and sweets. Read the labels here too for the fiber content—it's usually really low, even if the food is low in fat. Look for "Good source of fiber" or "High source of fiber" printed on the box.

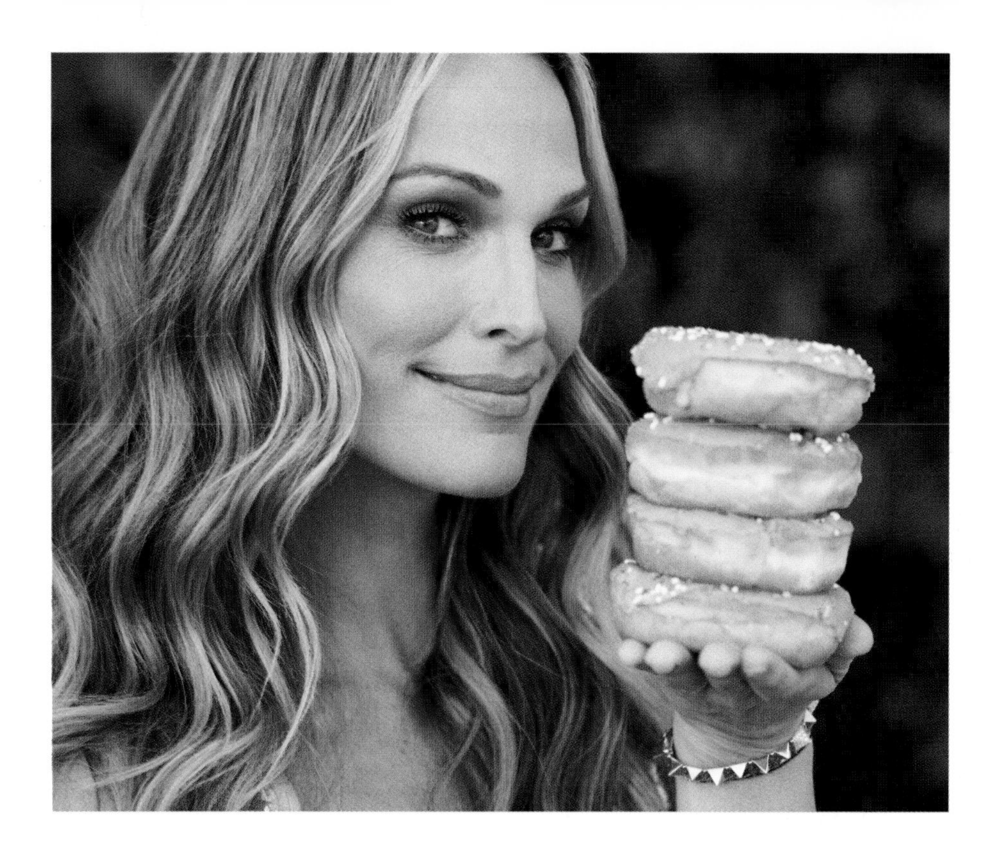

let's talk about sugar, baby

I used to eat *a lot* of sugar. I'd snack on gummy bears because they were low fat. Same goes for breath mints, Skittles, jelly candies. But guess what? Studies have revealed that sugar is as addictive as a drug. High-sugar diets have been found to contribute to binge eating because eating sugar releases the pleasure hormone in your body—and you'll want more. And more. And MORE! All those extra calories add up—and deliver *zilch* nutritionally. Not to mention, sugar is proven to contribute to inflammation in the body and to a myriad of health woes, including diabetes and other chronic diseases.

And don't be fooled—if you think putting that packet of brown cane sugar in your coffee is better for you than the white, think again. To your body, they are identical. Similarly, don't go buck-wild with agave or honey just because they are "natural." They are still sugar, are about 4 calories per gram, and are fiber flatliners. *Easy does it.* When using sweeteners, I like Stevia and Xylitol. Both are as sweet, are plant derived, and are significantly lower in calories than the regular old white stuff.

your fiber-focused menu

MY DAILY DIET TO GET AISLE READY

Here is exactly what I ate for breakfast, lunch, dinner—and in between—in prep for the wedding march. Generally speaking, I lost three to four pounds a week and within six weeks, I had reached my goal, "fit into my Marchesa wedding gown," weight.

BREAKFAST

CHOOSE ONE OF THE THREE OPTIONS

1. 1 small container 0% plain Greek yogurt (you can sweeten it with Stevia) with one of the following cereals:
   - Kellogg's All-Bran Buds (⅓ cup serving)
   - Fiber One, Original (½ cup serving)
   - Cereal of choice: must be 100 calories or less and 12 net carb or less
2. Up to 16 ounces of detox smoothie—this will also count as your serving of fruit for the day.
3. 3 fiber-rich bran crackers with your choice of one of the toppings listed on the next page.

OPTIONAL: Have your single fruit serving for the day now, or anytime as a snack.

BEVERAGE: black coffee, tea, or water

Rebecca's Detox Smoothie

yield: *Four 1-cup servings*

INGREDIENTS:

- 1 bunch fresh spinach leaves
- ½ a head of romaine lettuce, leaves torn up
- 1 small scoop, Sunwarrior Vegan Protein Powder
- 2 cups water
- 2 stalks of celery or 1 cucumber, peeled
- 1 apple or pear, cored
- ½ banana (frozen gives it a creamy texture)
- Juice of ½ a lemon

DIRECTIONS:

In a blender add the spinach, romaine lettuce, protein powder, and water. Blend until smooth. Next add the celery or cucumber and blend. Then add the apple or pear and blend. Finally add the banana and lemon juice and blend until creamy.

Nutritional Content for Journaling = 21 g carbs, 15 g fiber

fiber-rich CRACKER TOPPERS!

* 2–3 ounces low-fat cheese. Optional: top with tomatoes or other veggies
* 4 egg whites (hard-boiled, omelet, scrambled). Optional: add sautéed veggies and 1 ounce low-fat cheese
* ½ cup 1% fat cottage cheese
* A few slices of avocado
* 1 small container 0% plain Greek yogurt (you can sweeten it with Stevia) Optional: add sliced fruit on top
* 1 ounce low-fat cream cheese or 1–2 Laughing Cow light cheese wedges with 2 ounces smoked salmon. Optional: add tomato, capers, and onion
* 2–3 ounces, all-natural, organic deli meats (turkey, roast beef, ham) Optional: top with lettuce, tomato, mustard, low-fat mayo

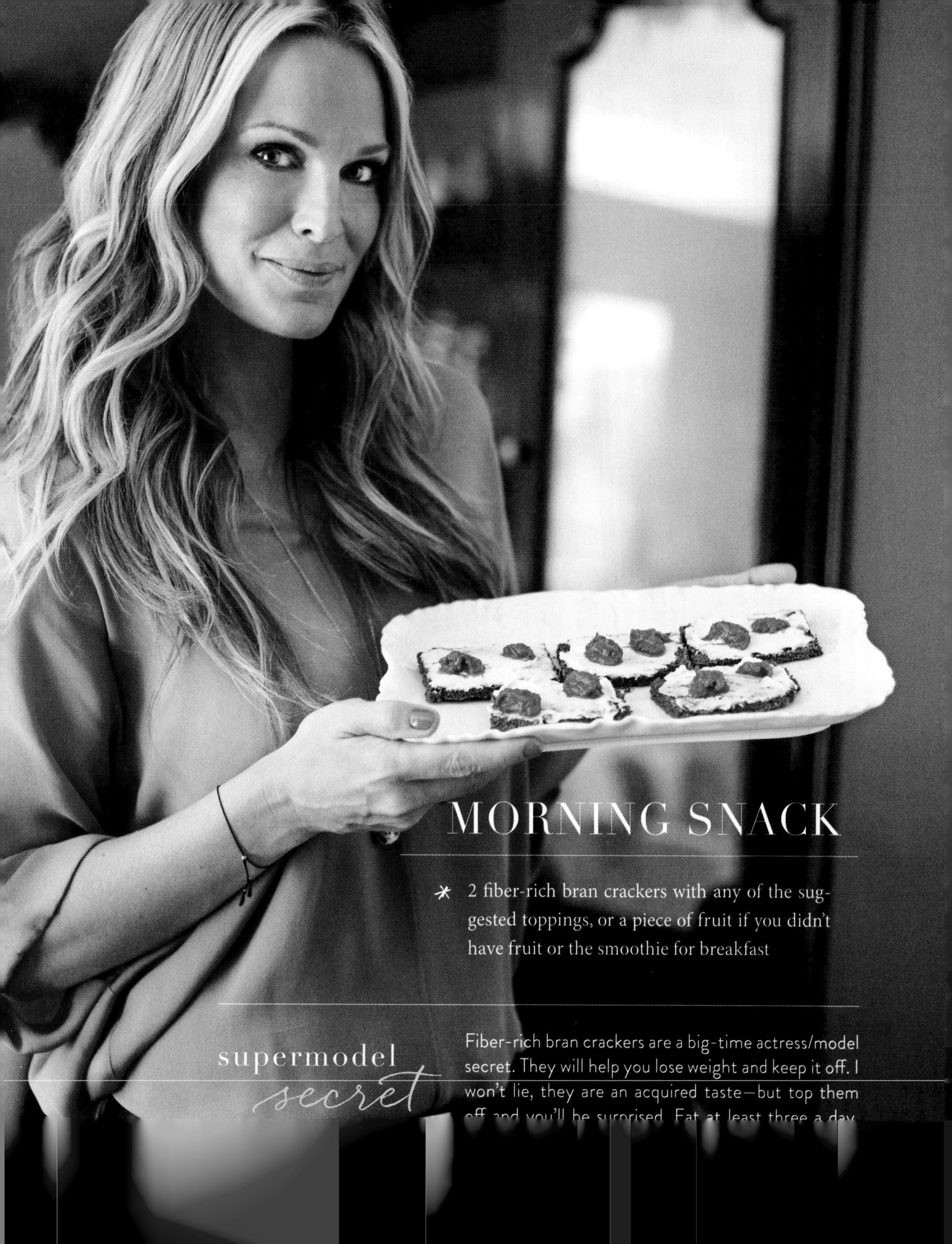

MORNING SNACK

* 2 fiber-rich bran crackers with any of the suggested toppings, or a piece of fruit if you didn't have fruit or the smoothie for breakfast

supermodel *secret*

Fiber-rich bran crackers are a big-time actress/model secret. They will help you lose weight and keep it off. I won't lie, they are an acquired taste—but top them off and you'll be surprised. Eat at least three a day

LUNCH

CHOOSE ONE OF THE FOUR OPTIONS

1. An everyday supermodel salad
   - Large vegetable-filled salad topped with lean protein. (Feel free to include as many nonstarchy vegetables in your salad as you want. Top your salad with 2–3 ounces of lean protein—no more than the size of a deck of cards.)
   - **DRESSING:** Any vinegar or lemon/grapefruit/orange juices are fine, or have low-fat, low-calorie dressing on the side and use sparingly. If out for lunch, ask your server for a side of vinegar.
   - Steer clear of going overboard on salad toppings that can add up to unwanted calories, like excess beans, nuts, seeds, cheeses, avocado, dried fruit, and corn. These toppers have healthy properties but are also calorically dense—so just a sprinkle!

2. Sushi Lunch
   - Miso soup, green salad with ginger dressing with your choice of one of the following:
   - Sashimi (up to six pieces)
   - Hand rolls WITHOUT RICE (up to three rolls)
   - **COMBO:** one hand roll without rice and up to three pieces of sashimi
   - Naruto roll/cucumber-wrapped roll without rice (one Naruto roll only)

   SUSHI RULES: Skip white rice. No mayoized anything, crunchy fried onions, or tempura. Avoid appetite-stimulating soy sauce and instead ask for low-salt/low-fat dressings/sauces.

3. 2–3 ounces lean protein and vegetables
   - Lean proteins can be grilled, steamed, poached/boiled, or baked.
   - Try adding one teaspoon of Parmesan cheese to steamed vegetables to add flavor.

4. Soup and salad
   - 1 cup broth or vegetable-based soup such as chicken and vegetable, miso, gazpacho, or vegetable soup

   BEVERAGE: black coffee, tea, or water (or have one glass of wine or a spunky spirit!)

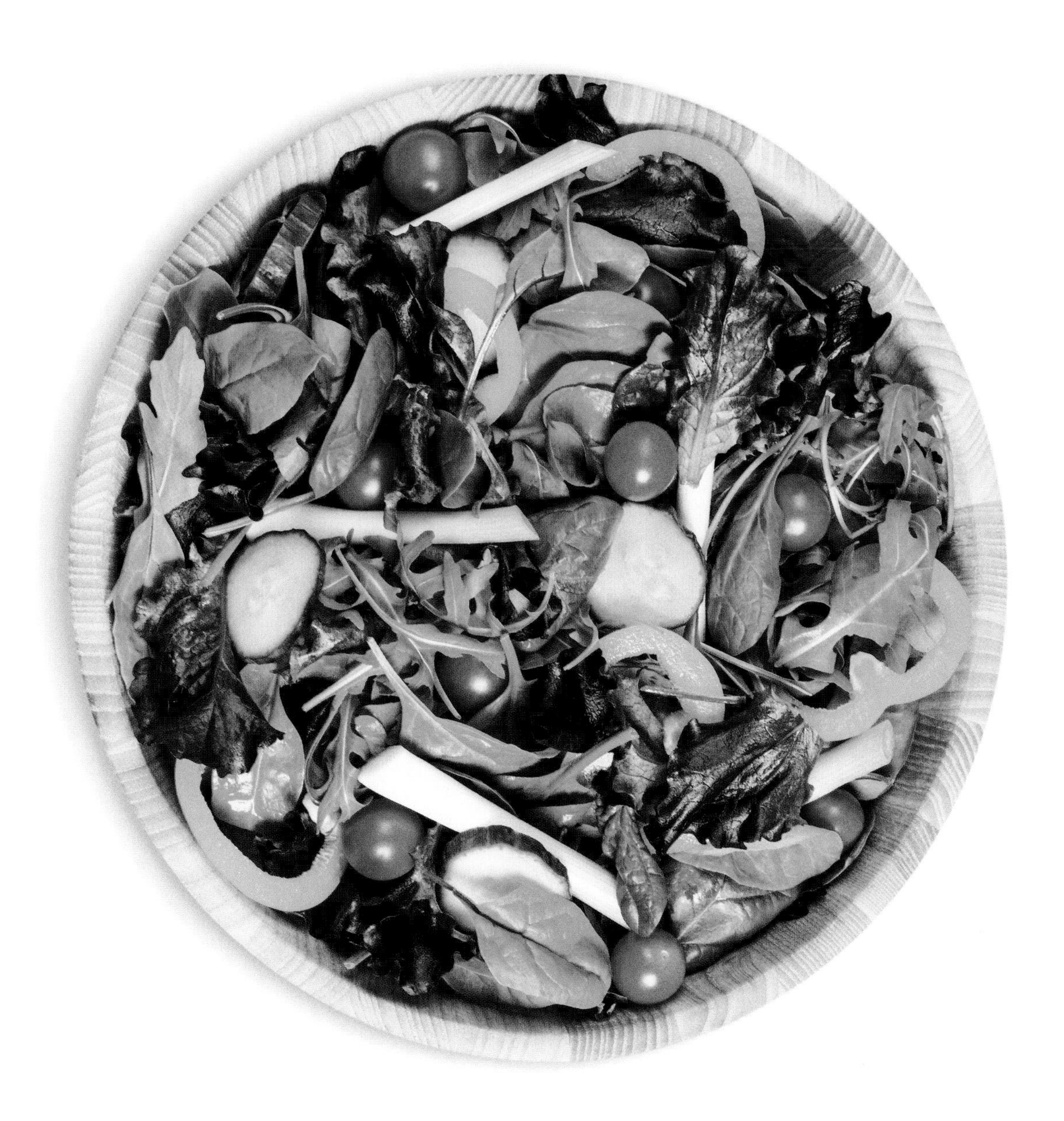

rebecca's *rule*

Create the illusion of more food. We eat with our eyes. You can have pasta. But choose a whole-grain version . . . and switch the ratio. The veggies should be the bulk of the dish, and your pasta the topper. All the extra fiber will fill you up and you'll hardly miss the garlic bread!

AFTERNOON SNACK

CHOOSE ONE OF THE FOUR OPTIONS

1. 2 fiber rich bran crackers with a topping
2. Cucumber or carrot slices with a little hummus or tzatziki dip
3. 1 small container 0% plain Greek yogurt or 1% cottage cheese with vegetables like carrots, celery, tomatoes, peppers, and green beans
4. Up to 16 ounces of detox smoothie

DINNER

CHOOSE ONE OPTION

WHEN COOKING AT HOME: Generally, I follow the same plan as lunch, choosing one of these options:

1. An *everyday supermodel* salad (lots of veggies topped with 2–3 ounces of lean protein)
2. A serving of lean protein and veggies
3. Soup and salad. I ate Chef Gavan's green soup like it was going out of style! (Recipe included later.)

WHEN DINING OUT: Stick with a similar game plan. Choose one of the following three options:

1. Salad and protein appetizer
    - Choose any kind of salad with nonstarchy vegetables: tricolor salad, arugula salad, green salad, artichokes, mushrooms, or chopped salad. Dressing on the side.

- Protein appetizers can include: carpaccio, braseola, raw oysters, clams, mussels, lobster, shrimp, scallops, tuna tartar, or other raw fish appetizers.

2. Protein appetizer and steamed vegetables
   - Remember, if vegetables are not steamed (perhaps they are sautéed instead) only eat half the serving.
3. Sushi dinner
   - Play by the same rules as lunch. No kamikaze rolls stuffed with mayo. Tip: some places will do a cucumber-wrapped roll rather than rice. Just ask!

BEVERAGE: black coffee, tea, or water of course. And guess what? A small glass of white wine, prosecco, or a vodka/soda with a twist! If you must sweeten it up, add just a splash of your favorite juice. But absolutely no high-calorie, sugary mixers.
DESSERT: Yes. You. CAN!! Amen. Rule is, keep the calorie count in check. I try not to go above 100 calories.

- A cup of hot chocolate
- A small square of something decadent, like dark chocolate. I love Choco-Rite Calcium Bites. Chocolatey goodness and 500 mg of calcium. I keep them in my freezer for extra crunch.
- Fudgsicle or Creamsicle
- Small serving of fruit—I love a handful of frozen grapes or blueberries!
- Anything that satisfies your craving—*but no more than three bites!* Play by the 3 BITE RULE with dessert *always,* whether eating out or at home.

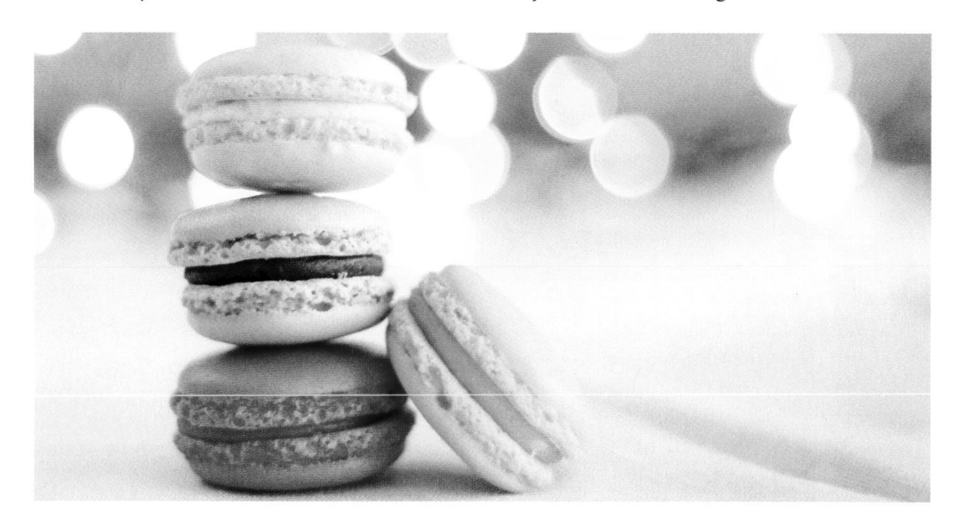

Green Veggie Soup by Chef Gavan Murphy

I ate this soup almost every day while I was fiber-focusing my way to a wedding-ready body—either for lunch or dinner. It's the perfect light meal, is packed with vitamins and minerals, and is low on calories . . . with no fat. (We obviously need some fat, but I get my healthy fats elsewhere.) And, ladies . . . it's absolutely perfect for dinner if you have to put on something tight/hit the town afterward. The hubby and I feed it to our toddler and believe it or not he's Baby Gaga for it.

yield: *4 servings*

INGREDIENTS:

2 cups raw broccoli
1 head kale—stems removed
1 bag spinach
2 garlic cloves—minced
4 cups low-sodium vegetable broth

DIRECTIONS:

Put everything except the spinach in a soup pot and bring to a boil. Cook, partially covered with lid for 15 minutes or until broccoli is softened. Blend in batches while adding fresh spinach. Return to another pot once blended and add more broth or water to desired consistency. This soup can also be made with chicken broth. Taste and season with a pinch of salt and pepper, and even a teaspoon of grated parmesan. As my baby, Brooks, would say, "Num, num!"

TIP: To boost the protein ratio, Rebecca suggests blending a serving of silken tofu into the soup (or any veggie soup for that matter). The added protein adds weight to the soup and will make you feel fuller longer. Believe it or not, tofu makes for a deliciously creamy texture à la cream of broccoli soup.

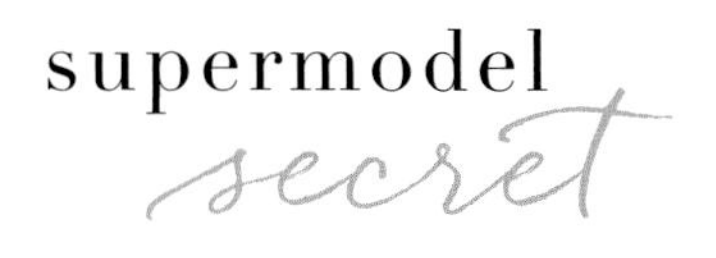

Changing your eating habits isn't about being perfect in the week and then binging on the weekend. One day of indulging might not make you gain weight, but an entire weekend, *every weekend,* will. Our plan is about making healthy choices *every day* and those healthy choices INCLUDE allowing yourself treats along the way. It's about treating . . . not cheating. If you love pizza, have a slice every now and again, that way you won't binge or overeat on a "cheat" day. Pair ONE slice of pizza with a hulking, fiber-filled salad and you'll be satisfied.

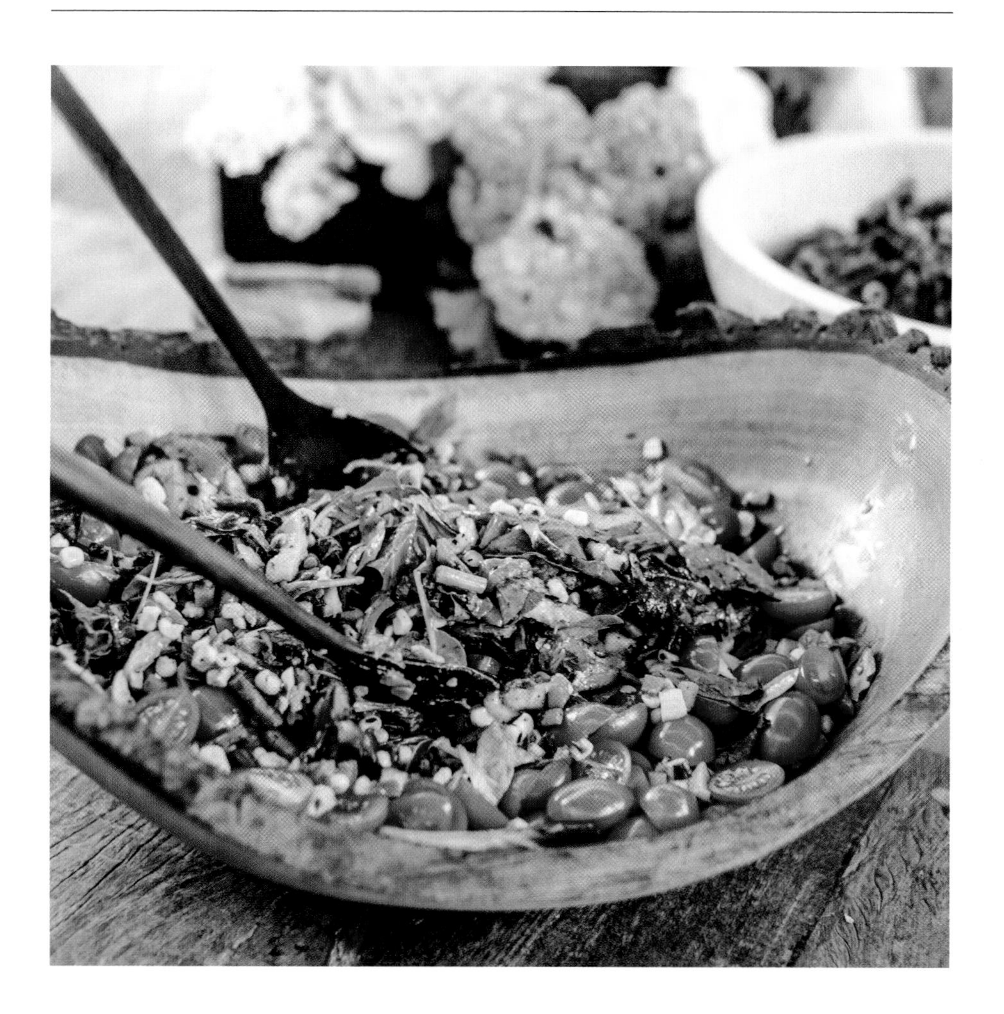

foods that are *fakers*

There are so many "health foods" out there that are fakers. They are high in sugar or calories or unhealthy fats, even though they're labeled "diet" or "low-fat." Here are a few to avoid:

1. **FRUIT SMOOTHIES:** Is a fruit smoothie better for you than a cheeseburger? Not always! Many of the bottled ones sold in stores or served at fast-food restaurants are outrageously high in calories and added sweeteners! Make your own (Rebecca's detox smoothie or Fergie's combo). A homemade, greens-based smoothie is a delicious way to trick yourself (and your family) into eating more veggies.

2. **GRANOLA/GRANOLA-STYLE BARS:** Store-bought granolas can be swimming in fats, oils, sugar, and salt. The dried fruit alone can add up to a ton of calories. Instead, make your own raw trail mix to satisfy the urge to crunch. Combine a few raw walnuts, almonds, sunflower and pumpkin seeds, and a pinch of dried coconut for an occasional sweet surprise. (Udi's gluten-free granola is a healthy store-bought option.)

3. **SWEETENED YOGURT:** Brightly lit shelves of this are all over your grocery store. These sweetened yogurts pack a sugary punch. Some brands have over 17 grams of sugar and major carb count. Instead, have plain Greek with a swirl of agave or honey, that way *you* control the sugar. Top it off with a few berries and a dash of flax seeds for skin-friendly antioxidants and heart-healthy essential fatty acids.

4. **FROZEN YOGURT SHOPS:** Is this actually considered food? By now we should all know that fat-free does not necessarily mean calorie-free. A medium serving of this frozen fakey-food can have tons of calories and sugars and then when you add the toppings . . . #fugetaboutit! You wind up with more calories (and chemicals) than a scoop of ice cream. Just say no!

5. **FAT-FREE MUFFINS, BREADS, AND BAGELS:** These are just butt expanders. Even bran ones. Some have one-third of the average daily recommended dose of calories in them—all in one stupid muffin. And there is no nutritional value. Zippo! Oh, and that NY bagel you love to eat? IT'S LIKE EATING SIX PIECES OF WHITE TOAST. Is it really worth it? Damn. There are always bagels on-set. *Always.*

6. **CATCHPHRASE PHONIES:** Just because it's labeled "low-cal" or "gluten-free" or "vegan" or "fat-free" or "organic" doesn't necessarily mean it's "good for you." Remember, french fries are technically "vegan." While sometimes it's a healthy choice, often enough they are packed with sodium, sugar, or other yucky additives or allergens. Get beyond the front of the box and learn to read labels and recognize no-no ingredients.

7. **HEALTHY "EXTRAS":** You might think that one extra scoop of pine nuts on your salad, or a few *more* slices of avocado on your turkey wrap are no big deal, *because they are healthy*! BUT even healthy foods add up. That *extra* spoonful of almond butter will make its way onto your butt. Once I started cutting out all the little "extras" I really began to see a difference in my weight. I am convinced this alone is what has helped me get off this last, stubborn bit of baby bulge.

Something that has changed my life is starting off every day with a green smoothie that includes kale, spinach, romaine, celery, banana, apple, and pear. It gives me an energy boost to start the day, while cleaning out my digestive system from the previous day. I used to have a hearty breakfast, but now I earn my meal by finishing the smoothie and waiting until I am hungry. It gives me great energy to work out without feeling heavy. But, I do admit, ordering room-service breakfast in bed on vacation with my husband is now a big, fun splurge!

—FERGIE

---

let's talk about salt, baby

Salt, like sugar, is as addictive as nicotine. And like sugar, it releases dopamine in the body. You will crave more. Salt increases both hunger and thirst. Research shows a link between salt consumption and an increased intake of sugary, calorie-heavy drinks. More bad news? Some studies suggest that a high-salt diet boosts insulin production, telling your body to store more fat. NO bueno. Safe guidelines recommend no more than one teaspoon of salt (2,300 mg) a day. For African Americans, people over fifty, or people with chronic diseases, the recommendation is even less.

I suggest chucking your basic table salt in the trash. Why? It's totally denatured and stripped of all the natural benefits. Try Celtic gray salt or Himalayan pink salt. Both are alive with minerals and better for you. But remember, the suggested intake stays the same. In general, be salt savvy: packaged foods can have stiletto-high sodium levels. And forget the salt-rimmed margarita and tortilla chips. I love both, but when I indulge—I always pay. Before my wedding and after the baby, I personally chose to cut out all salt because I bloat like the Goodyear Blimp.

---

supermomma secret

Feeding your little ones high-sugar foods and salty snacks will set them up for food failure. According to Rebecca, young palates are highly sensitive, and the little buggers get addicted easily and early on. They will crave these foods and be desensitized to nature's true candy. If you want an *everyday superbaby*, feed them natural treats, such as fruits and low-salt foods. You will help them establish a healthy palate that will serve them for years to come.

My *everyday supermodel* strategy to shed and shred long term.

When Rebecca and I met, I found out I was eating way too much protein. It's because I was *so terrified* of carbs before—even the good carbs in healthy fruits, brown rice, beans, and veggies. So I ate a lot of meat—turkey and chicken—all the time. While I was on her program, I did eat lean protein, but cut back on the amount of animal protein (ate smaller portions) and started adding more vegetarian-sourced protein to my meals. I have learned that eating more plant foods is essential for staying fit and healthy.

The fact is: we do not need to eat meat for every meal, every day. That is the old way of thinking. And to be clear, I'm not a vegetarian or a vegan, but I do work to incorporate vegetarian (or plant-based) meals into my diet, because it's good for me—it's good for all of us. Going all vegetarian isn't sustainable for me—and that is certainly not what I'm advocating (although that may be the right choice for some)—but going *a little more veggie* is! More and more clinical research tells us that pledging to go a little more veg is good for our body and our overall health. Let's explore the what's and why's of more plant-based eating.

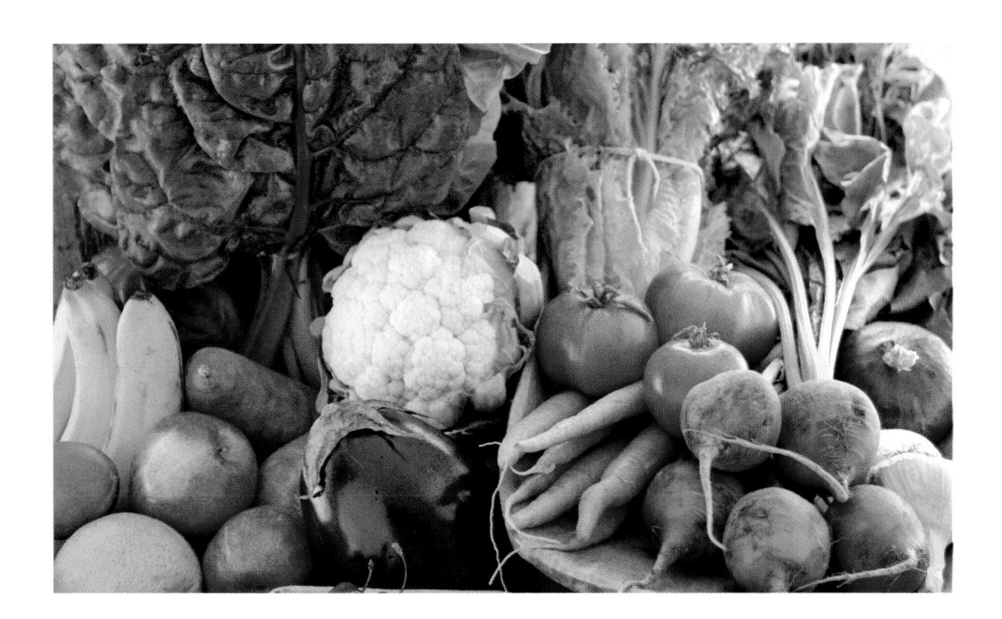

The *basics*

* You don't eat anything with eyes, mouth, or a brain. Or that came out of something with eyes, mouth, or a brain. (Plant-based eating means no dairy either—so no eggs, milk, and cheeses).
* You eat whole grains, legumes, nuts, seeds, vegetables (even sea veggies!) and fruits.
* Your protein sources are plant based.

The *benefits*

* Naturally low-cal and fat-free! Most plant foods—fruits, veggies, legumes, and grains—contain no fat. (Avocados, coconuts, nuts, and seeds are the exception.) And most are lower in calories than meat and dairy products. So you can eat as much as you want. Few restrictions here!
* Fruits and veggies are at least 90 percent water. Research shows that those who eat foods that have a higher water content have a lower body mass index and slimmer waists.
* Most vegetarian sources of fat are high in the "good" fat and low in the "bad" fats. Even the few that are high in "bad" or saturated fats, such as macadamia and brazil nuts, or coconut, are still relatively low when compared to dairy and meat products.
* Plant-based eating motivates your bowel movements and boosts your metabolism. The plant fiber is like a giant broom moving through your organs—your liver, kidneys, and intestines.
* No cellulite? Whaaaaaaaaaaat?! Less cholesterol in our bodies means fewer toxins and less fat stored in our blood and tissues. When adding more plant-based foods and meals into my eating plan I've found my body to be firmer and my skin to be smoother and more elastic. Your cellulite will improve. I've noticed this firsthand. That's reason alone to go more veggie, soul sister.
* Studies tell us that dairy can lead to inflammation in the body and create excess mucus. Dairy can aggravate irritable bowel syndrome and is believed by many to be the source of numerous allergies, not to mention it frequently houses unhealthy hormones, antibiotics, and even pesticides.

It's up to you, but I do *limit* my dairy. (I'm not overboard on this, but when I eat dairy, I try to choose organic options.)

Other general benefits

- Eating more greens means more vitamins and minerals, and more energy. Think green = machine!
- Studies show that diets high in leafy greens and healthy fats boost memory, fact recall, motor skills, and more.
- Plant foods are easier to digest than meats, so they give your body processes and organs a minivacation.
- Studies suggest vegetarians have a reduced risk of heart disease, cancer, diabetes, obesity, and *live longer*. I'm not advocating that a strict vegetarian diet is for everyone, but these stats convince me that eating more veggies is a form of preventative health.
- Eating plant foods is better for the environment. Growing fruits and veggies uses significantly fewer resources than producing meats for market. It also contributes *way* less to environmental pollution—even more so if you shop local!

let's talk about fats, baby

Remember when every diet and weight-management program seemed to say we should avoid any and every fat? I did! And remember the wonders of chemical cocktails like Olestra that were marketed to us? We all know how that ended. *In a Hail Mary sprint to the toilet.*

I used to eat like that: absolutely no fats, *no exceptions.* Then I'd go and eat no-fat crap food. Not anymore. After working with Rebecca, I know now that we need healthy fats in our diet. They are good for you! Let's break down the "good," the "bad," and the "ugly" when it comes to fats, an essential macronutrient.

GOOD FATS: These are unsaturated fats, including omega essential fatty acids (EFAs), monounsaturated and polyunsaturated fats. Our body needs these fats for *everyday supermodel* skin and a whole lot of other necessary body processes. They are liquid at room temperature and mostly sourced from plant-based foods.

- Some nutrients, including vitamins A, D, E, and K, are fat-soluble, meaning we NEED fat to absorb them! Good fats are essential for the development of healthy skin, eyesight, and brain function.
- Good fats help to *lower the bad cholesterol* (LDL) levels in our bodies AND *raise the good cholesterol* (HDL) levels.
- Studies show that people with lower LDL and higher HDL have significantly less risk for heart attacks and cardiovascular disease and a significantly reduced risk of other chronic diseases.

Where to Find These *good fats*

- Plant foods such as avocados, olives, almonds, walnuts, hazelnuts
- Any oils from these plants or nuts, such as olive oil, walnut oil, and grapeseed oil
- Many seeds, including sesame, sunflower, pumpkin, and chia
- Fish, including salmon, sea bass, and all oily fish (FYI: lean meats, such as chicken, turkey, or beef, do not contain healthy fats)

BAD FATS: These are some saturated fats and trans fats (yucky man-made fats). Saturated fats are solid at room temperature and are mainly from animal sources. Most trans fats are man-made from oils through a food-processing method called partial hydrogenation and are also solid at room temp. Studies show both saturated and trans fats clog arteries and contribute to poor health and increased body fat.

- The Mayo Clinic states "Saturated fat raises total blood cholesterol levels and low-density lipoprotein (LDL) cholesterol levels, which can increase your risk of cardiovascular disease. Saturated fat may also increase your risk of type 2 diabetes."
- Bad fats are proven to contribute to weight gain.

Where You'll Find *bad fats*

- Nonlean animal products
- Most full-fat dairy products, including eggs, cheese, and butter
- Anything fried
- Packaged and processed food can be full of bad fats so *always read the labels*. This can even be the case for so-called packaged "health" foods.

supermodel *secret*

Remember, if you are *trying to lose weight,* the more fats you eat—good or bad ones—the more calories you are taking in. Fats are calorie dense. Always keep portion control in mind with all foods, but especially when it comes to fats and even healthy fats. Avoid "salad-drenching" with excess oil or eating *more than* a small handful of heart-healthy nuts.

what about protein?

Protein is undoubtedly crucial for a healthy body. But research suggests that *too much animal protein* may have negative effects, including increasing the acidity of our bodies, leaching calcium from our bones to neutralize that acidity, and being tough on our kidneys. The Mayo Clinic website says to, "emphasize plant sources of protein, such as beans, lentils, soy products, and unsalted nuts. These high-protein foods have the added bonus of being higher in health-enhancing nutrients than are animal sources of protein."

So how much protein do we actually need? Well, there are different schools of thought. You will have to compare research and be the judge for yourself. On Rebecca's plan, she had me eat between 8 and 10 ounces a day, or about 55–65 grams. According to the U.S. Recommended Daily Allowance (US RDA) a woman needs about 46 grams per day. The Mayo Clinic says to get 10 to 35 percent of your total daily calories from protein. Protein has four calories a gram. Based on a 2,000-calorie-a-day diet, this amounts to about 200 to 700 calories a day, or about 50 to 175 grams a day. (Don't forget, 7 grams of protein equals an ounce). In his book *Eat to Live,* Dr. Joel Fuhrman suggests a helpful formula specific to you. Multiply .36 by your body weight to find your recommended protein intake. If you are 120 pounds, you need 44 grams of protein daily. 150 pounds? You need 54 grams.

supermomma secret

If you are pregnant or breast-feeding, you must up your protein. The US RDA suggests eating 71 grams daily to support healthy growth of the bugger in your belly.

Where Can You Find *plant-based protein*

- **QUINOA:** 11 grams per cup
- **LENTILS:** 19.9 grams per cup
- **BEANS:** 12–15 grams per cup
- **SPIRULINA:** 6 grams per cup
- **TOFU:** 10 grams per ½ cup

HOW TO EAT A MORE PLANT-FOCUSED DIET: First, start just by adding more vegetables and healthy grains/legumes to your diet when you can. Start gradually. When you feel comfortable, try replacing at least one full meal a day with a plant-based option. Here are some tips for going more veggie:

- Remember, dinner does *not* have to have meat! Try a healthy stir-fry over a small serving of brown rice or a home-cooked soup as hearty dinner fare.
- Go online or to vegetarian cookbooks for inspiration. Try out some new recipes that highlight plant-based main ingredients.
- Chef Gavan says to experiment with healthy sauces, spices, and seasonings as you venture into plant-based eating. They really up the ante on vegetarian dishes and add savory quality so you don't miss the meat.

Try making one full day a week all veggie, baby. I love the idea of Meatless Mondays—and it's become so widely embraced that it's turned into an international campaign. Today, there are tons of sources for easy, meat-free meals. My girlfriend, actress Ali Larter, has a cooking and entertaining book, *Kitchen Revelry,* filled with outrageously delicious veggie-based dishes. I love her pesto and vegan truffle recipes. Check it out!

molly-fied *meatless* monday

BREAKFAST

Rethink eggs and yogurt for breakfast—mix it up and eat a veggie soup. If you miss your daily yogurt, there are now scrumptious soy and almond versions. Sprinkled with fresh berries, a few walnuts and chia seeds, it's delish.

LUNCH

Everyday supermodel salad with all the veggie fixin's (tomatoes, a few slices of avocado, crunchy carrots, and a sprinkle of sunflower seeds), a few beans for added protein, and a light drizzle of olive oil/balsamic vinaigrette.

DINNER

Quinoa lentil salad for dinner with vegetable consommé or squash noodle pasta. (See recipe from Chef Gavan.)

SNACKS

Graze on carrots, a green apple with touch of almond butter, or our detox smoothie.

Quinoa Lentil Salad by Gavan Murphy

This is a delicious hearty salad, packed with protein and fiber; it is totally plant based and will leave you feeling satisfied.

yield: *6 servings*

INGREDIENTS:

1 cup lentils (I used regular green lentils)
1 cup quinoa (I used red quinoa)
3 tablespoons white-wine vinegar
2 teaspoon salt
3 tablespoons extra-virgin olive oil
½ cup fresh mint, finely chopped
2 tablespoons lemon zest
Salt and pepper to taste

DIRECTIONS:

Rinse the lentils. In a small saucepan add enough water to cover the lentils by 2 inches, add 1 teaspoon salt and simmer until tender but not falling apart, about 15 minutes.

Meanwhile, place quinoa, 2 cups water, and 1 teaspoon salt in another saucepan and bring to a boil. Reduce to simmer, cover, and cook until all water is absorbed, about 15 minutes.

When lentils are done, drain well. Remove hot lentils to a large mixing bowl and stir in 1 tablespoons of vinegar, salt and pepper to taste. Cool lentils completely, stirring occasionally.

When quinoa is cooked, drain any excess liquid. Cool and add to lentils in mixing bowl.

In a small bowl whisk together remaining 2 tablespoons vinegar, oil, salt, and pepper to taste.

Combine lentils, quinoa, and dressing. Add in mint and zest. Mix well. Cover and chill until ready to serve.

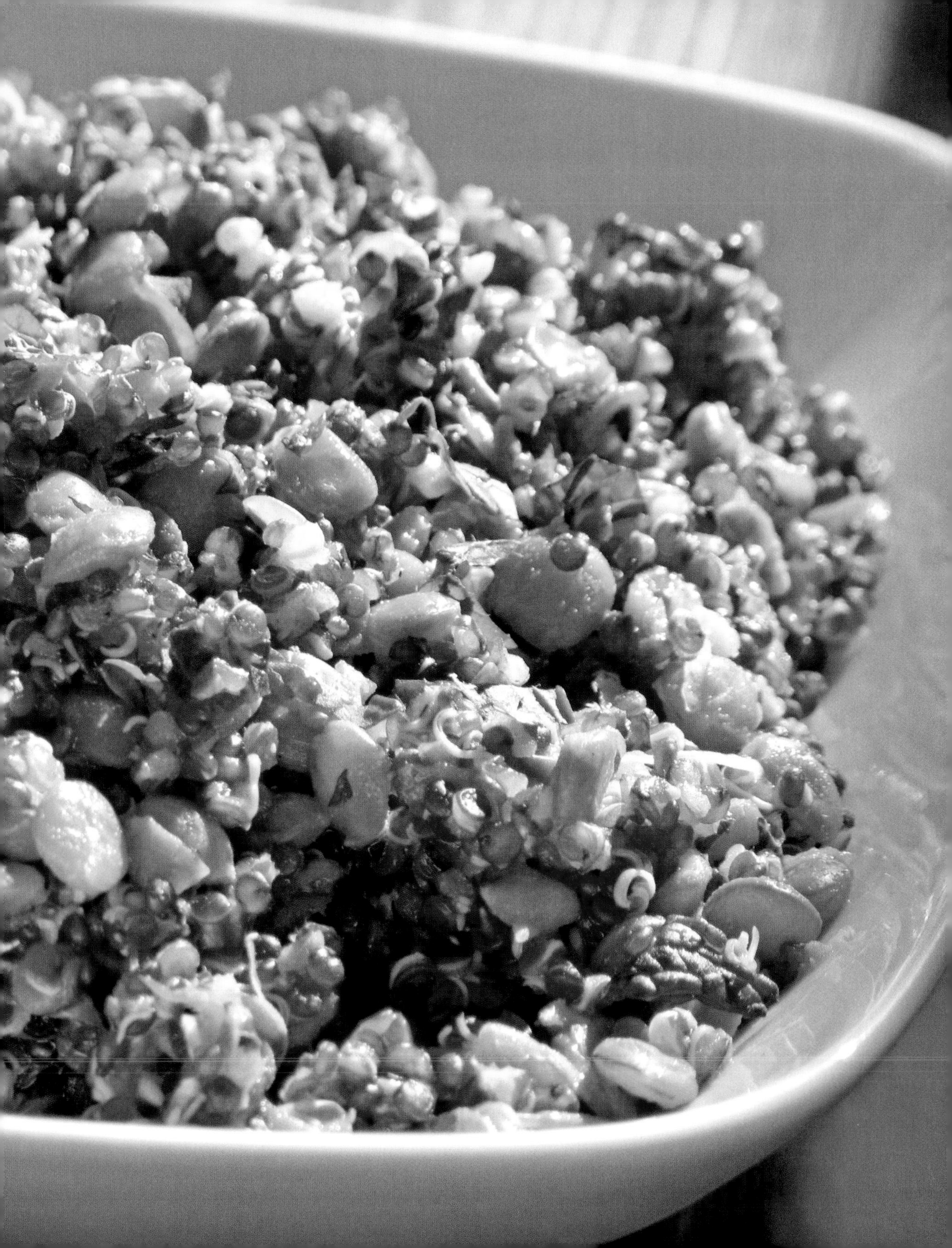

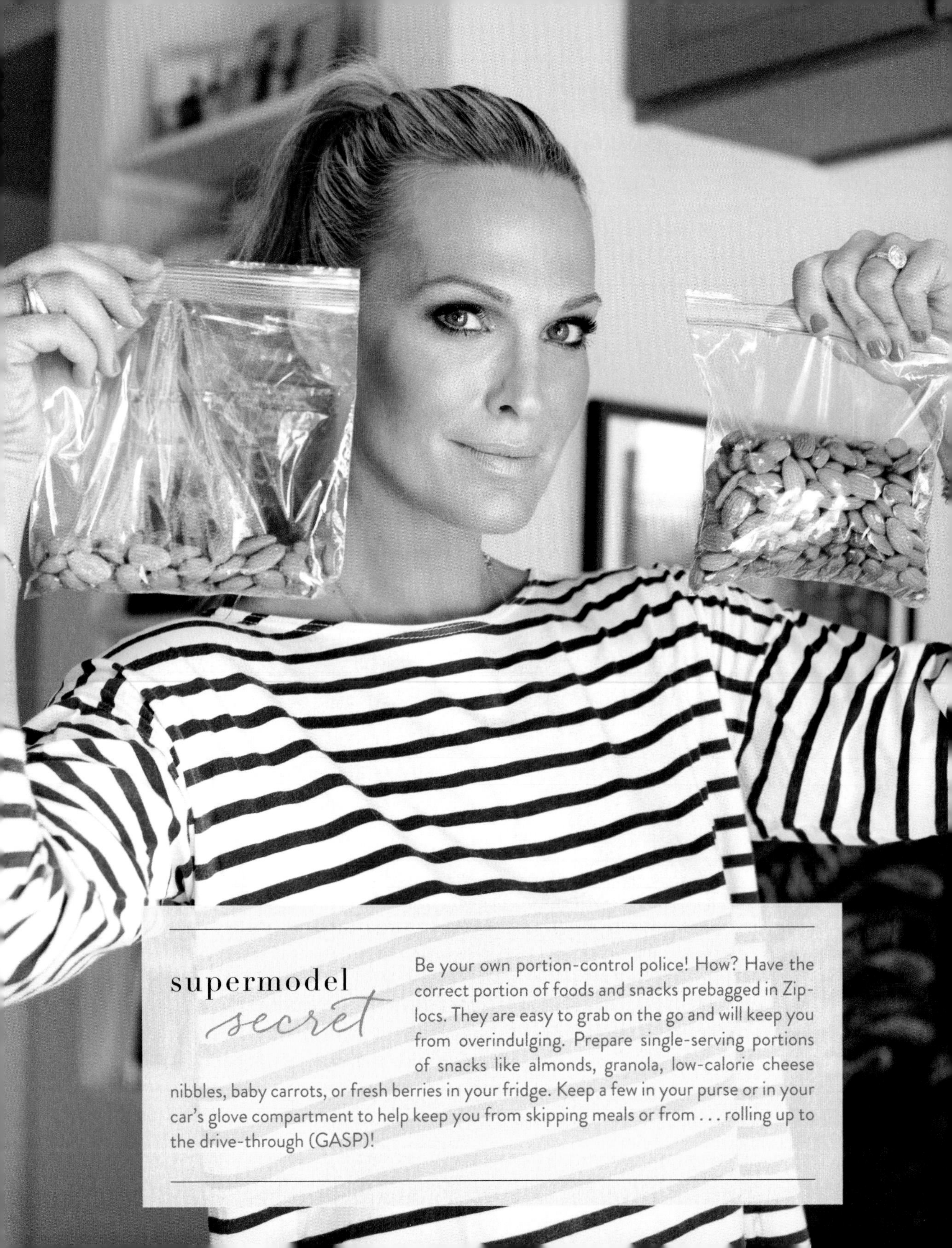

supermodel *secret*

Be your own portion-control police! How? Have the correct portion of foods and snacks prebagged in Ziplocs. They are easy to grab on the go and will keep you from overindulging. Prepare single-serving portions of snacks like almonds, granola, low-calorie cheese nibbles, baby carrots, or fresh berries in your fridge. Keep a few in your purse or in your car's glove compartment to help keep you from skipping meals or from . . . rolling up to the drive-through (GASP)!

LET'S TALK *raw* AND WHY IS IT ALL THE RAGE?

Raw basically means no cooking required. No cooking means less time in the kitchen. Preparing raw meals is basically assembly, so it is fantastic if you are short on time. You can chop foods up and prepare them in advance too. Well, I can get behind that! Raw foods are great to work into your plant-based diet for a fitter figure.

Raw foods have more living enzymes in them than cooked foods (most packaged foods have zero), because cooking breaks these enzymes down. For example some cancer-fighting compounds in broccoli are greatly reduced when broccoli is cooked. Certain vitamins, such as vitamin C and folate, are also destroyed when cooked. (That's important to know when you are trying to get the right amount of folate when pregnant.) That doesn't go for *all* veggies, but generally speaking, cooking frequently causes a reduction in nutritional value. Cooking can also promote the formation of potentially harmful (even cancer-causing) compounds in food during high-heat cooking. All the more reason to give raw eating a go! Fresh veggie juices are an easy way to add raw food and living enzymes to your diet. These do not include the ones you can buy bottled at Starbucks or at the grocery store—sorry! Those have been heated and processed (pasteurized) so the enzymes have been squelched. Try a local juice bar, juicing at home, or even a juice delivery service and go raw, even for just a snack.

---

supermodel *secret*

MY THOUGHTS ON EATING RAW OR GOING VEGAN. I know a lot of models and actresses who go raw or vegan and they look great. Recently raw/vegan diets seem to be the rage; they are all over the media and are hailed, by some, as the be-all and end-all to losing weight. I do think it can be a successful strategy to weight loss and improved health—*if you do it right*. But for me, it's about incorporating it into my lifestyle. Not making it my lifestyle. For a very brief period, I followed a strictly raw, vegan diet. It was too restrictive for me personally, and I found that I didn't have the energy I normally do. But what I learned in the process was to work the occasional vegan or raw meal into my diet because I know it's good for me—enzymes! Some of the salads I eat are both vegan and raw. If you choose to eat a raw or vegan diet, do the necessary research and consult a doctor or nutritionist to do it safely. Be sure to supplement with the necessary amino acids, B vitamins, and iron that you don't get when eating raw or vegan.

---

more *tips* for PLANT-BASED eating

1. **BUY ORGANIC WHEN IT COUNTS.** It's a fact; conventional farming practices use unhealthy pesticides and other unsafe, or unproven, practices when growing our foods. Organic food is becoming more accessible and more affordable than ever before, but I know that it is still more expensive—especially when you are buying for a family. For many of us, it isn't financially realistic to buy exclusively organic, so be smart about which fruits and veggies you do spend extra for. A helpful guide is "The Clean 15" and the "Dirty Dozen Plus" (see the accompanying box here). "The Clean 15" are the fruits and veggies that don't tend to carry as much pesticide/chemical residue. The "Dirty Dozen Plus" generally have the most pesticide/chemical residue. Avocados are part of the "Clean 15," so you might choose not to splurge on organic for those green guys. However, 30 percent of conventionally grown strawberries test positively for pesticides and top the list of the "Dirty Dozen Plus." Strawberries are definitely worth the splurge. If you can't spend the extra cash on organic, buy conventionally grown fruits and veggies but remember to wash them well and peel those that you can (like cucumbers).

2. **AVOID ANY PROCESSING.** Our food has been so processed that some of it is barely recognizable. Research suggests that highly processed foods may not satisfy hunger as well as less-processed, higher-fiber foods. That goes for the soy-based products too, like seitan and all the fake meats out there. Even if they're technically plant based, keep 'em to a minimum.

THE CLEAN 15: Asparagus, avocados, cabbage, cantaloupe, sweet corn, eggplant, grapefruit, kiwi, mangos, cauliflower, onions, papayas, pineapple, sweet peas (frozen), sweet potatoes.

THE DIRTY DOZEN PLUS: Apples, celery, cherry tomatoes, cucumbers, grapes, hot peppers, nectarines, peaches, potatoes, spinach, strawberries, bell peppers, kale/collard greens, snap peas.

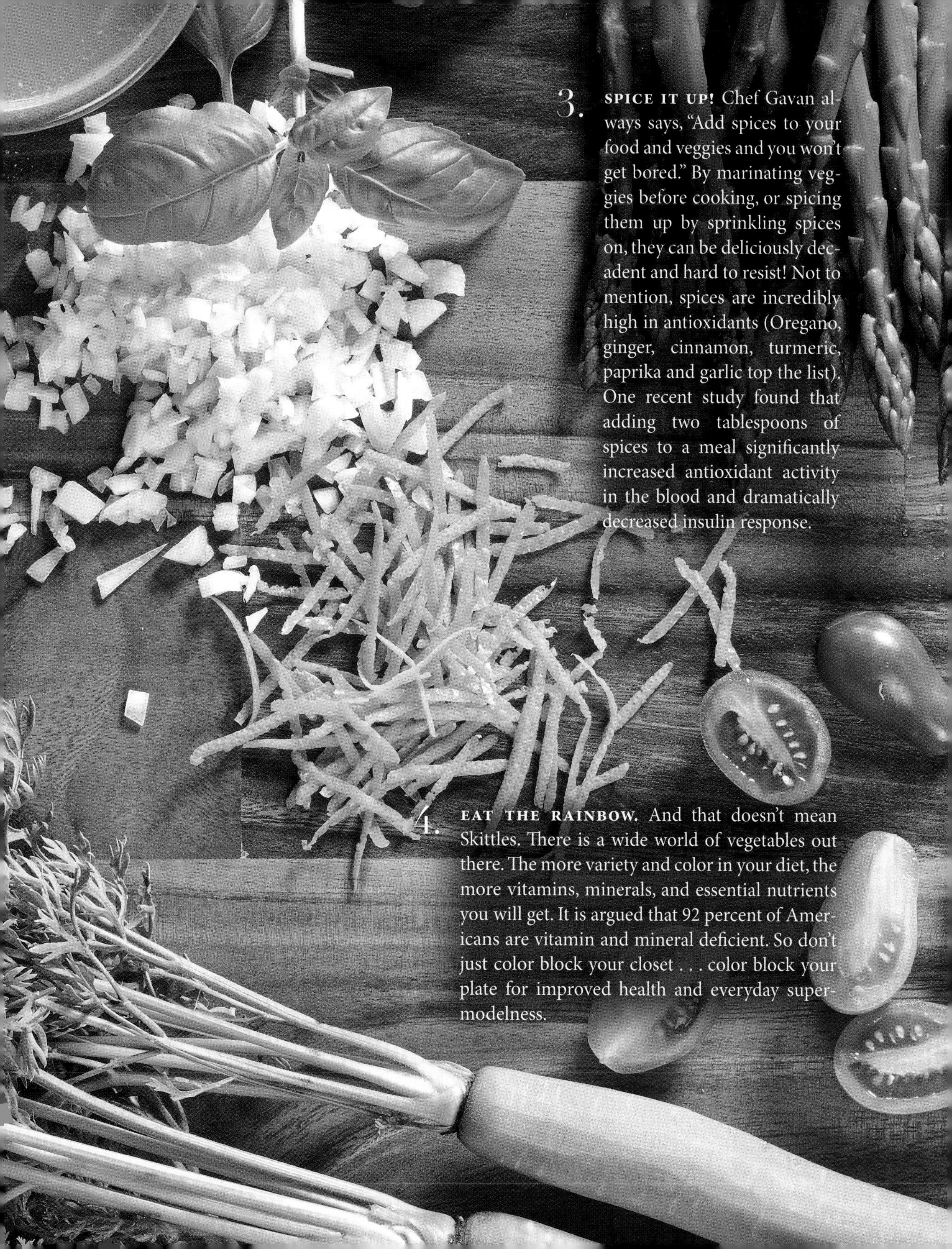

3. **SPICE IT UP!** Chef Gavan always says, "Add spices to your food and veggies and you won't get bored." By marinating veggies before cooking, or spicing them up by sprinkling spices on, they can be deliciously decadent and hard to resist! Not to mention, spices are incredibly high in antioxidants (Oregano, ginger, cinnamon, turmeric, paprika and garlic top the list). One recent study found that adding two tablespoons of spices to a meal significantly increased antioxidant activity in the blood and dramatically decreased insulin response.

4. **EAT THE RAINBOW.** And that doesn't mean Skittles. There is a wide world of vegetables out there. The more variety and color in your diet, the more vitamins, minerals, and essential nutrients you will get. It is argued that 92 percent of Americans are vitamin and mineral deficient. So don't just color block your closet . . . color block your plate for improved health and everyday supermodelness.

How I got inside the pages of *Sports Illustrated*

When I was twenty-six , after I'd been modeling about six years, I received a life-changing (holy sh*t!) call from my modeling agent, Leigh Crystal. She had gotten me a meeting with Diane Smith, the legend behind the *Sports Illustrated* swimsuit edition. To be in the pages of *Sports Illustrated* was (still is) a highly coveted gig among models. I wasn't going to just show up to that meeting. I was going to show up looking and feeling *the best I had ever looked and felt in my entire life.* I wanted *Sports Illustrated* more than I'd wanted anything else in my modeling career.

To prepare for the meeting, I flew out to California and spent seven days at the Ashram. The Ashram is a hard-core, seven-day retreat where you hike in the mountains, do yoga, eat 100 percent vegetarian, and basically get a total mind and body makeover. Here's how they describe it: "A combination of simple spirituality, loving punishment, and camp-like congeniality." It was tough, but in a good, positive, strength-building way. I highly recommend it for anyone who needs a mind/body retreat—CEOs, celebs, teachers, accountants—and *everyday supermodels.*

I left the Ashram looking and feeling fantastic. My mind and body were in the best shape they've ever been. I felt like I could do anything and meet any challenge. I was confident and knew I could get that job if I wanted it. The Ashram is tough and isn't accessible to everyone. But what is accessible is the lesson I learned there—commit to something hard and challenge yourself to stick to it. You can create your own seven-day at-home Ashram. Commit to seven days of demanding exercise, healthy eating, and meditation. See how you feel afterward. Do it with a friend and hold each other accountable.

I met with Diane in New York feeling GREAT and soon after the meeting, we got the call. *Sports Illustrated wanted to shoot me.* This could change everything. I knew I had to be in tip-top condition to feel good in front of that lens. A friend of mine told me about a detox and fasting retreat in California called We Care. We Care supports you through a seven-day liquid fast and promotes healthy, effective weight loss if that is your goal. I'd never tried fasting before, but my friend loved it, and another model I knew had just been through it. I decided to go and do the We Care Cleanse & Detox program one week before my shoot date with *SI.* It

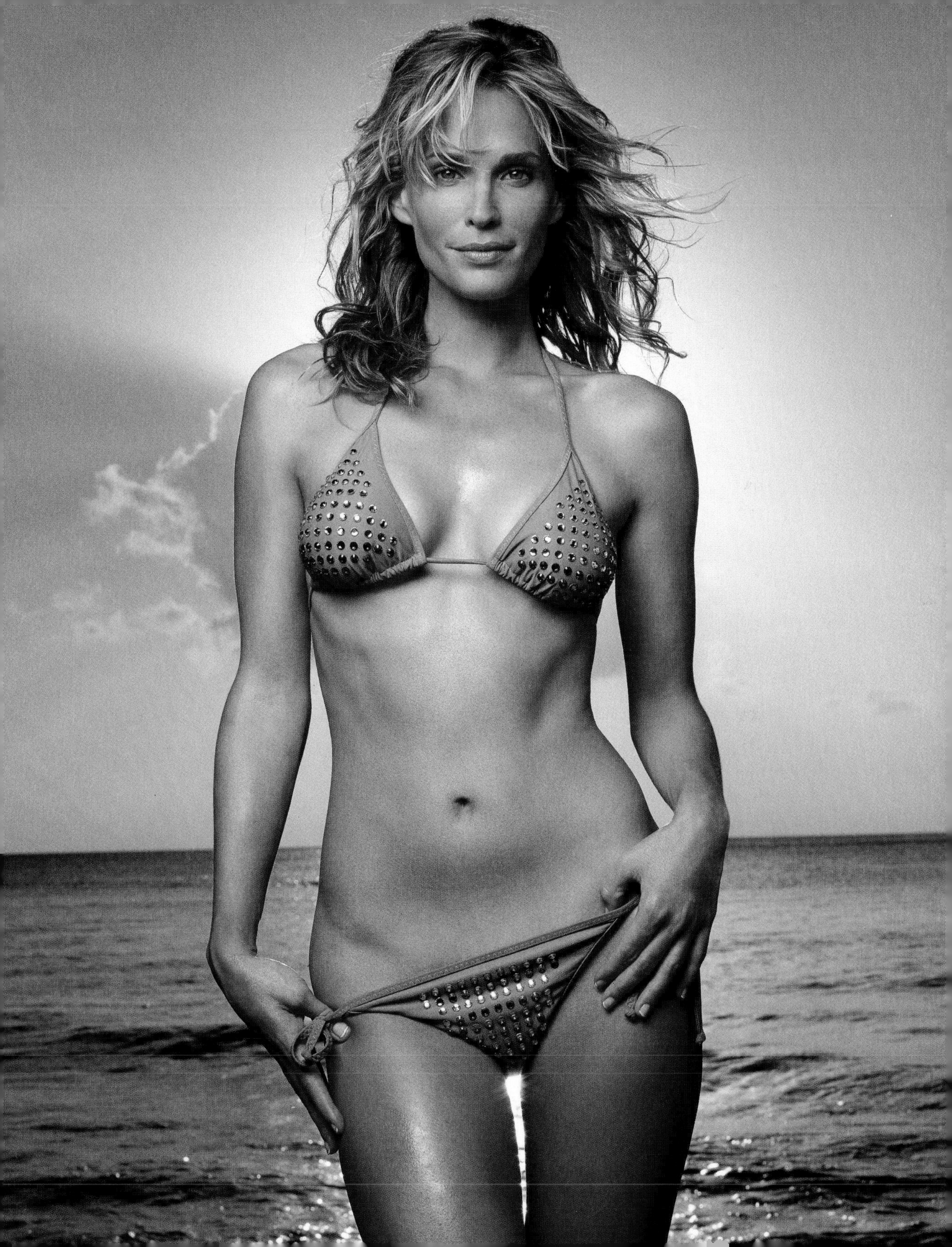

changed my life—and my understanding of how fasting can play a role in your total health plan.

After seven days at We Care, I flew to Hawaii and shot with photographer Walter Chin. With *SI,* just because you do a shoot doesn't mean your photos are automatically selected for the magazine. No one knows who will make the final cut. So I waited. And waited. I wanted to make it in more than anything. And somehow, some way . . . my photos made it in. It was a huge break in my career. My time at the Ashram and We Care absolutely helped prepare me physically and emotionally to make it happen.

That feels like a million years ago now, but to this day, I still go to We Care once a year, sometimes twice. For those who can do it, a liquid fast every season is great for the mind *and the behind*. Early in my career I could do a full seven-day cleanse, but now when I do a liquid fast, I don't do more than three days. I usually go to We Care after the holidays when my mind and body need a break and to rejuvenate. If you have to get into amazing shape, or just need to do something to clear things out—We Care or an accredited and supervised retreat in your area is a good way to go. There are also great at-home options for juice cleanses I list later in the chapter. If you are generally really fit, a longer fast is okay. But if you aren't, start with something short, no longer than three days. Either way, if you are feeling the pull, take the plunge to see if a cleanse or fasting plan is right for you and your body. I swear by it. But I'm aware it's not for everyone.

WHAT EXACTLY IS FASTING? During a fast there is no chomping of anything. It's all liquid, baby. And lots of it. Fasts are believed to get the junk stuck in the body—mucus, toxins, waste, bad bacteria—the hell out! If you've never fasted, fasts should be monitored by a certified doctor or nutritionist.

The *basics*

- **LIQUIDS:** While you fast you should only be consuming liquids. Those liquids can be water, juice, tea, or coconut water. The Master Cleanse is a popular fast and involves making a drink from cayenne pepper, agave, water and lemon juice. I've never done it, but my girlfriend Marguerite swears by it.
- **TIMING:** You can fast for one meal, say breakfast, or one day, as in just liquids all day. Or longer. Remember, that every body is different
- **BODY CHANGES:** You are detoxing, so some people first experience minor breakouts, headaches, and lethargy, but then break through and

have clearer skin, a clearer head, and more energy. The first day or two of a fast, I'm a zombie, but by the third day, I feel better.

- **EASE IN AND EASE OUT:** Don't go from eating burgers and fries every day to a seven-day cleanse and then immediately go back to eating burgers and fries. A week or two before you start your monitored cleanse, make an effort to eat lots of veggies and drink a lot of water. Start to cut processed foods out of your diet. Same goes for after your cleanse is completed. Don't sink your teeth into a slice of pizza and an ice cream sundae the day you are done. Start by incorporating soups and foods that are easy to digest.
- **MONITOR:** Always consult with a nutritionist or doctor before beginning any fast that is longer than a day, and make sure you are being properly monitored throughout the process.
- **KNOW THIS:** You might not feel well. You might even feel sick. Feverish. Just plain yucky. Some people feel like they are on the top of the world, others like they just watched Miley Cyrus on the MTV Music Awards . . . nauseous and disturbed. Know that a lot of reactions are normal. That's why you need to be monitored!

IS A FAST SAFE? According to Dr. Joel Fuhrman: "To fast is to abstain from food while one possesses adequate reserves to nourish vital tissues; to starve is to abstain from food after reserves have been exhausted so that vital tissues are sacrificed." In normal people words, yes, a fast is safe—if you have "adequate reserves." If you have extra weight on you . . . *you have adequate reserves.* But again, always check first with your doc or accredited nutritionist.

THE *benefits*

That plateau you've hit? That weight that just isn't budging? Adios! Fasting can help to break through that blockage and improve metabolism function. Something even more valuable in for the long run? Fasting can help reset our taste buds and shift unhealthy cravings for things like sugar and fat, to healthier ones. This is one of the most powerful, long-term benefits of a fast. It can even help us kick addictions. I honestly found that I craved less salt and sugar after I finished my first fast. Fasting also allows your organs to rest, because the digestive system doesn't have as much work to do. Fasting fanatics argue that the abilities of our detox organs, such as our skin, kidneys, liver, and lungs, to process waste and eliminate toxins greatly increases.

A *typical day* for Me at We Care

Generally, the idea is to consume liquids about every hour, or every hour and a half. The order might go something like this:

1. Distilled water with 1 squeezed lemon
2. 1 tablespoon chlorophyll and a glass of water (liquid chlorophyll can be found at most health food stores)
3. 1 cup green veggie juice (see Gavan's recipe)
4. First detox drink—water with apple juice and fiber cleanser (fiber flax/psyllium supplements can be found at most health food stores in pills or a loose form that can be added to water)
5. 1 pint veggie juice
6. Second detox drink—water/apple juice and fiber cleanser
7. 1 cup lemon water
8. 1 cup green tea or yerba mate
9. 1 cup tea for liver and kidneys
10. Third detox drink—water with apple juice and fiber cleanser

---

At the beginning of every year, I like to do a cleanse. Usually that means eating really clean, drinking lots of fresh veggie juices, reducing salts and sugars in my diet, and even limiting meat. After the holidays, I always renew my vow to be healthier and physically fit.

—ALI LARTER, actress and author

My Favorite Green Juice by Chef Gavan

Ever since doing We Care, I try to drink a fresh veggie juice every day. Packed with vitamins, minerals, and nutrition, loaded with live enzymes and soluble fiber, it gives me a ton of energy—and does a brain and body good. You can liquid fast for just one meal a day with your green juice.

yield: ***2 ½ pints of supersized nutrition***

INGREDIENTS:

- 1 bunch Swiss chard
- 2 small bunches of spinach
- 2 small gala apples
- 6 stalks of celery
- 1 small piece fresh ginger, peeled

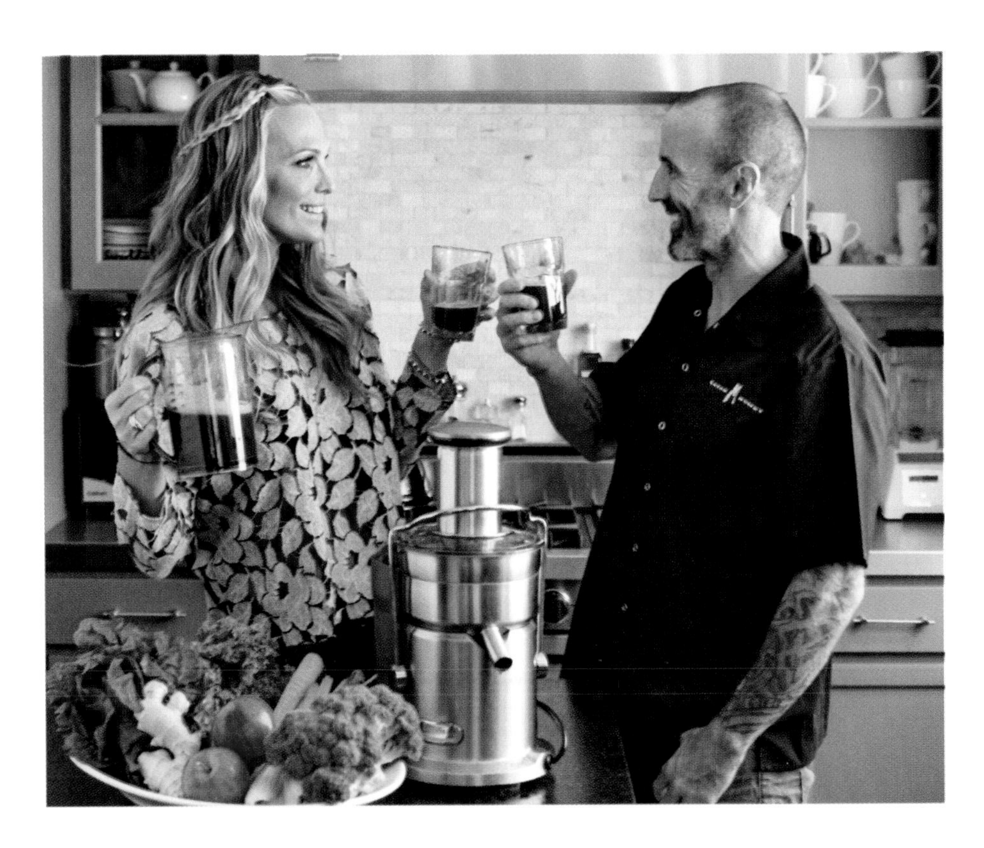

supermodel *secret*

I wasn't raised in Berkeley, California, where the slow-food movement and hippie-health stuff started ages ago. I'm from Kentucky. Our idea of health food is fried okra. The Ashram and We Care were enlightening experiences for me. Why? They gave me my first real understanding of the wider world of health and wellness. Opening my mind to new, and sometimes unconventional, ideas has helped me to better understand my body and has provided me with strategies that have worked for me. The takeaway here is, be open and don't be afraid to try new things. Do your research and make sure they are safe for you and then go for it.

AT-HOME JUICE CLEANSES AND FASTS: Plenty of companies offer liquid fasts and delivered-to-your-doorstep cleanses. Although they often aren't cheap, they are convenient. I believe a short cleanse can help kick-start your health-engine and are a good investment in YOU. Here are a few.

- **BLUEPRINT CLEANSE:** This was one of the first, original home-delivery cleanses. The program is highly customizable and ships all over the United States. A three-day cleanse is about $200. (www.BlueprintCleanse.com)
- **PRESSED JUICERY:** This is a local L.A. company for me and the one I use there. It has cleanses and monthly subscriptions for juice delivery. A three-day cleanse is about $180. (www.PressedJuicery.com)
- **JUICE PRESS:** An NYC-based one I just discovered and love. Locations all over the city, everywhere you turn. (www.JuicePress.com)
- **URBAN REMEDY:** Like the cleanses above, this company has programs suited to first timers or veterans or to specific issues. A bonus—it has healthy food delivery too! It's about $60 a day for each cleanse. (www.UrbanRemedy.com)

ADDITIONAL DETOXERS: At We Care, in addition to the liquid fast, other tactics are recommended that help assist in a healthy and effective detox. A total program would include the following:

1. PROBIOTICS: These help establish good bacteria in our body, assist in fighting disease, and contribute to healthy digestion. I take Florastor and Align brands. Dr. Ohira brand doesn't need to be refrigerated and is convenient for travel.

2. MASSAGE: Because you are going through a detox phase, massage is an excellent manual way to stimulate the circulation and help move toxins stored in the tissue and blood out.

3. COLONICS: These slightly awkward and uncomfortable procedures are believed to clear out stubborn debris from the intestines. Be sure to get a recommendation and find an accredited practitioner to perform your colonic.

4. SKIN BRUSHING: Our skin is a detox organ—it serves as both a barrier in and an exit out. Skin brushing therefore helps get lymphatic fluid moving and grooving.

5. MEDITATION: Meditation can be tough, especially when your brain goes a million miles a minute like mine. Getting control of your mind lowers stress hormones in the body and increases feel-good chemicals that strengthen your immune function. If you have trouble on your own, try a guided audio meditation.

FINAL *thoughts* ON FASTING

Fasting doesn't have to be scary. For me, it's part of being healthy and reboots my system when I get off track. It reminds me to slow down, have patience, and get a handle on cravings and desires. And while our bodies and organs are generally efficient at detoxifying, I believe giving them a little R&R is a good thing. Fasting is something I do, but I understand it might feel too extreme or challenging for some—and that's okay. There's still a lot of great information above about detoxing the body and improving your health, even if *fasting* is not your cup of tea.

My *everyday supermomma* pregnancy program

I packed on the pounds when I was pregnant with Brooks (seventy-two, remember?). Momma bear was BIG. One reason I gained so much: I had a pregnancy-induced thyroid issue. Another reason? I started retaining a ton of water early on. There were days I didn't want to leave my house or be seen in public. For someone whose career often depends on looking a certain way, pregnancy proved to be a difficult experience for me. My younger self would have freaked out. But it was up to me to stay focused on a healthy, balanced diet, and not worry about the weight. It would come off. After all, I felt so blessed to be pregnant.

Being an older mother (I was thirty-eight when I got pregnant with my first), I felt tremendous gratitude. It already felt like a miracle getting here—I wasn't about to screw it up! I started working with Lori Bregman, a fertility and wellness coach and doula, a few months before my wedding in order to prepare my body for pregnancy and boost my fertility—and I continued to work with her throughout my pregnancy. In her Rooted for Life Program (www.rootedforlife.com), she provides wellness and coaching strategies to support the optimal health of momma bear and baby bear for every stage of pregnancy. She incorporates diet, lifestyle, and general wellness strategies. And it must have worked. On June 19, 2012, I became a supermomma to the healthy, happy, and handsome seven-pound, two-ounce Brooks Alan Stuber! Here's a look at what we did to get there.

My *get* Pregnant and *be* Healthy While Pregnant Plan

1. **FERTILITY SMOOTHIE:** One thing I had almost every single day when prepping to get pregnant and while pregnant was Lori's fertility smoothie. It's supercharged with vitamins, minerals, antioxidants and is specifically formulated to enhance fertility. I started drinking it a few months before I conceived and stopped a few months after giving birth. The ridiculously good-tasting recipe is included on p. 58.

2. **MASSAGE:** When trying to get pregnant, being calm and relaxed is key—some research suggests that stress reduces fertility. Lori recommended regular massage, so I allowed myself to indulge! And then, once pregnant, I experienced intense back pain and other weird body pains, so again, massage was important. Lori stresses the importance of reducing physical pain and other stress while pregnant, for the benefit of the baby's developing nervous and immune systems. Massage is proven to lower cortisol levels (stress hormones) and comfort the body, which will indirectly transfer to your baby. If a regular massage is out of your budget, ask your partner to give a helping hand if he wants a happy momma and calm baby!

3. **ACUPUNCTURE:** To prep my body for pregnancy and once I was pregnant, I got weekly acupuncture from Dr. Jing at the TCM Healing Center in Santa Monica. I believe in it. No way to prove it boosted my fertility—but I promise you, it definitely reduced my back pain big-time! A lot of medications that reduce pain are off-limits when you are with baby, and acupuncture is a proven drug-free pain reducer. FYI: Acupuncture is also helpful in reducing morning sickness, anxiety, and depression. For those experiencing postpartum syndrome and are still breast-feeding, many studies have found that acupuncture improves symptoms. Go to a licensed acupuncturist and specifically search for a clinic that is certified and does not reuse instruments.

4. **EXERCISE:** I kept up with my regular workouts, which I talk about in the fitness chapter, but made adjustments for pregnancy courtesy of my trainers and recommendations from my doctor. Weekly yoga was on Lori's list of things I must do. I explored poses that help to calm the body and help open up the hips for childbirth, which I outline in the fitness chapter. Post pregnancy, I needed to work out to relieve new momma anxiety and to help with energy and—of course—the wicked witch of baby-weight

5. **SUPPLEMENTS:** Prior to conceiving, I consulted a fertility specialist, Dr. Shahin Ghadir, and here's what he told me to do, so I did it! "All women should be on a multivitamin, and if they are in the reproductive-age category, I recommend being on a prenatal vitamin. If the egg reserve also has shown a decline, then the female patient should consult with a fertility specialist and consider also taking CoQ10 and also DHEA." I followed that supplement plan and also took vitamin D because I was deficient.

Lori Bergman's Fertility Smoothie

This nutrient-rich and delish beverage has been custom designed to get you pregnant and keep you and baby healthy while in womb. It's packed with vitamins and minerals, omegas to stabilize mood and regulate the menstrual cycle, antioxidants for enhanced immunity and vitality—in addition to ingredients that may help keep FSH levels (the hormone that decreases your chance for fertility) low.

INGREDIENTS:

- Frozen, mixed, organic berries (⅔ cup) (antioxidant rich!)
- Almond or rice milk (⅔ cup)
- Protein powder (something natural and clean, without a lot of additives or soy) (See your powder for dosage—promotes healthy tissue development.)
- 2 shots of wheatgrass (I use a frozen one by Evergreen, but you can use powder or fresh shots—helps lower FSH levels and create a more alkaline pH—better for sperm to squirm.)
- Frozen acai berry (½ cup) (antioxidant rich)
- Mixed powdered greens (1 teaspoon) (to nourish the blood and promote healthy cell growth)
- Maca root (1 teaspoon) (for increased libido, energy, and healthier endocrine system)
- Royal jelly* (½ teaspoon) (for balanced hormones, stress reduction, and higher estrogen levels)
- Bee pollen* (½ teaspoon) (a natural aphrodisiac, helps produce healthy eggs and is vitamin rich!)
- Liquid omegas (See product for dosage) (for balanced hormones, helps to regulate menstrual cycle and increased blood flow to uterus)

*(*Do not use if you have a bee allergy.)*

DIRECTIONS:

Read dose/serving information on back of each product. Mix everything together in a blender. Use more or less milk to achieve a desired consistency. You can always add water as well for blendability.

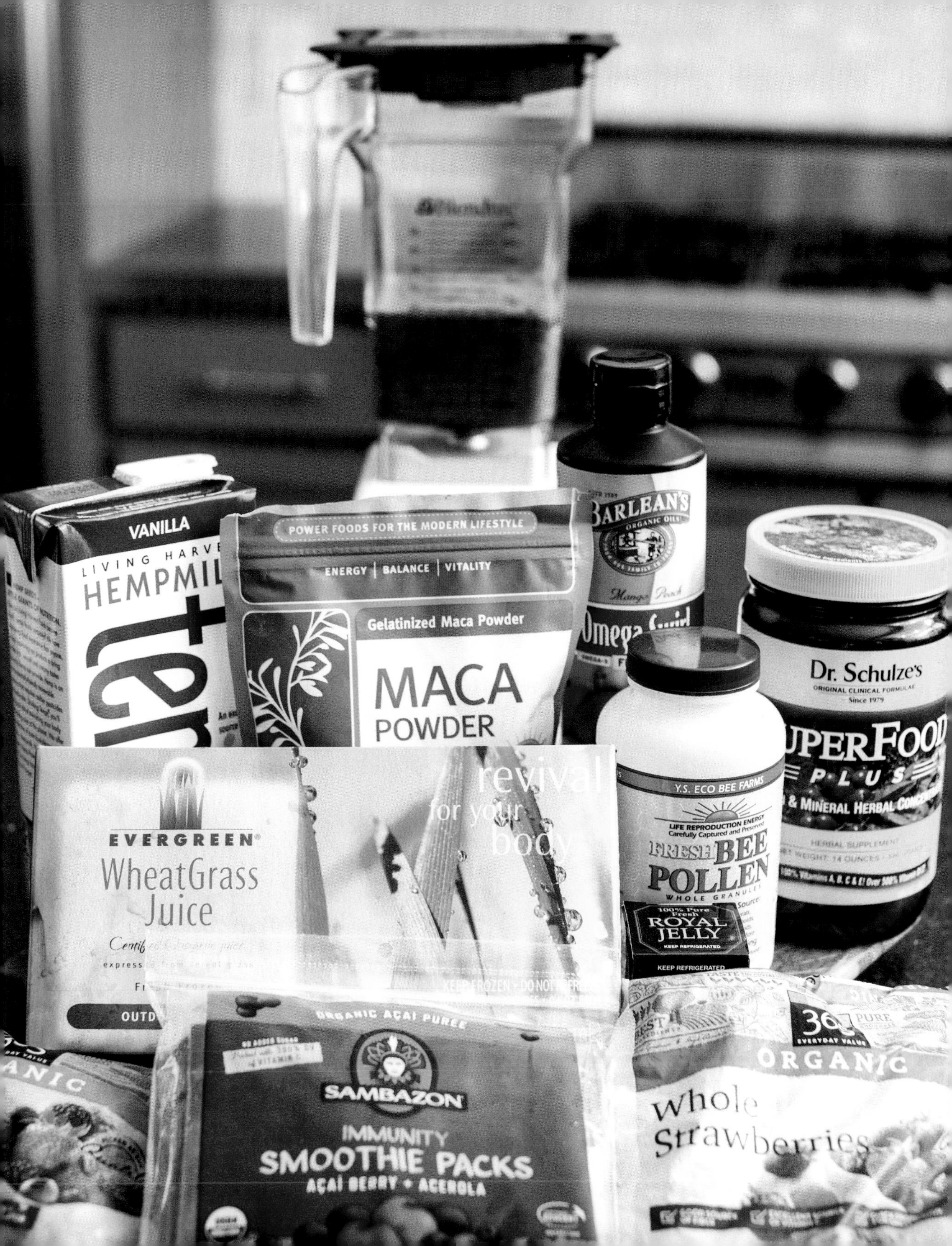
VANILLA
HEMPMIL
POWER FOODS FOR THE MODERN LIFESTYLE
ENERGY | BALANCE | VITALITY
Gelatinized Maca Powder
MACA
POWDER
BARLEAN'S
ORGANIC OILS
Mango Peach
Dr. Schulze's
ORIGINAL CLINICAL FORMULAE
Since 1979
PLUS
HERBAL SUPPLEMENT
EVERGREEN
WheatGrass
Juice
revival
for your
body
Y.S. ECO BEE FARMS
LIFE REPRODUCTION ENERGY
Carefully Captured and Preserved
FRESH BEE
POLLEN
WHOLE GRANULES
100% Pure
Fresh
ROYAL
JELLY
KEEP REFRIGERATED
KEEP REFRIGERATED
ORGANIC AÇAI PUREE
SAMBAZON
IMMUNITY
SMOOTHIE PACKS
AÇAI BERRY + ACEROLA
ORGANIC
Whole
Strawberries

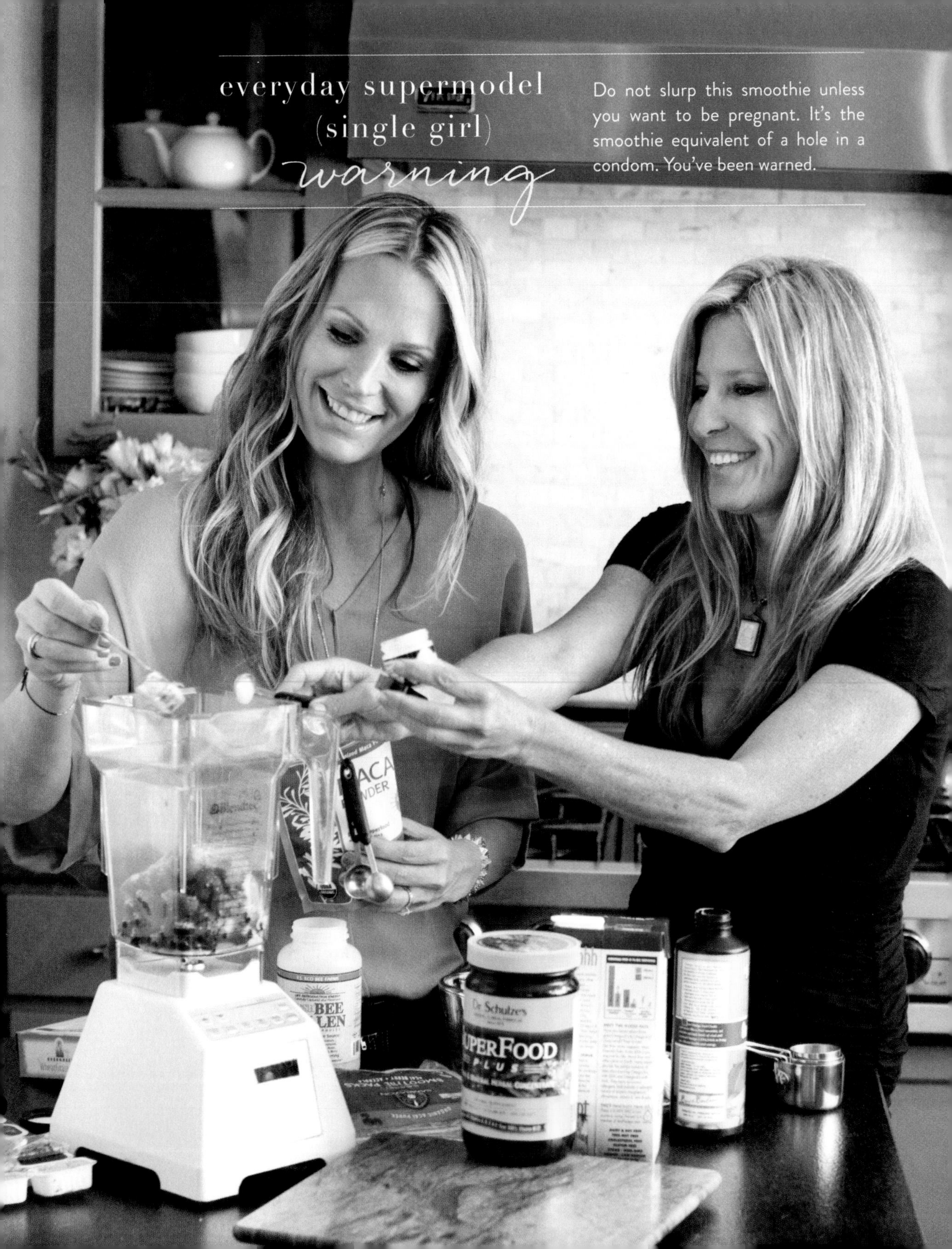

everyday supermodel (single girl) *warning*

Do not slurp this smoothie unless you want to be pregnant. It's the smoothie equivalent of a hole in a condom. You've been warned.

some everyday supermomma *secrets*

- Water your tadpole. You are growing, baby is growing, and you need to drink lots and lots of water. Hydrate your garden and your seed. Not only does it help keep the metabolism moving, but it's important because your body just gets and feels funky—for those who suffer swelling and even skin issues (I was soooo itchy!?)—water helps keep skin hydrated and can help reduce fluid retention and minor skin irritations.
- Lower your sugar intake while pregnant (even high-sugar fruits). It's important to reduce the risk of gestational diabetes.
- When I was pregnant, I read everything I could find about healthy habits. *Healthy Child, Healthy World* is a comprehensive book on how to make your life more eco- and baby-friendly. I emphasized an organic, whole-food diet and switched all the cleaning products in my house to nontoxic. Jessica Alba sent me a big box of goodies from her Honest Company that I love and still use today.
- Oh, and just because you are pregnant, that does not give you creative license to eat whatever you want. C'mon, sister, that just ain't allowed. Believe it or not, most dieticians will tell you we don't need a lot of additional calories while pregnant. According to Rebecca Baer, we're talking one extra apple with almond butter and a handful of crackers and hummus spread. That's about all the "extra" calories experts argue you need. You do need to increase your protein, as mentioned earlier. And eat as healthy as possible. I followed Lori's month-by-month diet plan, eating specific foods during each stage of my pregnancy to support my baby's healthy development.

WISDOM FROM MY OB/GYN (AND AUTHOR OF *EXPECTING 411: CLEAR ANSWERS AND SMART ADVICE FOR YOUR PREGNANCY*), DR. MICHELE HAKAKHA: "One of the most important things a woman can do when she finds out she is pregnant is to find a practitioner she trusts. And if that means interviewing seven different docs, do it! It's imperative to have someone taking care of you that is willing to listen, spend time, offer advice, and truly have a vested interest in you and your baby. In most pregnancies, things go very smoothly. But, on occasion, there is a bump in the road. When something unplanned arises, it is essential to be able to trust in what your practitioner is advising.

One more piece of advice for newly pregnant moms is to be smart about your pregnancies, but not crazy. There are so many things that can be obsessed over during pregnancy . . . It's important to know the big do's and don'ts, but don't sweat the small things. Most babies will be just fine following simple rules. Enjoy your pregnancy, it only lasts nine and a half months."

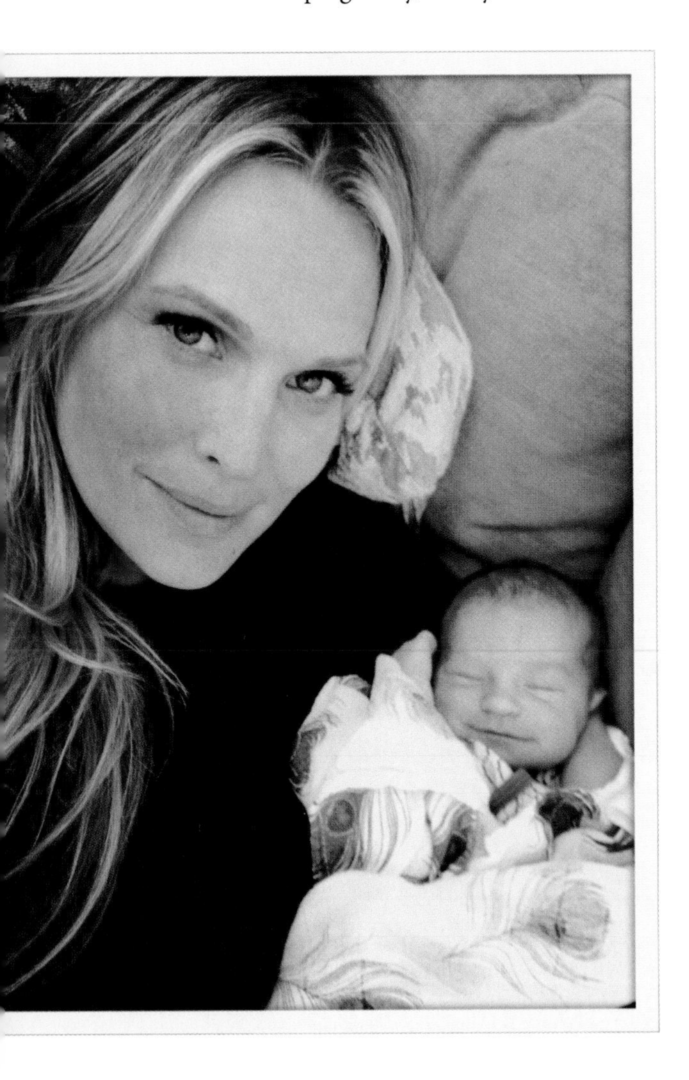

POSTPARTUM, NOT EXACTLY A PARTY: After Brooks was born, I was elated. We were parents—I had fulfilled my lifetime dream of becoming a momma. But at the very same time I was faced with so many changes, that I sometimes felt sad and out of control. I had trouble with my milk coming in, so I couldn't breast-feed. Nothin'! I felt inadequate. Many moms who experience breast-feeding issues feel like failures, and I was one of them. On top of it, like all new parents I was sleep deprived and scared I might do something wrong. Comedian Louis C.K. put it best in one of his bits: Kids are a big responsibility. My kid is "someone I have to make not die."

And then, there was my weight gain to deal with. Honest to God, I was terrified it would be there FOREVER and I experienced plummeting self-esteem. There is so much pressure for all women, models or not, to snap back to our skinny, sexy prepregnancy selves in a few short months. For some women it's possible (aliens!), but for most of us, it's not realistic. Thankfully, my husband was so supportive. I tried at first to lose the weight on my own, but it wasn't budging, so a few months after giving birth I reached out to Rebecca Baer and got back on her weight-loss program. It took me over a year to lose the bulk of it, but I got there. My advice is: Be good to yourself. Don't beat yourself up. But if you are having trouble with the weight loss, do yourself a favor and find a nutritionist or program to help, even if it comes off slowly. The happier you are in your skin, the happier your baby will be.

supermodel *secret*

Before I was married, I'd never really cooked in my life. I could have survived with Hasbro's "Easy Bake Oven." So when I found out I was pregnant with Brooks, I decided to take some cooking classes. Today, I'm no Martha Stewart, but I have some simple dishes I like to make for my family and healthy, homemade go-tos for my growing toddler. I do all right! We make meals not out of packages or cans, but healthy snacks like mashed avocado and black beans on gluten-free toast—it's one of his favorites—and soooo easy. On Sundays, when I plan the meals for the week, I plan his out too.

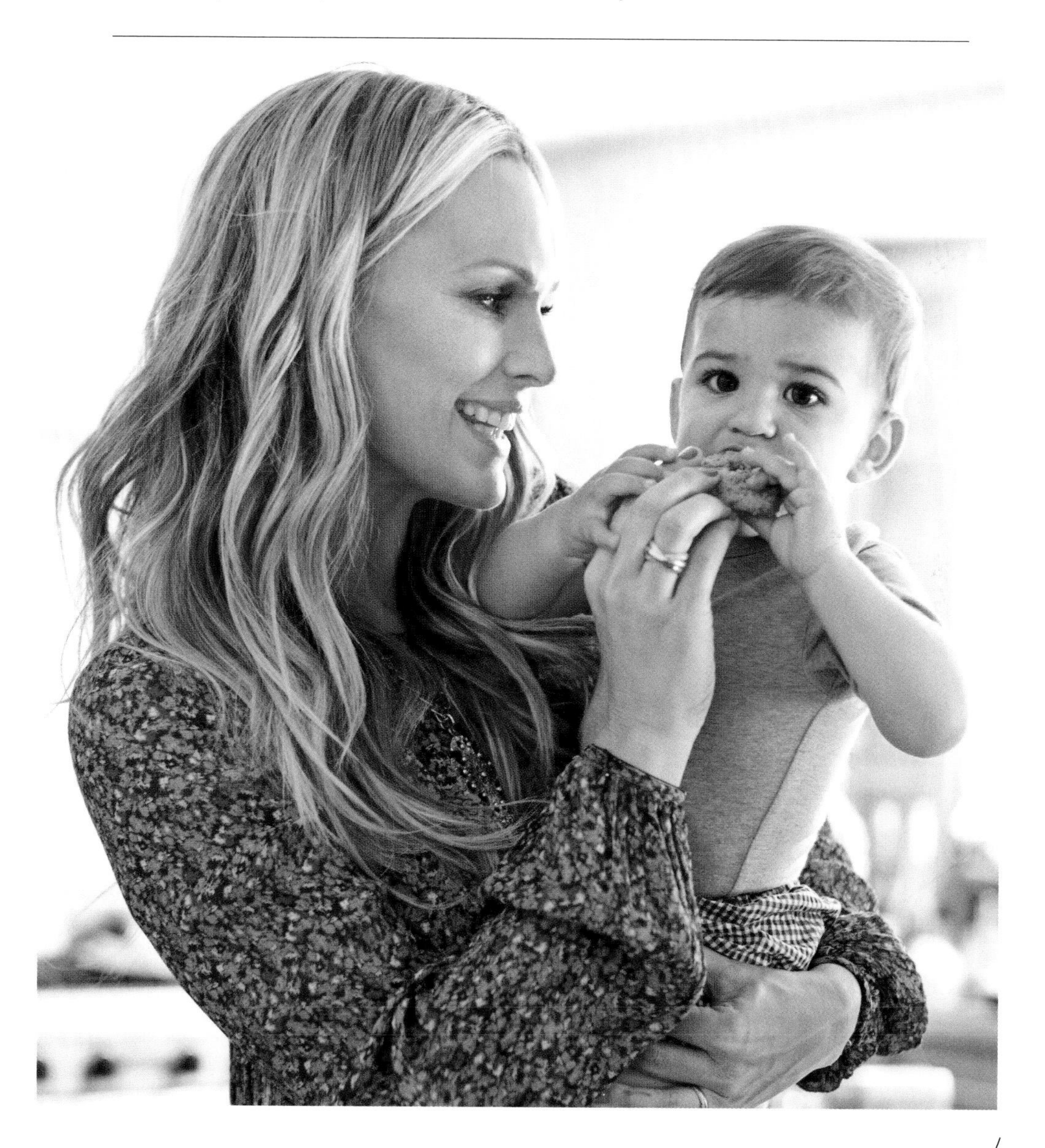

BRINGING IT ALL TOGETHER

AVOIDING PITFALLS: It's so easy to revert to old, unhealthy ways of eating—but don't. You can do this! We've got to stay focused, people, and work smarter. Practice these tips below and escape slimming slipups.

- KEEP IT HEALTHY AT HOME: *Don't buy crap!* Just don't do it. You have a growing teenager or a hungry, hungry hippo of a husband? Fine if they have the unhealthy food—but make them hide it.
- PREPARE IN ADVANCE: Chef Gavan suggests using Sunday night (or whatever night works for you) to cut up veggies and prepare healthy go-to snacks and meals for you and the fam in advance. When you plan and prepare, you don't leave anything up to chance!
- GET CREATIVE: Don't make all social events around meals. Period.
- GRAZE DON'T GORGE: Gia, my friend and the talented photographer for this book, is the queen of eating healthy snacks all day long. It's a great way to stay satiated, get your five servings of fruits and veggies . . . and not binge on bad stuff.
- NEVER DINE OR SHOP HUNGRY: Do not go to the grocery store—or out to eat for that matter—hungry. We all know this. When feeling famished, we are more vulnerable to unhealthy cravings and bad choices. You'll likely end up with Cheetos in your grocery cart or a cheese enchilada on your plate! Have a healthy snack before these kind of outings.
- DON'T SKIP: Don't do it. Don't skip meals. And always eat breakfast. This will help to encourage a healthy metabolism. Skipping meals creates unhealthy spikes and drops in blood sugar and whacks out your metabolism. Research confirms five to seven small, regularly timed meals a day is best when working towards weight-loss and maintenance.
- SLOW & STEADY: And finally, make a few changes at a time. It doesn't have to be all or nothing. But do start.

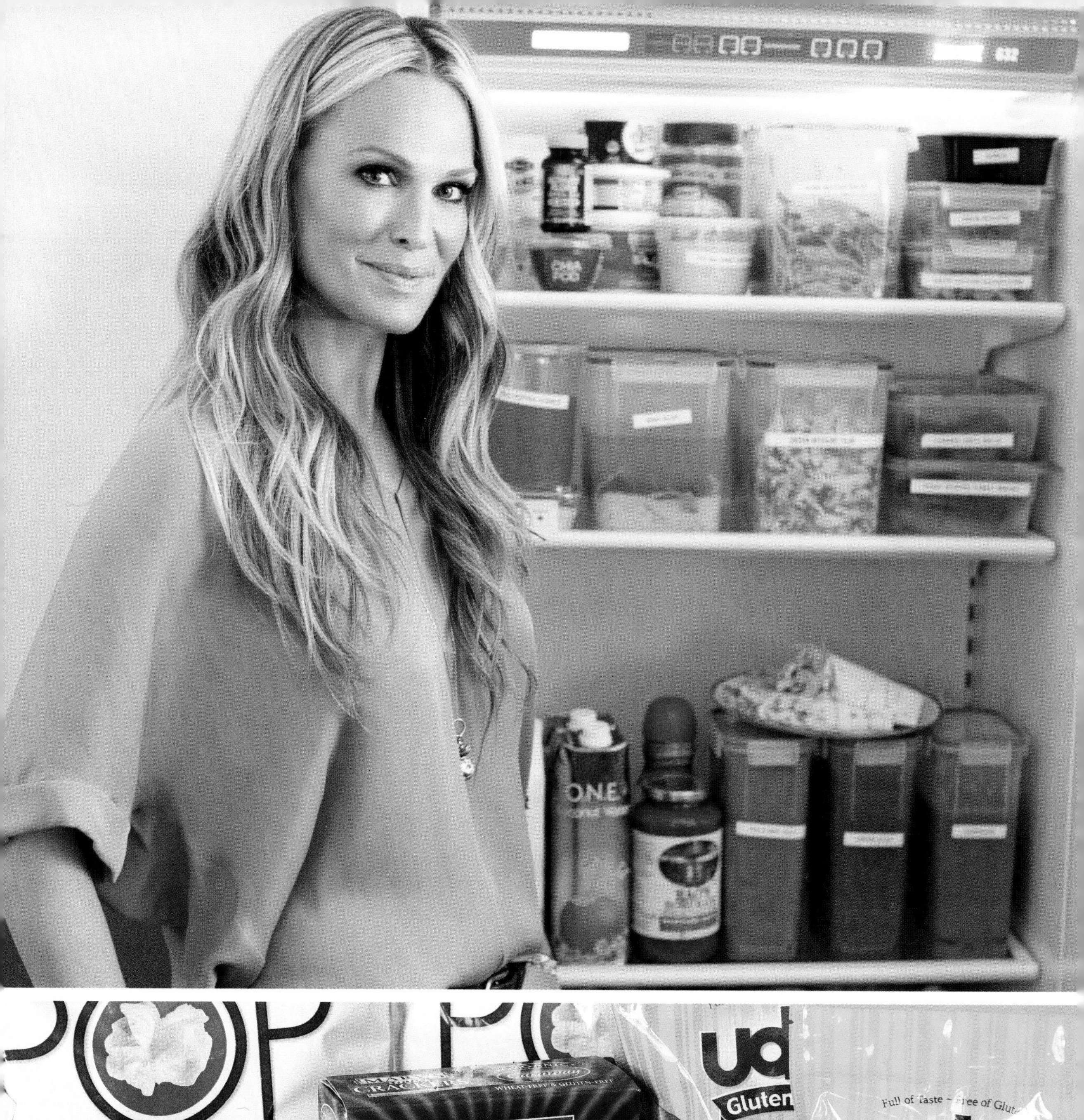

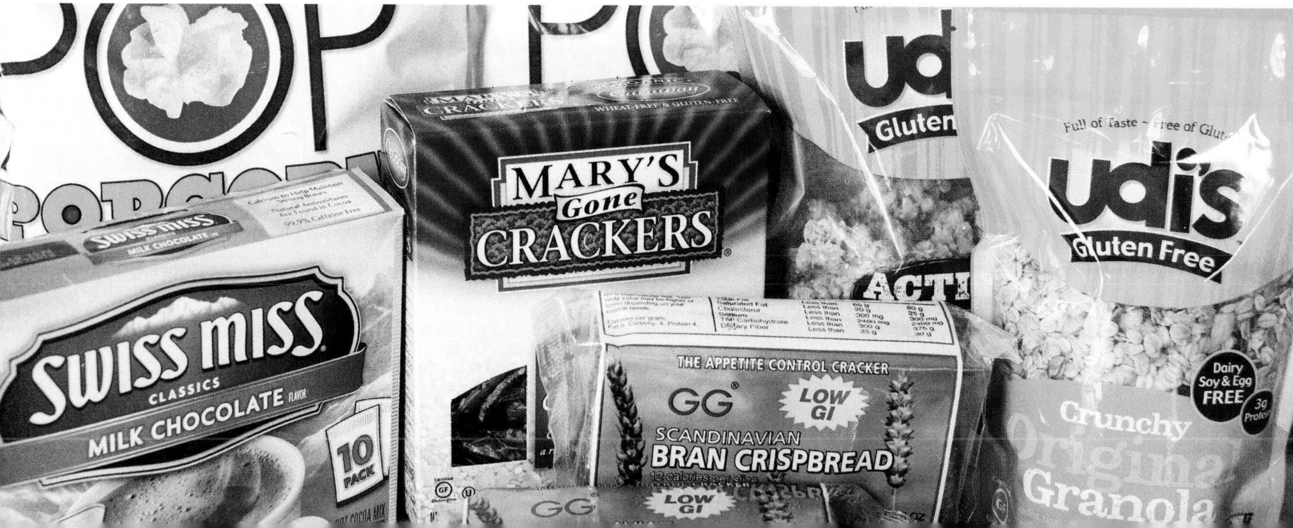
MARY'S
Gone
CRACKERS
SWISS MISS
CLASSICS
MILK CHOCOLATE
10 PACK
udi's
Gluten Free
THE APPETITE CONTROL CRACKER
GG
LOW GI
SCANDINAVIAN
BRAN CRISPBREAD
Dairy Soy & Egg FREE
Crunchy

healthy swaps

All snacks have a good twin and a bad twin. Swap high-calorie-fat-sugar choices for their leaner twins. Check out the chart opposite, and learn to swap the angels for the devils.

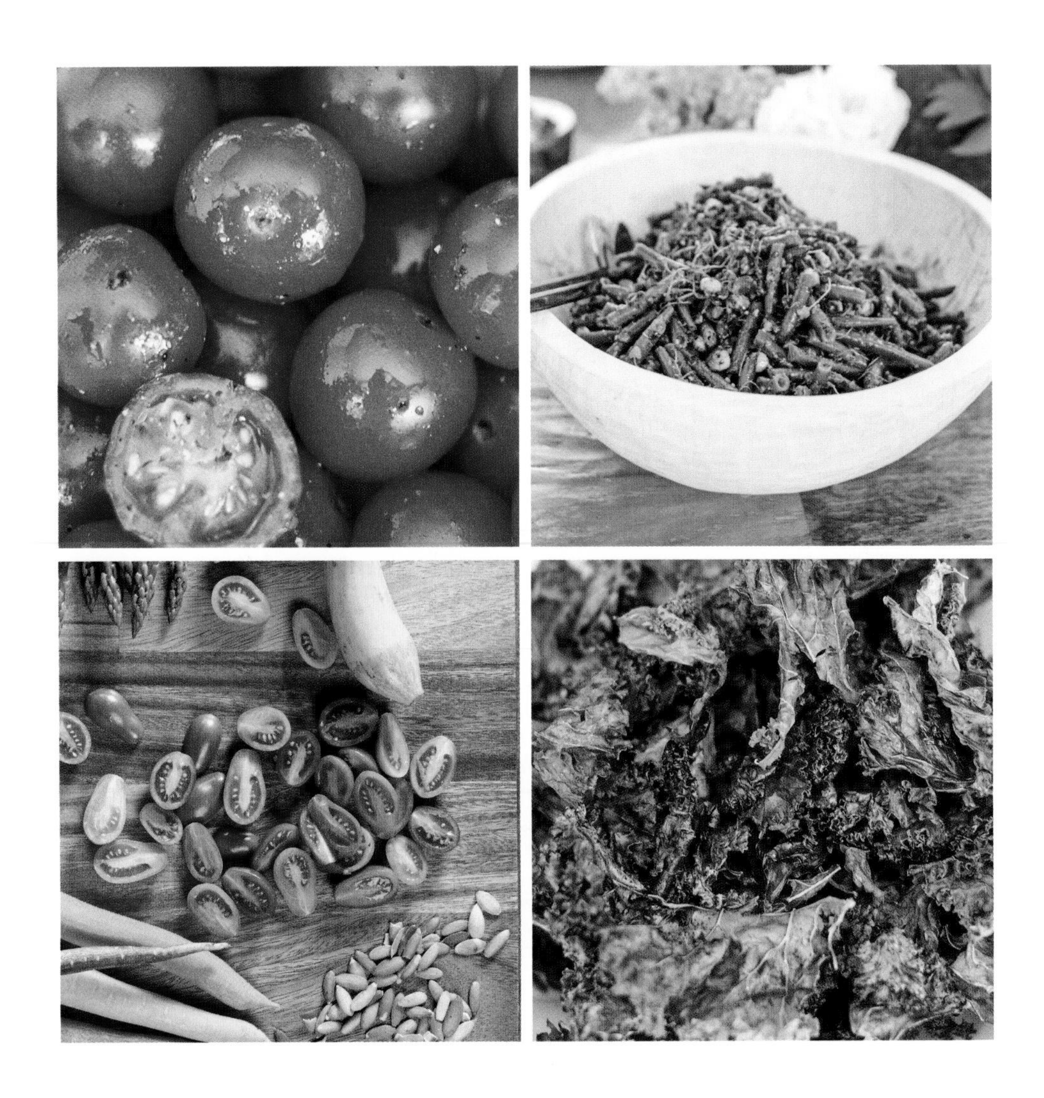

CHOOSE THE *angels*		OVER THE *devils*
Low-fat cheeses and cheese bites	>	High-calorie Brie and other high-fat cheeses
Xylitol and Stevia sweeteners	>	White, brown, or cane sugar
Sparkling water with a splash of juice, sprig of mint, or citrus	>	Carbonated sodas
High-fiber crackers	>	High-carb/low-fiber breads and crackers
Green apple, berries, orange slices	>	Candy, sugary snacks
Prosecco or wine spritzer	>	High-calorie margarita or mixed drinks
Low-calorie hot chocolate	>	Brownie
Herb-sprinkled heirloom tomatoes (or Skinny Pop—LOVE!)	>	Buttery popcorn
Kale chips	>	Potato chips
Healthy, green smoothie	>	High-calorie, blended coffee drink or sugary fruit smoothie
Greek yogurt with chia seeds or walnuts	>	Ice cream sundae with sprinkles
Extra-virgin olive oil or coconut oil	>	Canola or vegetable oil
Squash noodles or veggies	>	Pasta (All those empty carbs in pasta? Who needs 'em! Get yourself a spiralizer, available online on the cheap, and turn almost any sturdy veggie into supernutritional noodles.)
Toasted sunflower seeds or pine nuts	>	Bacon Bits
Herbal and green teas	>	Fruit juices or high-calorie beverages

supermodel *secret*

I looooooooooove fried chicken, coleslaw, biscuits and gravy as much *(if not more!)* as any tailgatin', country-music-lovin,' church-goin' southern girl. And I absolutely do indulge in the occasional down-home meal like this when I'm in Kentucky. But when I'm not back home— I just don't. However, sometimes I do get homesick and crave a taste of the South. Bless his heart, Chef Gavan created a healthy swap version of this classic "southern comfort" fried chicken dinner. It's an *everyday supermodel* version! It's just as southern comfortable, I promise, minus the "extra cushion." The recipe and all the fixin's are on my website, mollysims.com. Y'all try it out, now, and let me know what you think. My grandma's mouth-watering-biscuits and gravy are there too!

Dining Out *dos & don'ts*

Eating meals out can be a danger zone. Here are some savvy tips to staying safe and slim.

* Breadbasket be GONE! Tortilla chips—Adios! NO bread. NO chips. NO way. Period.
* You book the rezzie. Be in charge and pick healthy dining destinations. If you aren't in the driver's seat, scout the menu first online and select what's on your eating plan and stick to it.
* Order first. That way, your three-cheese-quesadilla-ordering friend won't tempt a change in your healthy selection.
* Always share a dessert (and remember the three-bite rule) or . . . forgo dessert and opt for tea.
* Avoid words like *cream, fried, panfried,* and even *sautéed* and look for words like *steamed* and *baked* instead.
* Order main courses from the à la carte or appetizer menu. The portions are almost always smaller.
* If at a buffet, serve yourself up on a smaller plate and put the heathier foods on your plate first. Studies show you eat more if your plate is larger, and that we tend to put more of the first three foods we select onto our plates. So pick healthy ones.
* Be high maintenance. Ask your server if the chef can steam instead of cream the spinach. Ask to substitute bacon in the Cobb salad with sunflower seeds. The lean lesson: It never hurts to ask.

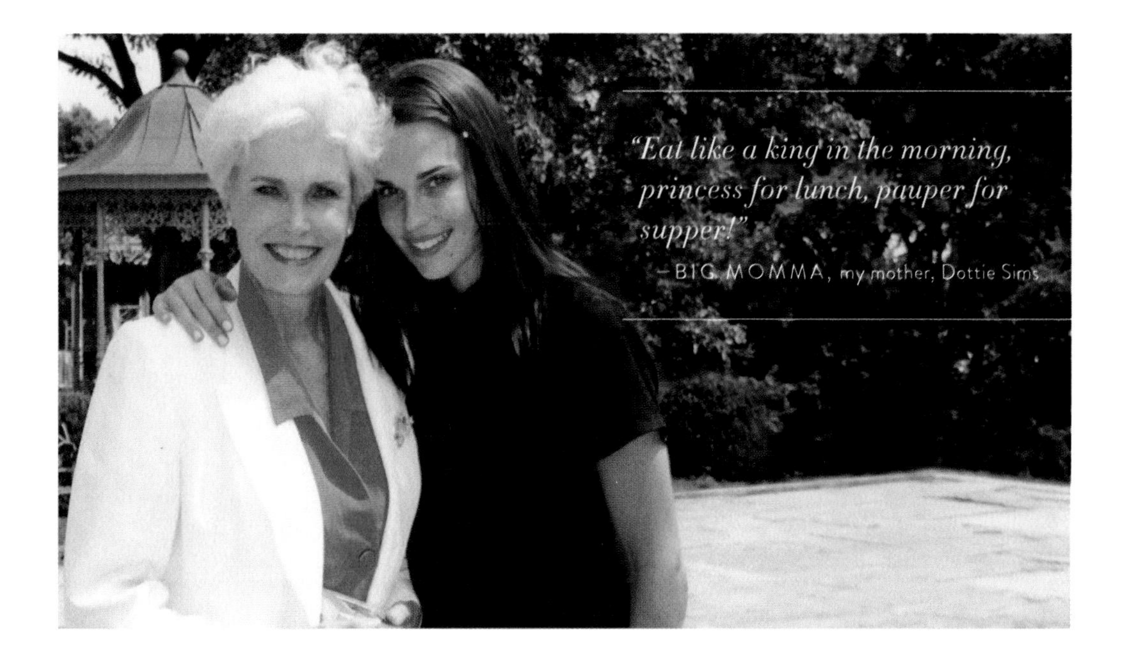

supermodel *soapbox*

SAY BYE-BYE TO THE "BUTS"

They go something like this:

1. I really want to eat better, *but I just don't have any time.* (Really? Why don't you make time?)
2. I try to eat healthy, *but my husband eats like crap.* (Do you and your husband share a mouth?)
3. I do my best to eat healthy, *but then lose motivation.* (Seriously? Who doesn't!?)

I've heard it all and I can relate. But it's time to stop the excuses. If you aren't happy with where you are, where your health is, or the state of your belly or behind—consider this a call to action. You work so hard for your boss. Why don't you work as hard for yourself? Get to work on yourself for yourself. Make YOU your number one priority. You can be healthier if you put your mind *and mouth* to it. Bury those weak excuses like a dog does a bone.

Whether trying to lose weight or maintain a healthy weight, my eating plan is always lean protein and *fiber focused*, incorporates *plant-based meals*, and uses the occasional *juice cleanse and fast*. I avoid starchy carbs and excess salt, sugar, and bad fats like the plague. I drink a ton of water. I treat myself here and there, but I stick like glue to the plan—at home and away. I truly believe these strategies are the reason for my success.

Of course, food is only one component as fitness is also key, which we discuss in the next chapter. If you go through a dramatic weight gain, be it because of pregnancy or something else, or just can't get the weight you want off, do yourself a favor and get professional guidance. If you don't have the funds for a nutritionist or wellness/weight loss doctor, invest in a onetime consultation from someone accredited (you can even get Skype consultations these days!), get an outline of targeted strategies focused on you and then get started.

When it comes to an *everyday supermodel* bod, I promise, I am no different than you. There is no way around it—it takes work. But I believe it's worthwhile work and contributes to our health, happiness, and self-esteem. Start making changes and healthy choices today. A healthier body does not have to be a fantasy. It can feel good to respect yourself and be good to yourself by tackling weight loss and maintenance in a healthy way!

the *everyday* supermodel TOP 10 takeaways

1. Get fiber focused and stop fiber flatlining. Don't avoid carbs like the plague; instead, eat a balanced diet, and choose carbs that are good for you and high in fiber—think healthy grains, fruits, and veggies!

2. Absolutely drink more water—drink it all day long. Creates the feeling of fullness, helps flush the fiber, and it contributes to a healthier metabolism. There is no downside to drinking more water.

3. Choose lean proteins and avoid fattier meats or high-cholesterol seafood, like shrimp and lobster.

4. Treat, don't cheat. Eating foods like sweets or chips shouldn't be "cheat" food. Allow yourself a small portion (think the three-bite rule) here and there. That is a healthier way of thinking than striving for perfection during the week and binging on weekends.

5. Avoid faker foods that claim health benefits but are really salt-filled, sugar-filled, or just empty calories—granola, bagels, fruit-packed smoothies.

6. Portion control always. Eat good fats, but in small amounts. Keep sugar and salt to a minimum. Calorie count, but don't let it control you.

7. Add vegetarian meals into your diet. Try to replace a meat-based meal with a vegetarian one a few times a week. And spice it up.

8. Juice boost! It's great for detoxing, getting good enzymes, and filling your body with overall goodness and nutrients. Try a liquid fast for one meal with Gavan's Green Juice. It's delish.

9. Try to buy organic and local whenever you can. Pay attention to the Clean 15 and the Dirty Dozen. Learn to be a kitchen vixen and cook up your goodies for your friends, kids, and family.

10. Make healthy swaps, stop making excuses, and do your body good—you deserve it.

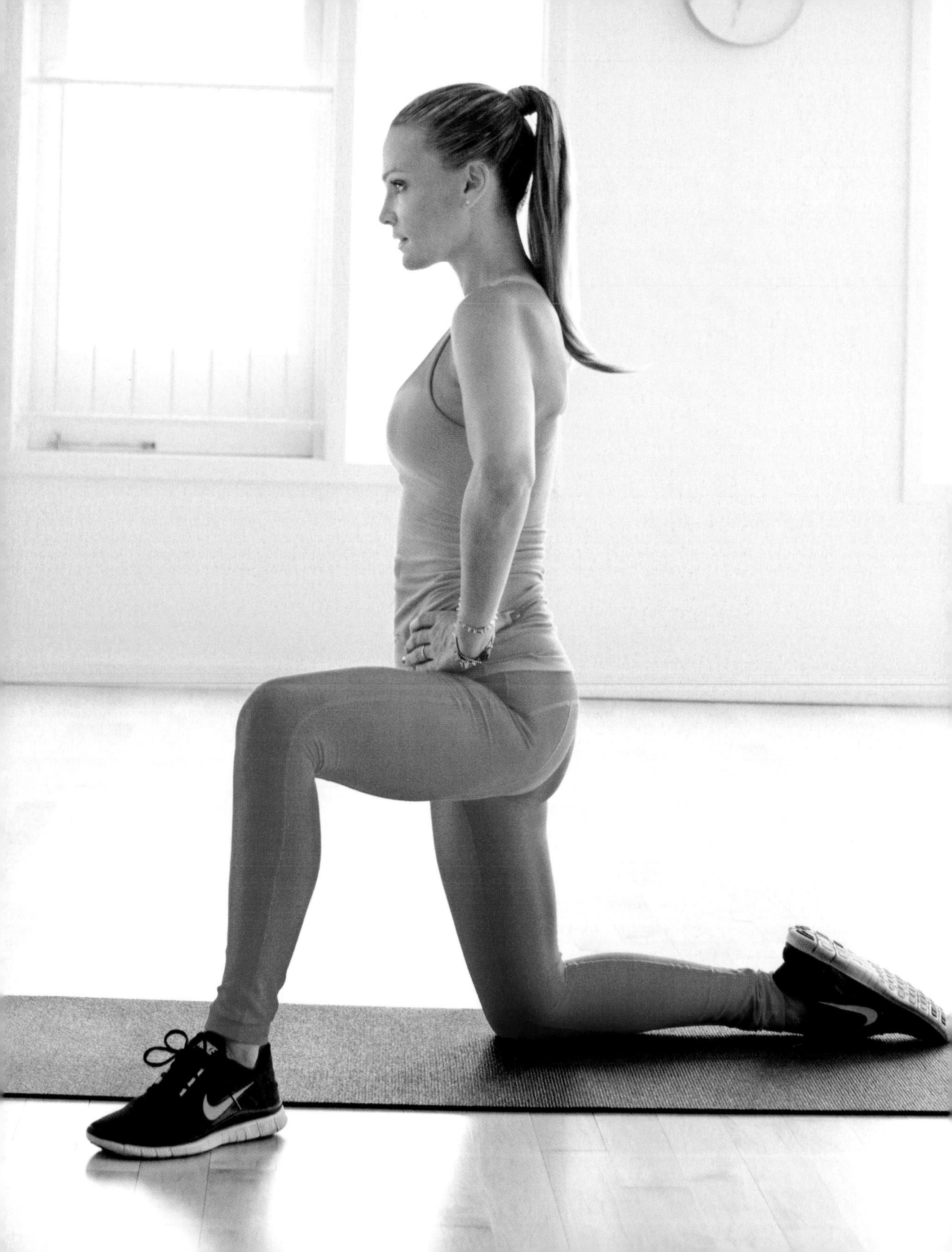

ch/2

let's get physical

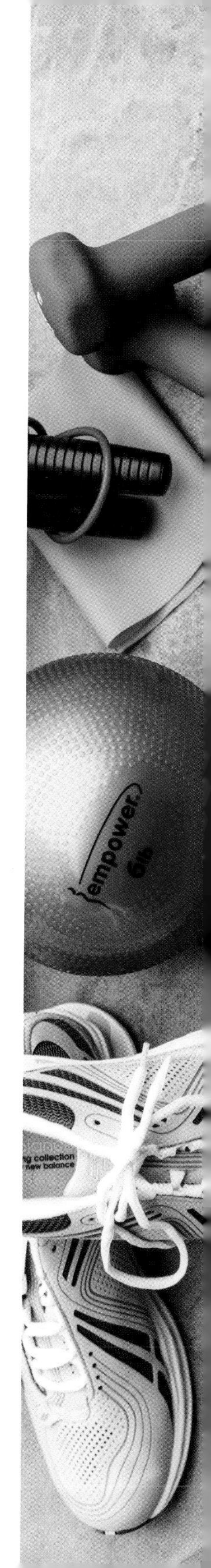

Folks, get used to it. Fitness keeps fat on the run! All the time I hear, *I bet you don't need to work out.* Does a parasite need a host? Does a groupie need a rock star? **Yes, I need to work out.** I've had to work out (and continue to) for every inch and ounce I've ever lost or kept off. Unless you are naturally long, lanky, toned, and trim like my friend Jess, whom I modeled with in Europe (and let's face it, almost none of us are), you are like me. And you will have to eat healthy AND work out to stay fit and firm.

I learned early on in my career that I was considered a *bigger girl.* I know that may sound crazy to everyone outside the modeling industry. I wasn't a size 0. I was a swimmer in high school. I have broad shoulders, sturdy legs, and I build muscle very easily. It's great for swimming. Not as great for supermodeling. Truth be told: I am TERRIFIED of bulking up. I can relate to almost every *woe-is-me* feeling you may be having about your figure. Your problem area might be your tummy. I've never liked my legs. Believe it or not, at one point I went to see a plastic surgeon about my "curvy" calves. Yes, *my calves.* I thought they were too big.

Although my career began on the heels of Cindy Crawford and Christie Brinkley (when women were allowed to have muscle and curves), at the height of my career the waif look was in. I was never going to be a waif, nor did I want to be—but that meant I'd have to be as lean as possible if I wanted to get hired. I could not bulk up.

Recently, I've had a new, different kind of struggle with weight. As I've mentioned, after my first pregnancy, the baby blubber would not budge. *Crapcrapcrapcrapcrap!!* I was so depressed. I knew something wasn't right; I was working out as much as I had prebaby, staying fiber focused and . . . *nothin'.* What on earth was going on? I went to an endocrinologist and got my answer. My thyroid and hormone levels had gotten screwed up during pregnancy (as can happen). So my doc put me on a natural thyroid replacement program to regulate my hormones. I continued to work out sixty to ninety minutes a day, at least five times a week without fail, combining cardio and strength training. Slowly but surely . . . the bulge began to budge.

It was mentally and physically challenging. There were days I was so tired I could cry—and DID. I had a newborn and wasn't getting much rest, but I stayed committed because I wanted my body back. As a kid, I can remember my own supermomma going to the high school track every single morning in her workout suit and red bandana. She walked five miles a day, rain or shine, and Kentucky winters are cold. No matter how I feel, I get up and work out. *Fitness to me is the rule—not the exception.* It's a part of my everyday routine and can be a part of your daily schedule, too. It's mental—mind over matter—and you can do it. I schedule it in and don't look back.

Speaking of mind, I also do it for my mental health. I feel better every time I exercise, without fail. Fitness improves every aspect of my life. Studies prove this. Exercise improves mood and cognitive function, relieves stress, depression and anxiety, and inspires creativity and enthusiasm for life! There is simply no downside. Not to mention, it can increase life expectancy by up to seven years. Exercise sets us all up for a lifetime of better physical and mental health.

Over the past twenty years, I've done every fitness program known to man. I've been looking for that perfect storm—a program that helps to strengthen, tone, and build long lean muscle and assists with weight loss and weight management. My Hot Bod Squad and I are going to give you the lowdown on what has worked for me and why. We'll show you how to move, stretch, dance, spin, and sweat your way to Brazilian buns. If you want to lose weight and get your brain and bod in shape —you have got to work out! Period.

One thing to note. Whenever beginning any kind of new workout regimen, it's smart to assess your current level of fitness and start slow. No one starts running one day and then busts out a marathon the next. Be patient, measure your successes, and feel out different programs to find what's right for you. Okay, *everyday supermodels:* Let's get physical, physical. Let me hear your bodies talk.

Fitness for me is so important. I focus on longevity. I used to care just about today and tomorrow, but now I think about my physical strength when I'm in my sixties and build on it now.

—ABBEY LEE KERSHAW, model

My *hot bod* Squad

- **TRACY ANDERSON:** Tracy is the founder of the Tracy Anderson Method, and I've trained with her for years. Her program is to flab what garlic is to vampires.
- **MARIA KELLING:** Tracy Anderson's director of fitness, and my personal trainer. Hail Maria—full of good bod grace!
- **JULIE RICE AND ELIZABETH CUTLER:** Founders of SoulCycle studios. Their team of instructors are the superstars of indoor cycling.
- **NICOLE HONNIG:** Certified yoga instructor. Nicole has coached me, my friends, and other Angelenos into downward dog, warrior pose, and pigeon position with grace.
- **AMANDA FREEMAN:** Founder of SLT (Strength/Length/Tone) Studios in New York. She's known for downsizing "big" city girls into beach-ready babes.
- **ALYCEA UNGARO:** My first Pilates instructor ever, and the owner of Real Pilates in Manhattan. She used to train all the models back in the day. She is awesome and really knows her stuff.

WORKOUT #1: CARDIO MEETS STRENGTH TRAINING

I used to think balls-to-the-wall cardio was the way to lose weight. But I've learned over the years, and research now tells us, that combined cardio and strength or resistance training is the way to go for a sexy shape and fit figure. You get the cardiovascular and calorie-burning benefits of cardio, with the muscle strengthening and toning benefits of resistance work.

I started working out with Tracy Anderson when I was in my early thirties. My body was starting to shift, and gravity was taking hold (otherwise known as sag and flab). Her techniques combine cardio and strength training and are made to suck everything in and up. I have watched weight slide off women of all shapes and sizes like a firefighter down a flagpole. Her method works well for me because it puts my heart, my mind, and my muscles to work—and still keeps the bulk at bay! I used to sprint from any kind of weight training for fear of building muscle. Now I know, I can do it—as long as I do it right.

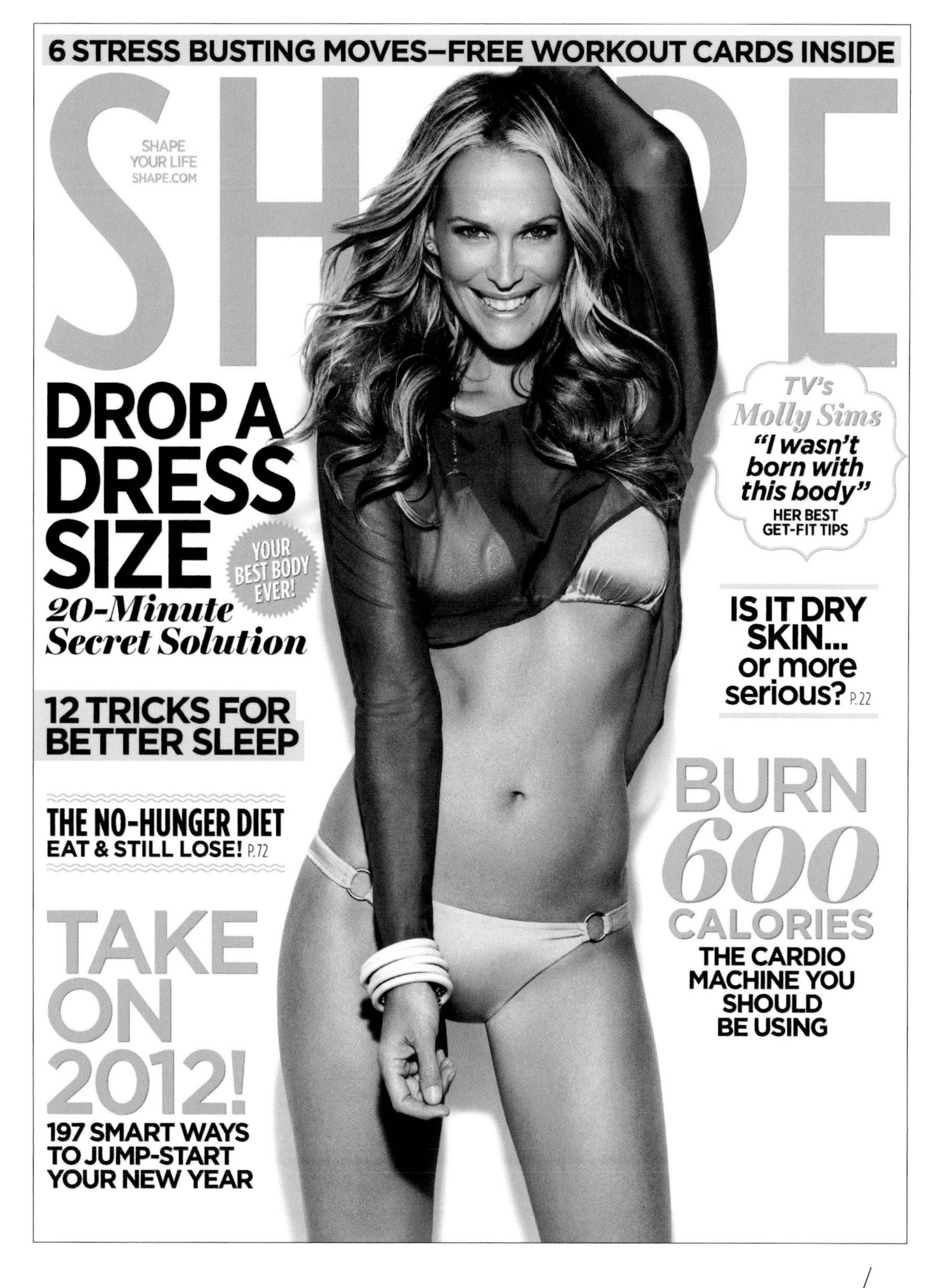
6 STRESS BUSTING MOVES—FREE WORKOUT CARDS INSIDE
SHAPE
SHAPE
YOUR LIFE
SHAPE.COM
DROP A
DRESS
SIZE
YOUR
BEST BODY
EVER!
20-Minute
Secret Solution
12 TRICKS FOR
BETTER SLEEP
THE NO-HUNGER DIET
EAT & STILL LOSE! P.72
TAKE
ON
2012!
197 SMART WAYS
TO JUMP-START
YOUR NEW YEAR
TV's
Molly Sims
"I wasn't
born with
this body"
HER BEST
GET-FIT TIPS
IS IT DRY
SKIN...
or more
serious? P.22
BURN
600
CALORIES
THE CARDIO
MACHINE YOU
SHOULD
BE USING

The *basics*

- Cardio (cardiovascular) fitness involves any activity that raises the heart rate, causing it to beat stronger and faster. It is also known as aerobic or endurance exercise, because it requires and refers to the use of oxygen to adequately meet energy demands during the length of exercise. Running, swimming, dance, and fast walking are all forms of cardio.
- Strength training fitness or resistance training is physical activity that uses resistance to induce muscular contraction, which builds the strength, anaerobic endurance and size of muscles.
- The Tracy Anderson Method is an example of a combined cardio/strength training workout. It combines Pilates, minor weight-lifting, and serious dance moves. At times, I feel like a Britney Spears backup dancer. Sometimes I just feel ridiculous. Who cares? It works.
- Tracy's program concentrates on the accessory muscles that lengthen, tighten, and sculpt—but *don't build mass.* Her studios are heated—but not too hot to handle.
- Certain drills introduce light weights, resistance bands, and tall step boxes, so it's never boring. My personal trainer changes up the workout every ten days to recruit different sets of muscles and encourage a balanced physique and weight loss.

Certain workouts can overdevelop specific muscle groups and completely ignore others. We've all seen really boxy abs and bulked-up quads. But Tracy's program is different. It not only gets you in top cardiovascular condition, but it's designed to create a sexy, feminine shape and sculpt curves.

—MARIA KELLING, Tracy Anderson trainer

The *benefits*

- In general, several studies show that combined cardio and strength training is the best exercise strategy for a reduction in body weight, fat mass and waist/hip ratio.
- Combined work creates longer, leaner ladies and gents rather than bulky Hulkies. Tracy's program is designed specifically to create a balanced and symmetrical bod.
- You can do it at home—I've included a workout for you! Also, Tracy's DVDs are damn good. The Metamorphosis program can be used at any skill level and is designed for four different body types. She also has a pregnancy, postpregnancy, and a ninety-day teen program.
- Workouts that combine cardio and strength are gaining in popularity and can be found almost anywhere! For other combined cardio and strength training classes, look for interval training or circuit training classes at your gym. Or create your own program. Go for a twenty minute run or walk the stairs at your community college track. Finish at home with a few sets of lunges and some work with 5 pound weights.

MY *daily* TRACY ANDERSON PROGRAM

Here's an upper and lower body breakdown of what my daily program often looks like. I'll do this at home with a trainer, or at a Tracy Anderson studio in L.A. or New York.

A NOTE ON REPETITIONS: Generally, do a set of reps until your muscles are on fire. By exhausting the muscle, you get the full benefit of the burn. A good rule of thumb is to do each exercise for at least a minute and up to three if you can handle the heat! When starting out, just do as long as your hardworking bod can stand. If that's only 30 seconds—that's still a good effort. If you do all the following exercises you should have about a 30-minute workout in the can for the day! Start with a short jog around the block or a few sets of jumping jacks to warm up.

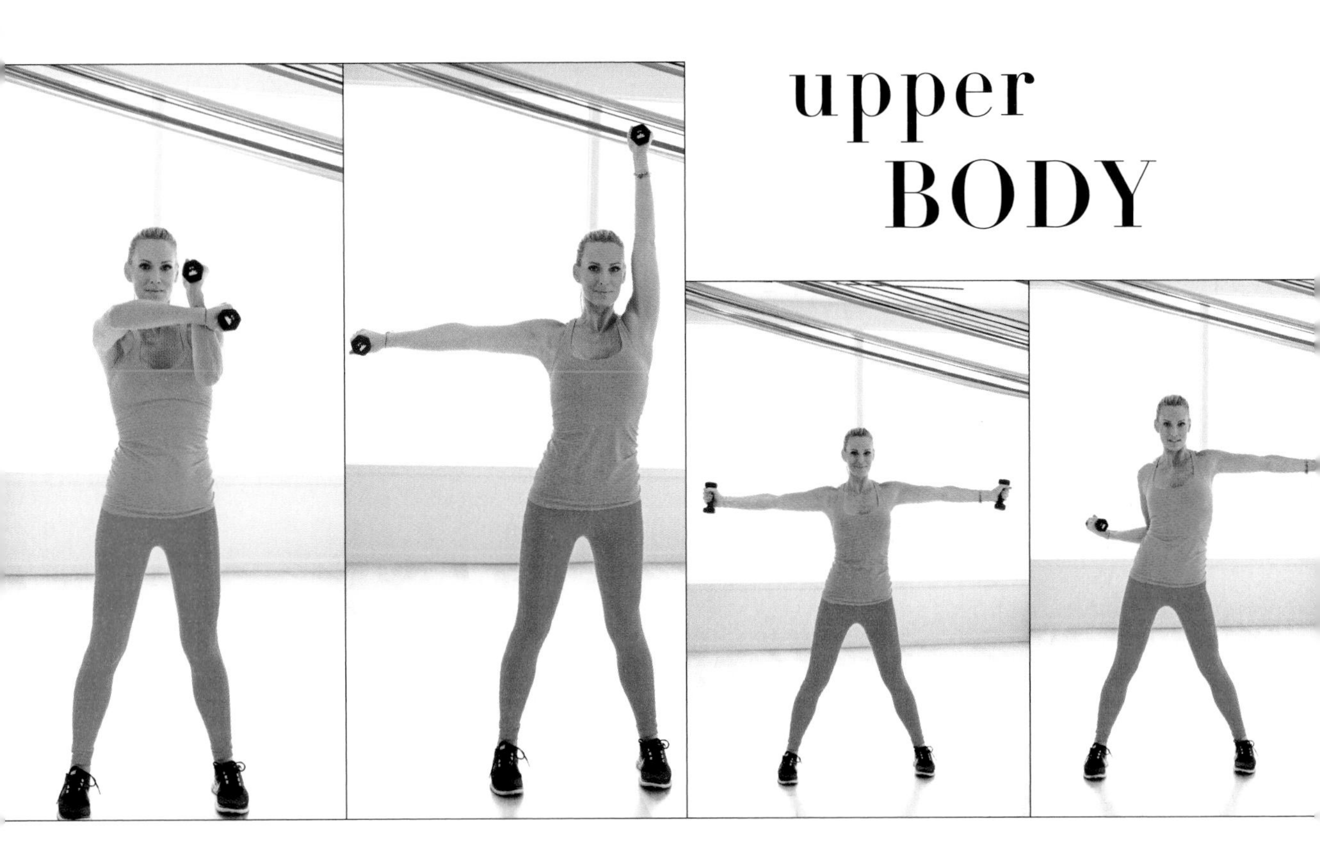

upper BODY

1. cross & punch

- Stand holding 3-pound hand weights both elbows bent.
- Cross one arm over the other arm with the elbow out to the side .
- Extend the crossed arm straight out to the side and the other arm straight up over head.
- Return to starting position.

2. side punch

- Stand holding 3-pound hand weights with both arms extended straight out to the side.
- Bend one arm so that the elbow is pulling behind the back, then extend that arm back out to the side.
- Nonworking arm will hold side position.

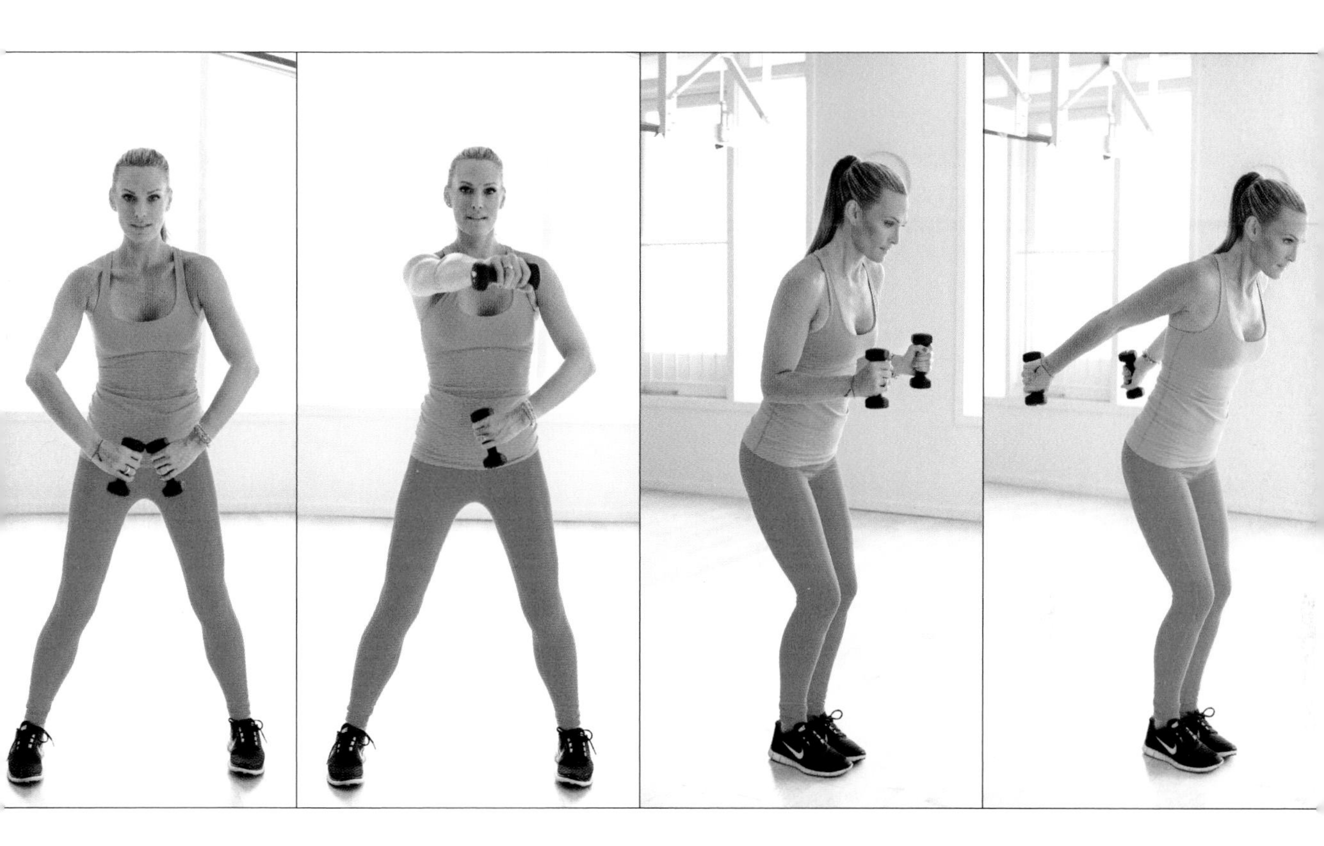

3. diamond punch out

- Standing holding 3-pound hand weights down by hip bones in a diamond shape.
- Lift one arm up and punch straight out in front of body.
- Return to starting position then repeat with the other arm.

4. triceps extend

- Standing with feet together knees slightly bent, holding 3-pound hand weights, hinged slightly at the waist.
- Hold weights and arms at 90-degree angle tight against body.
- Extend arms backward slowly and bring forward again to 90-degree angle.

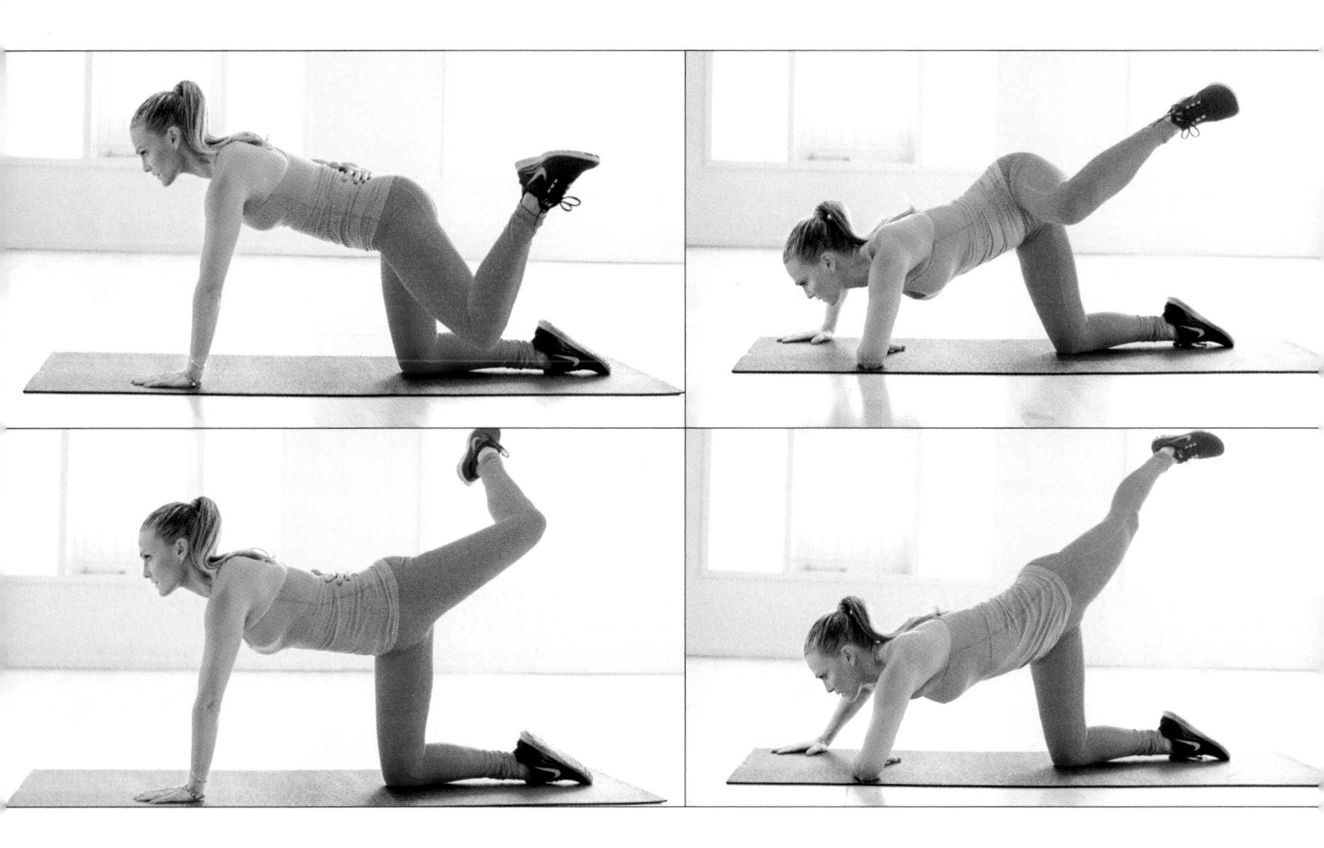

1. all fours inverted knee back lift

- Kneel on hands and knees, with the supporting side arm placed behind your back.
- The working side leg will start in an inverted position (the knee is facing inward and the foot is facing outward away from the body, with the lower part of the leg (shin) lifted up off the ground.
- Lifting with the glutes, pull the leg behind the body into an attitude position where the leg is bent at a 90-degree angle, with the knee facing out away from the body and the foot right behind body in line with the glute muscles.
- Return to the starting position and repeat.

2. elbow-down knee pull to high arabesque

- Kneel down on your hands and knees.
- The working side forearm will be down for support.
- Pull the working knee in toward the working side elbow with the knee open out to the side.
- Then extend the leg straight back behind the body reaching the foot high up toward the ceiling.

lower BODY

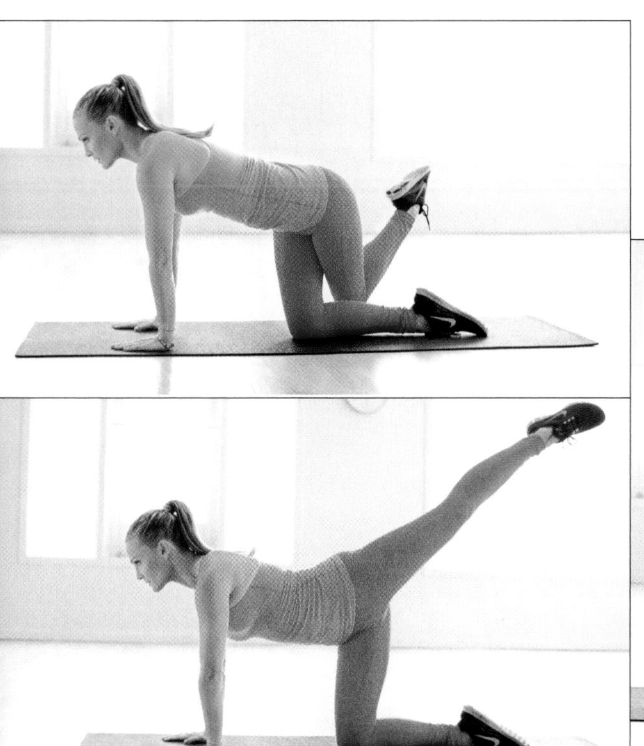

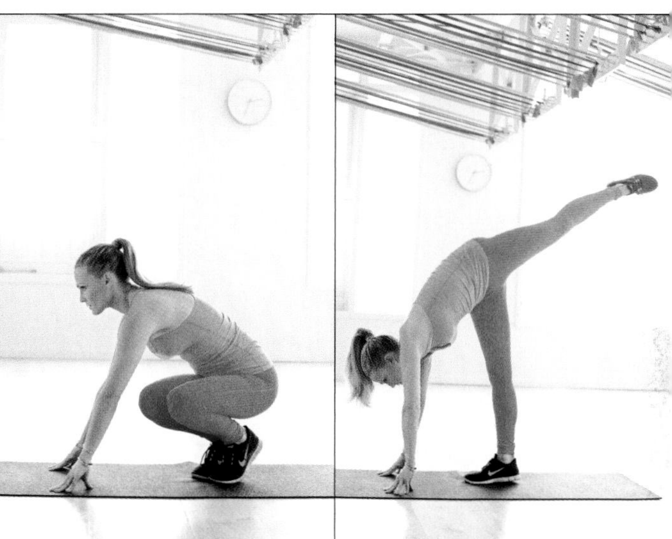

3. all fours knee pretzel to arabesque extend

- Kneel on your hands and knees.
- The working leg knee is bent and crossed over the supporting side leg.
- Straighten the working leg back behind body into arabesque.

4. all-fours kick mid-level and high level

- Kneel on hands and knees.
- Working leg is extended behind body at hip level.
- Slightly bend the knee as you lift the leg up higher past the hip level and extend out straight.
- Alternate midlevel and high level.

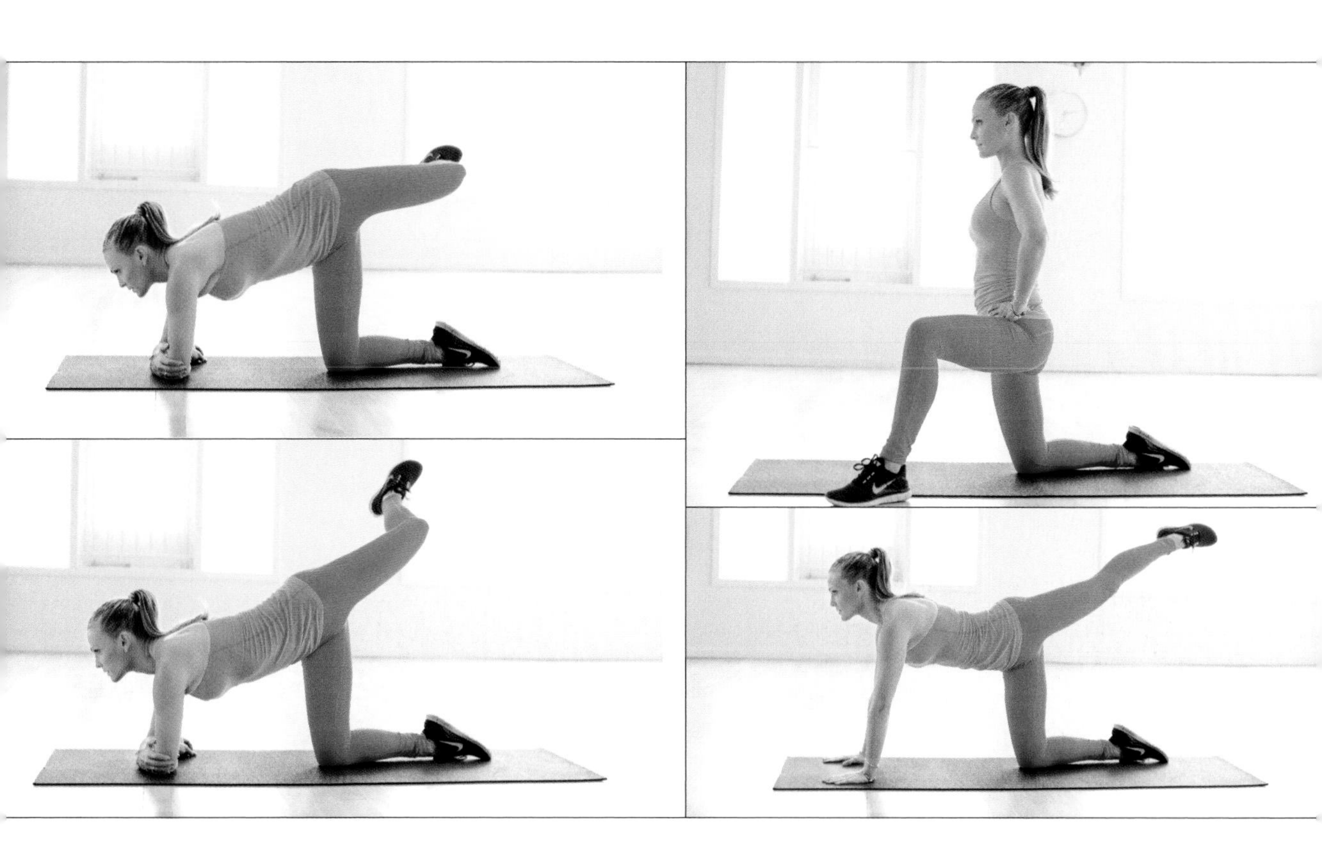

5. elbows-down attitude kick up

- Down on both forearms with the working leg behind the body in attitude at hip level.
- Extend the leg straight as you kick up higher toward the ceiling.
- Return to the starting position and repeat.

6. kneel high lunge to back arabesque

- Kneel up on your knees with the working leg out to the side with the foot on the ground.
- Lift the leg to extend back behind the body as you reach and place your hands on the ground.

7. standing abs (so much better than a crunch)

This is the perfect move to do *in privacy*—until you get it down. Then you can do it anywhere and everywhere! I'll do standing abs any old random time . . . like during commercial breaks or in the kitchen while I'm waiting for the coffee to percolate.

- Stand with legs slightly bent and shoulder-width apart with arms on hips.
- Shoulders move left while hips move right.
- Alternate side to side.

Be sure to keep your back straight and activate the core muscles. Go to mollysims.com for a tutorial!

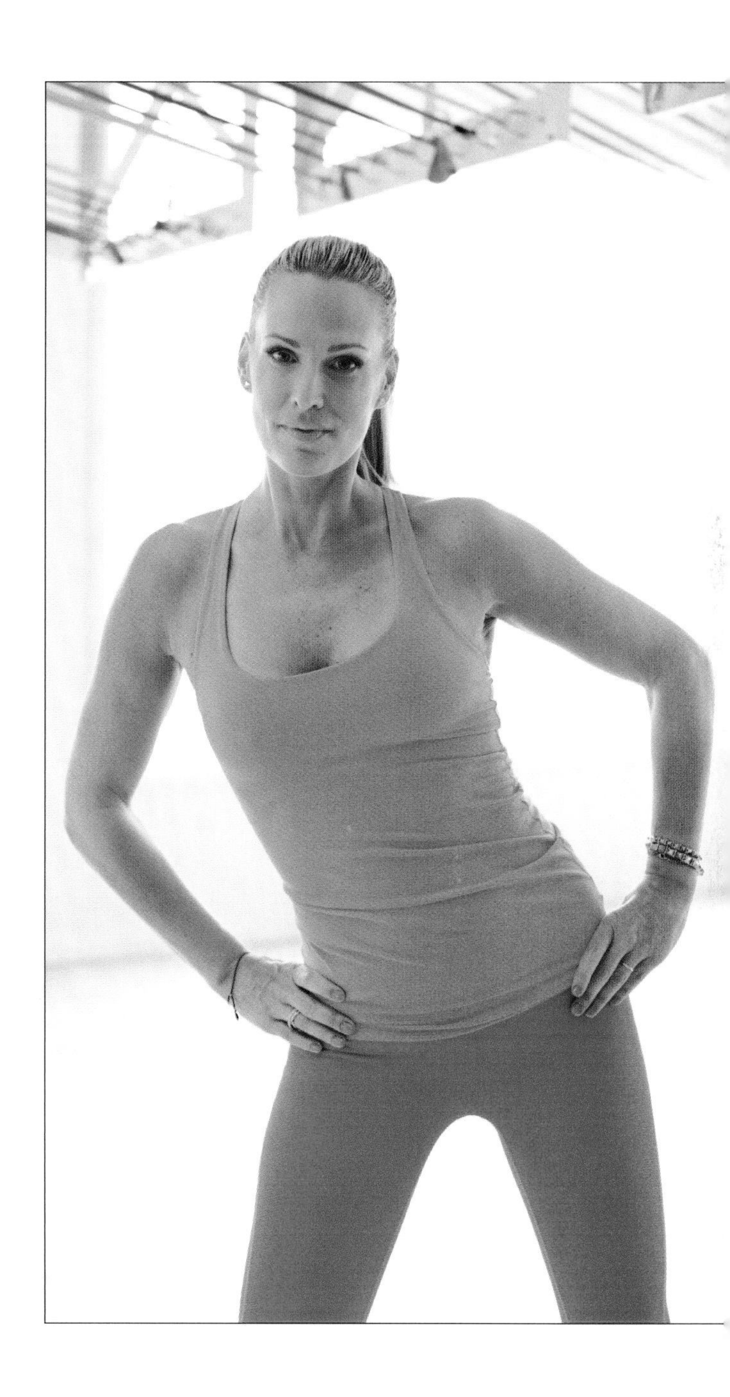

supermodel *secret*

I love Shakira, but my booty just doesn't shake like hers. When I first started with Tracy, it took me forever to get the choreography down. And then once I had it, she'd introduce new choreography! Motherf***er. But now, after years of doing her workouts, I am 100 percent more coordinated, and I pick up new routines much faster. Whatever workout you choose, don't allow embarrassment or frustration to get in the way of you going for it. Find instructors who are kind and willing to give you extra help and encouragement. Despite how awful I was early on, I kept at it, and it has really paid off for me.

TREADMILL TRICKS: I love to get tricky on a treadmill. There isn't a gym in the world that doesn't have one—so it's an easy go-to even when you're traveling. To maximize a treadmill workout go beyond "missionary style"—that is, walking or running—experiment, challenge yourself, and try out a few new moves. Start out slow. It just takes a little practice, concentration, and coordination.

Begin by walking at a slight incline for 5 minutes to warm up your legs and body. Once you are warmed up, try one of the following:

1. **SIDESTEP:** Yes, it looks funny. Yes, you will feel silly. But act like you own the place! Hold on to the front of the treadmill with both hands and face sideways on the treadmill, right foot in front. Begin to sidestep sideways. Do this for 5 minutes and then face the other direction, with the opposite leg forward, and sidestep for 5 minutes. Finish with a 5-minute cooldown, walking normally.
2. **SKIP:** Yep. You heard me. Just like it sounds. Hold the side arms of the treadmill for balance and get your skip on. It might take a little negotiating at first. Be careful. But you'll get it. Take breaks in between if you need. Finish with a 5-minute cooldown, walking normally.

These small tweaks and changes in technique help to work all the muscles in your body and you are guaranteed to feel the burn in places *you never have before*—guaranteed. This workout is especially good for the inner and outer thighs. Our entire treadmill workout is posted on YouTube: Google *Tracy Anderson Treadmill Workout with Molly Sims*. Start off doing just 15 minutes a day and eventually work up to 45 minutes.

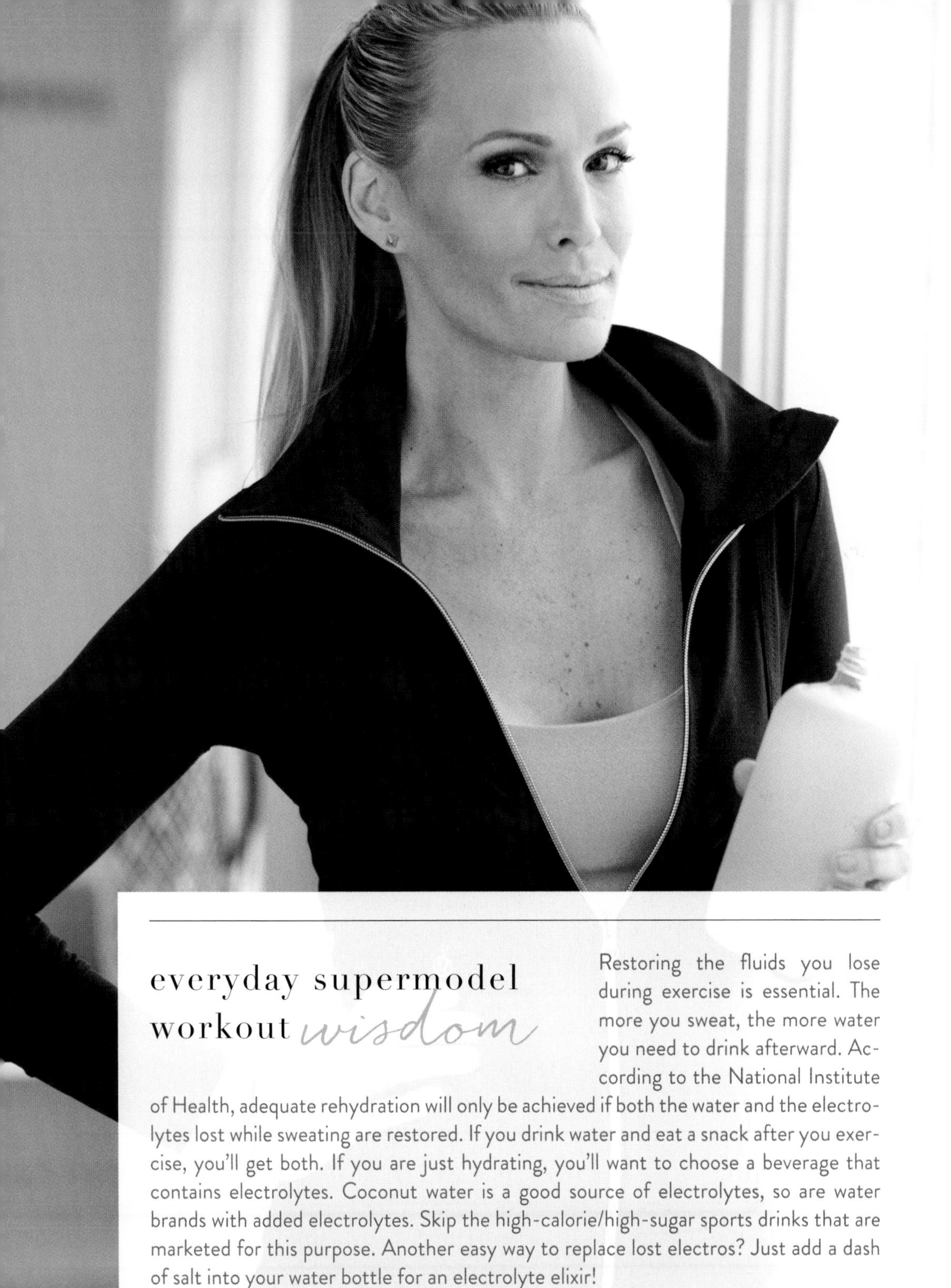

everyday supermodel workout *wisdom*

Restoring the fluids you lose during exercise is essential. The more you sweat, the more water you need to drink afterward. According to the National Institute of Health, adequate rehydration will only be achieved if both the water and the electrolytes lost while sweating are restored. If you drink water and eat a snack after you exercise, you'll get both. If you are just hydrating, you'll want to choose a beverage that contains electrolytes. Coconut water is a good source of electrolytes, so are water brands with added electrolytes. Skip the high-calorie/high-sugar sports drinks that are marketed for this purpose. Another easy way to replace lost electros? Just add a dash of salt into your water bottle for an electrolyte elixir!

WORKOUT #2: SPIN IT TO THIN IT—INDOOR CYCLING

Let's talk the science of spinning, or for you newbies, indoor cycling on a stationary bike. The bike is a taller, more upright version of the stationary bike of the past. Studios blast music, and good ones get you pumped! Not to mention, this workout will literally—kick—your—ass. That's why I do it. It's like a Brazilian butt lift from a bike!

But doesn't cycling bulk up the legs? *Yes, it can,* but it won't if you do it right. There are two keys. The first is to add cycling into your workout rotation once, maybe twice a week, not every day. And two, the setting on your bike is important. Not only for your personal comfort, but also so that you elongate the leg rather than contract it. The seat adjusts so you want it to be about as high as possible so you are ever so slightly reaching and stretching as you pump the pedals. All spin classes are not created equal. So when you are looking for a great spin class, experiment with instructors and locations until you find a class that will motivate you to the max.

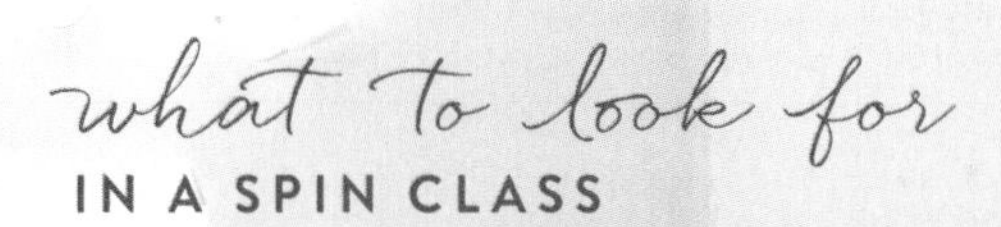

IN A SPIN CLASS

Imagine if Lance Armstrong, Avicii, Oprah, and *The Secret* all had a baby—*that baby would be SoulCycle*. I leave feeling alive, awake, passionate, capable, flush faced, and absolutely drenched in a sweat tsunami. I feel like I lose two pounds of fat and ten pounds of anxiety in every class. That is what you want in an indoor cycling class. This is not your average lunch-crunch workout, and you will need to shower posthaste. Bikes are close together and the room often feels warm and swampy. It's challenging as heck physically and therefore pushes you mentally and spiritually. The SoulCycle motto: "Aspire to Inspire." I always leave a good class feeling lighter, brighter, with my tush tighter. *Sweat, push, pedal—purge.* Let's do this people!

The *basics*

- A spin bike has fancy features and no brakes (you don't need them, it's not actually going anywhere!). From a knob on the bike you can easily control the spin resistance: you can increase resistance to mimic hill climbs, or lower it to simulate the flats.
- Some bikes have light weights attached for added arm exercises.
- At SoulCycle: add sexy (and flattering!) lighting, motivating playlists, and cream of the crop instructors who inspire. (I love, love, love Rique and Stacy, two trainers at the New York studio.)
- You are the only focus. And I promise, you will not think for a second about your to-do list, work e-mails, or changing the cat litter.
- Special note: You do need specific spin shoes. Some studios include them with the class, and at others you have to rent them. If you fall in spin-love, invest in your own pair.

The *benefits*

- According to the SoulCycle founders, you burn between 500 and 700 calories in 45 minutes of indoor cycling.
- Spin is a full-body workout so you can expect to see tighter abs, leaner arms and legs, and overall toning, as well as increased cardiovascular health.
- Your bigger muscles (i.e., the quads and glutes) are definitely activated in spin. When you work bigger muscles and more muscle groups, you burn more calories—not just during the workout, but for *days afterward.*
- Spin works both the fast- and slow-twitch muscle fibers (as does most cross-training or combined cardio/resistance training). Fast twitch are the muscles we use for explosive movements, like sprinting. Slow twitch are our endurance muscles, recruited in long-distance running. In spin, you alternate quick sprints (cardio work), with slow, steep climbs (resistance).
- Spin is a phenomenon. Every major and minor city had a studio. Beyond that—there isn't a gym in existence that doesn't have an upright stationary bike. Put on some tunes that get you juiced and get on that bike and ride. Alternate resistance; do climbs and fast straightaways. Be your own Rique and Stacy!

Everyday Supermodel *Tips*

1. Get the bike adjustment right. Ask your instructor or neighbor for help. Injuries happen when you aren't properly aligned. *So get it right.*

2. Don't bounce while on the bike, even though you'll want to. The way to engage the core is to stabilize your upper body and cycle your legs while keeping level.

3. Keep your shoulders down and don't scrunch. Contracting the body will create tension in the head, neck, and spine. Focus on elongating.

4. Oh, and look good, ladies! There is no shortage of Gosling-esque bachelors in spin classes. For realz.

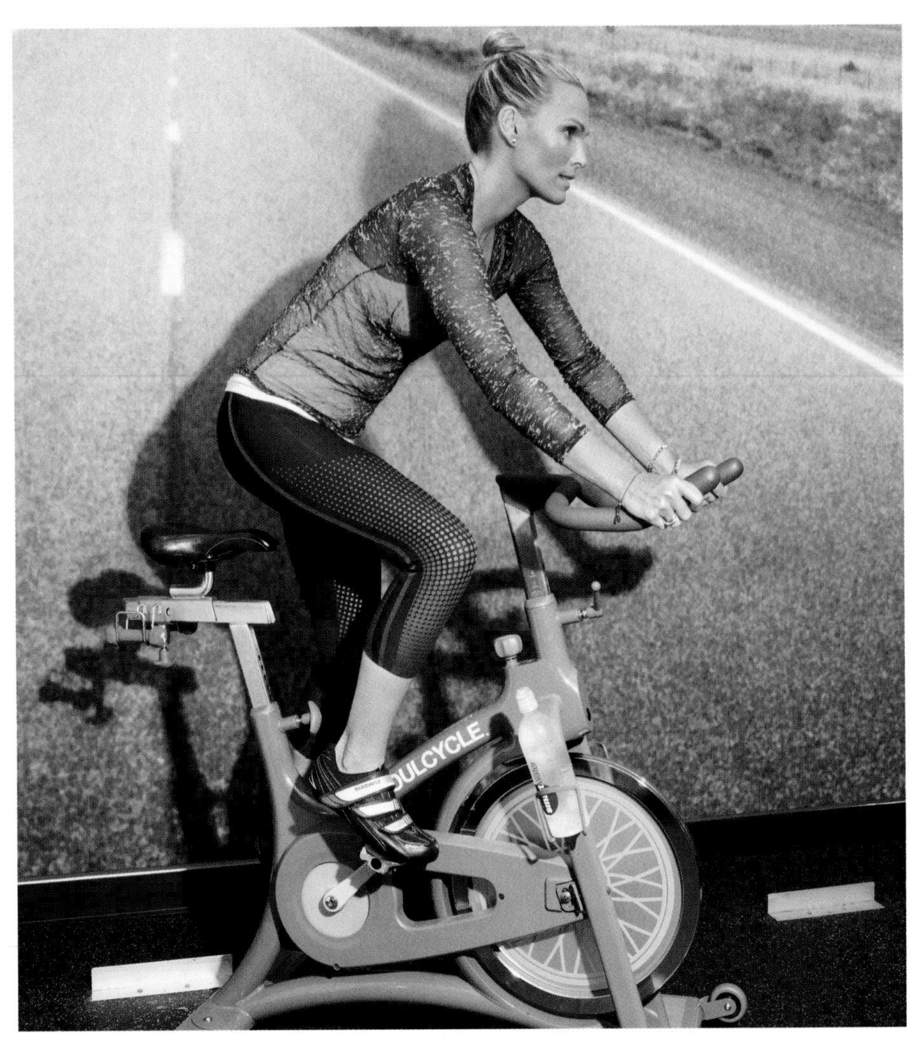

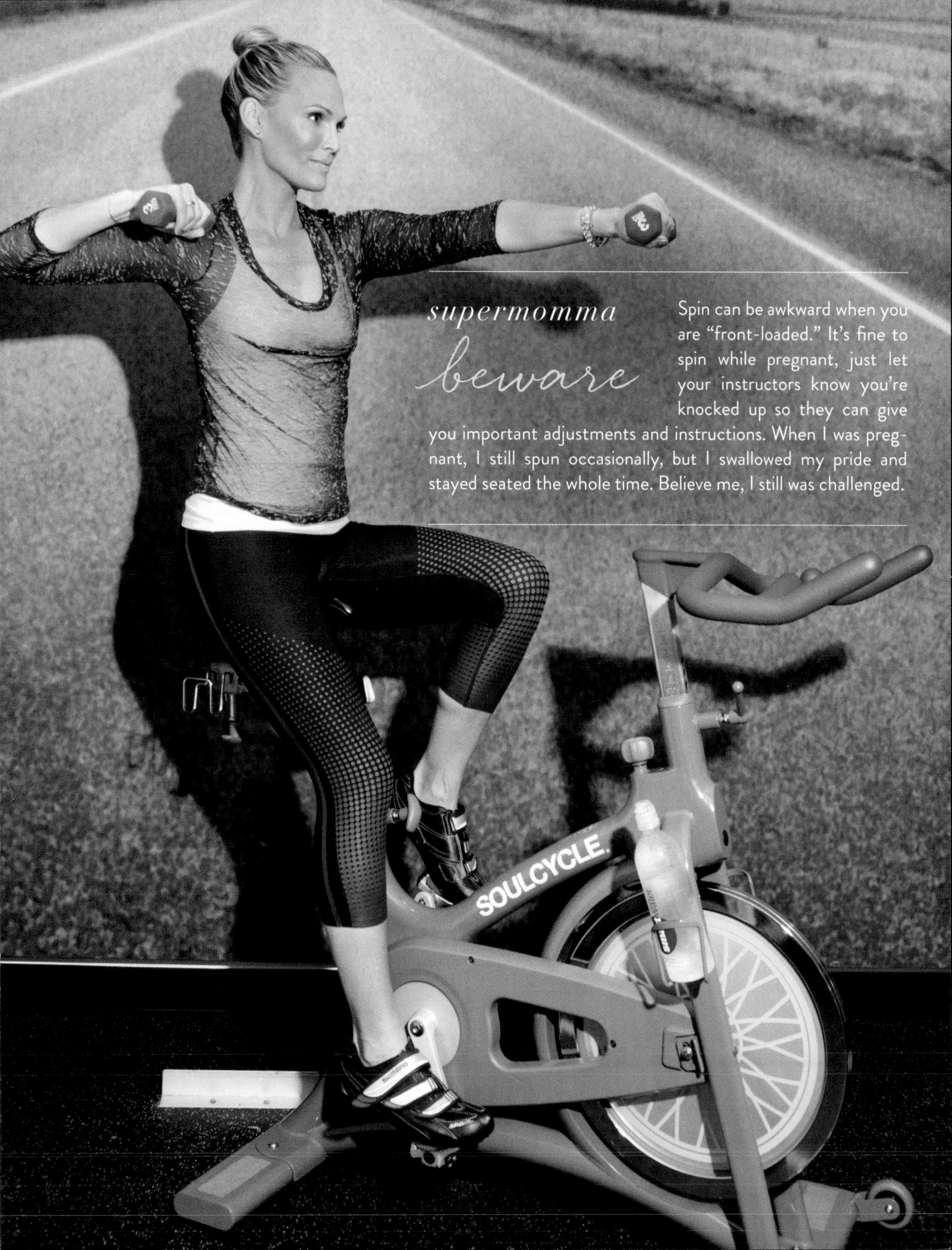

supermomma *beware*

Spin can be awkward when you are "front-loaded." It's fine to spin while pregnant, just let your instructors know you're knocked up so they can give you important adjustments and instructions. When I was pregnant, I still spun occasionally, but I swallowed my pride and stayed seated the whole time. Believe me, I still was challenged.

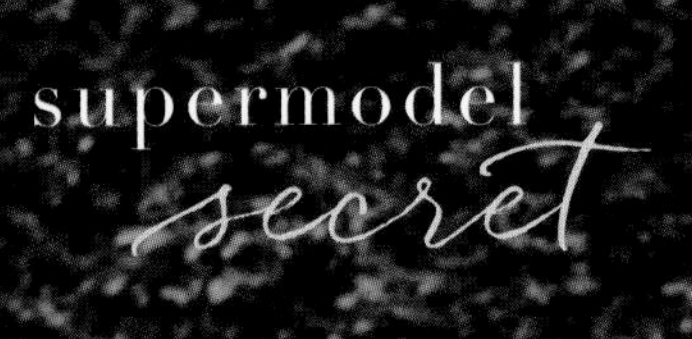

The benefits of exercise go far beyond the body and extend into every aspect of our lives—the psychological, spiritual, professional, personal. Exercise not only makes me feel body confident, but it makes confident in other areas of my life. Not to mention, it jump-starts my day and gives me extra motivation to get sh*t done! I don't know if I'd get anything accomplished without it.

Did you know studies reveal most people grossly underestimate how much they actually ENJOY exercising? Basically: When asked, people say they hate exercise. But then they exercise and are asked again, and after exercising—they say they love it! So focus on the high you are guaranteed to have afterward. Think of your daily workout as a daily deposit into your personal bank account of being healthy, happy, and hot. Make a small deposit every day. Over time, deposits add up!

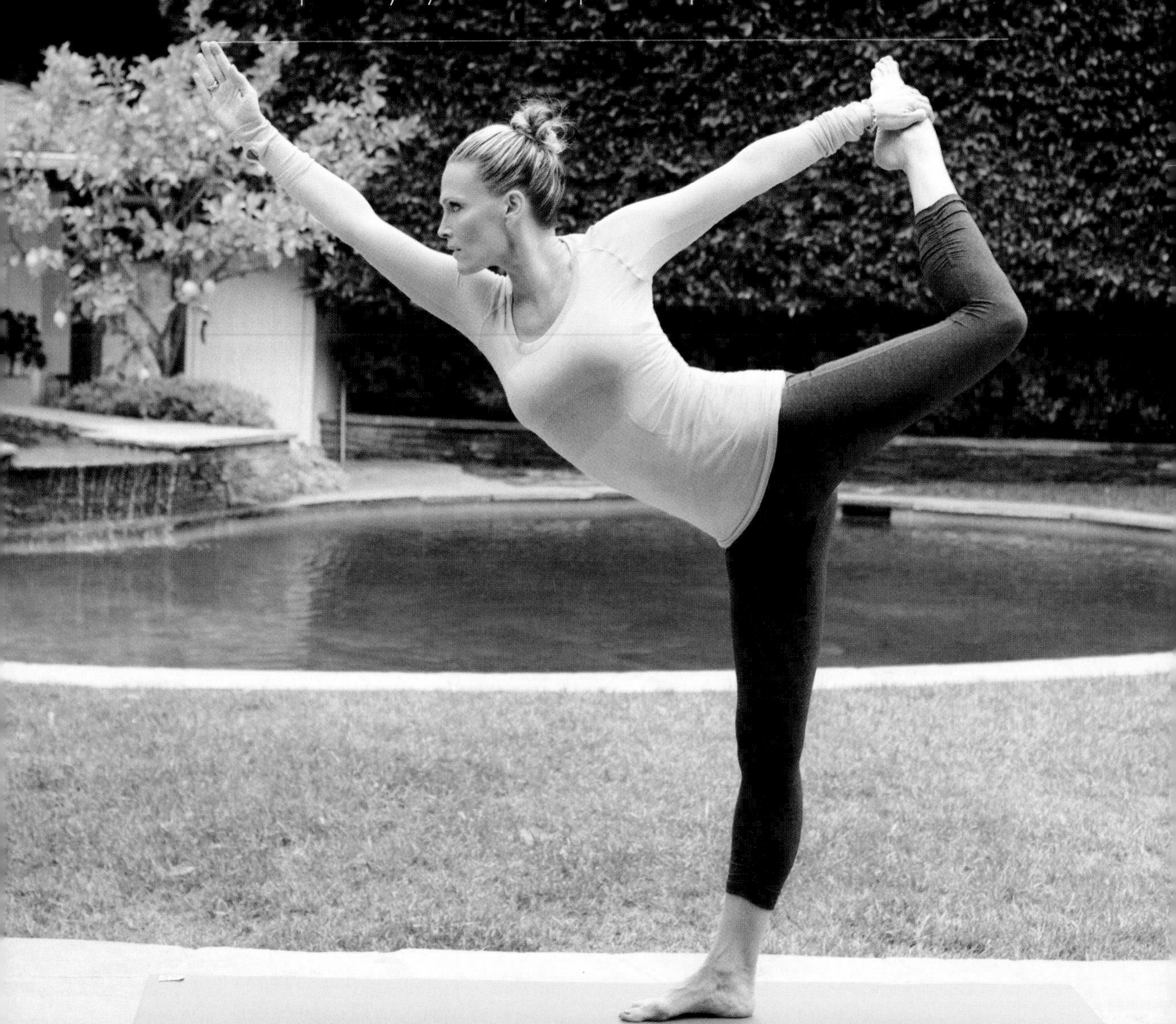

WORKOUT #3: YOGALICIOUS

I am not a yoga freak, but it's always been a part of my fitness plan. My instinct is always to go, go, go and move, move, move! So yoga helps to slow me down. I always finish feeling better. Whether you are ADD, OCD, or a member of the KGB, there is a yoga style right for you. While some forms aren't as physically demanding, other forms definitely are. In general, yoga is tremendous for improved balance, flexibility, fertility, depression, anxiety, and the list goes on. Not to mention, yoga is an ideal complement to almost any workout, especially to high impact exercise, such as running or muscle building work, such as weight-lifting. Yoga encourages the body to stretch, unwind, and expand. If you are a yoga newbie, here's a helpful cheat sheet from instructor Yogi Nicole Honnig. Namaste! May the light in me honor the light in you, *everyday supermodels*.

The *basics*

- Yoga is a body and mind practice that helps strengthen the physical, mental, emotional, and spiritual self.
- There are a variety of different yoga styles, traditions, and intensities. See our list of the most popular. Most styles consist of a series of movements and poses designed to increase focus, strength, and flexibility.
- Movements consist of both stationary poses, standing and sitting on the floor, in addition to flowing sequences. Some incorporate the use of straps, blocks, and other props to assist poses.
- In addition to physical work, yoga also incorporates breathing exercises and meditation techniques.
- Many practice yoga as a form of preventative medicine with complementary health benefits.

The *benefits*

- All styles improve overall flexibility, core strength, and balance.
- The more physically demanding styles, including Hot and Ashtanga, will burn the most calories and help more with weight loss.
- A significant body of research proves yoga reduces symptoms of depression and anxiety.
- Yoga has also been found to lower blood pressure, cholesterol, and heart rate, in addition to improving sleep quality and reducing insomnia.

Yoga *styles*

1. **VINYASA FLOW:** Kind of a potpourri class, focusing on flowing, continuous movement rather than long holds. It's very aerobic and focuses on breathing techniques.

2. **POWER YOGA:** Merges several styles of yoga, is physically demanding, and concentrates on strength building and flexibility. You'll encounter longer holds and warmer rooms. It can vary greatly from studio to studio and instructor to instructor.

3. **IYENGAR:** You might only do four or five poses per class, but the focus is on precision and correct body and breath alignment. Although it's very technical, Iyengar is a great choice for beginners, or for those with injuries, because teachers encourage the use of props, such as bolsters, pillows, straps, and blocks, to help with alignment and support.

4. **ASHTANGA:** Another very aerobic style of yoga. It's similar to Bikram in that it has a series of set sequences (rather than poses). The room is likely warm (not hot) and all the movements flow together to heat up the body and produce a detoxifying sweat.

5. **RESTORATIVE YOGA:** Almost all studios offer a restorative class. You do very few poses, most supported by props, and the poses are held for a long time. The focus is placed on calming the central nervous system. This is a great choice for those looking to reduce anxiety and relax body and mind.

6. **PRENATAL YOGA:** Despite its name, prenatal yoga is good prepregnancy, during pregnancy, and postpregnancy. It, of course, focuses on postures that women who are pregnant can do. You can go to a class and don't have to worry about modifying anything. Classes concentrate on helping reduce the discomforts of pregnancy, in addition to preparing the body for labor and motherhood. It also focuses on relaxation, deep breathing, and meditation. Calm mind and body equals a calm baby.

7. **BIKRAM OR HOT YOGA:** My personal favorite! Bikram is a set of the same twenty-six yoga postures. The postures never change (it's copywritten), so you know what you are getting every time, studio to studio, teacher to teacher—and it's in a HOT room. Hot yoga (also in a hot room, obviously) combines yoga styles and poses—but still delivers.

OUTER/INNER HOTTIE: When I finish a Hot yoga class, I feel like I've had a whole body orgasm. Detox, detox, DETOX! The amount of sweat that leaves your body is remarkable. You are basically a human sprinkler system. The "inner heat" stimulated by these styles is believed to burn away the six poisons of being human: *desire, anger, delusion, greed, envy,* and *sloth*. You know—when you are anxious, cranky, crazy, b*tchy, jealous, and lazy. As you breathe in and out of the poses and as you sweat—you are not only burning fat and toning flab, you are clearing your mind, body, and spirit for improved focus, strength, and joy. Basically, you are becoming a more evolved person.

Exercise is very important! Not only for your body, the way you look and feel, but also for your mind. You need to have a healthy fit body to think straight. I do a lot of running and mix in the gym and all kinds of styles of yoga.

—ANYA RUBIK, model

YOGA POSES FOR AN *EVERYDAY SUPERMODEL* SILHOUETTE: Yoga makes me feel calm and confident. And you can do it almost anywhere, anytime. If you are a rookie, my advice is to take a few classes first and consult the instructor to make sure you understand the proper alignment of each pose. Once you have a strong understanding—the yoga world is your "om" oyster. There isn't a city on this planet where you can't find yoga classes. Even better, most studios offer weekly free or donation-only community classes. Can't make it to class? There are plenty of high-quality online programs with top instructors, teachers you might not normally have access to in your hometown (checkout DoYogaWithMe.com or YogaGlo.com).

13 POSES 13 minutes

YOGI *nicole* put together a series of poses for you to yoga-cize at home. Hold each pose for approximately 5 to 10 deep breaths. The entire program can be anywhere from 13 to 30 minutes, depending on how long you hold each pose. Start with one minute. As long as you have a mat, you can do this just about anywhere. I love to do the sequence on the weekend in my backyard.

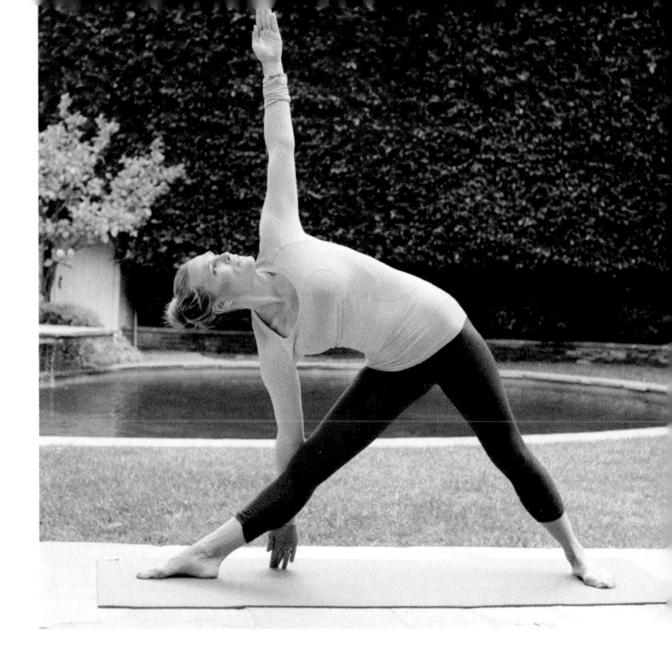

1. triangle pose

Stretches hips, inner thighs, hamstrings, shoulders, chest, and spine.

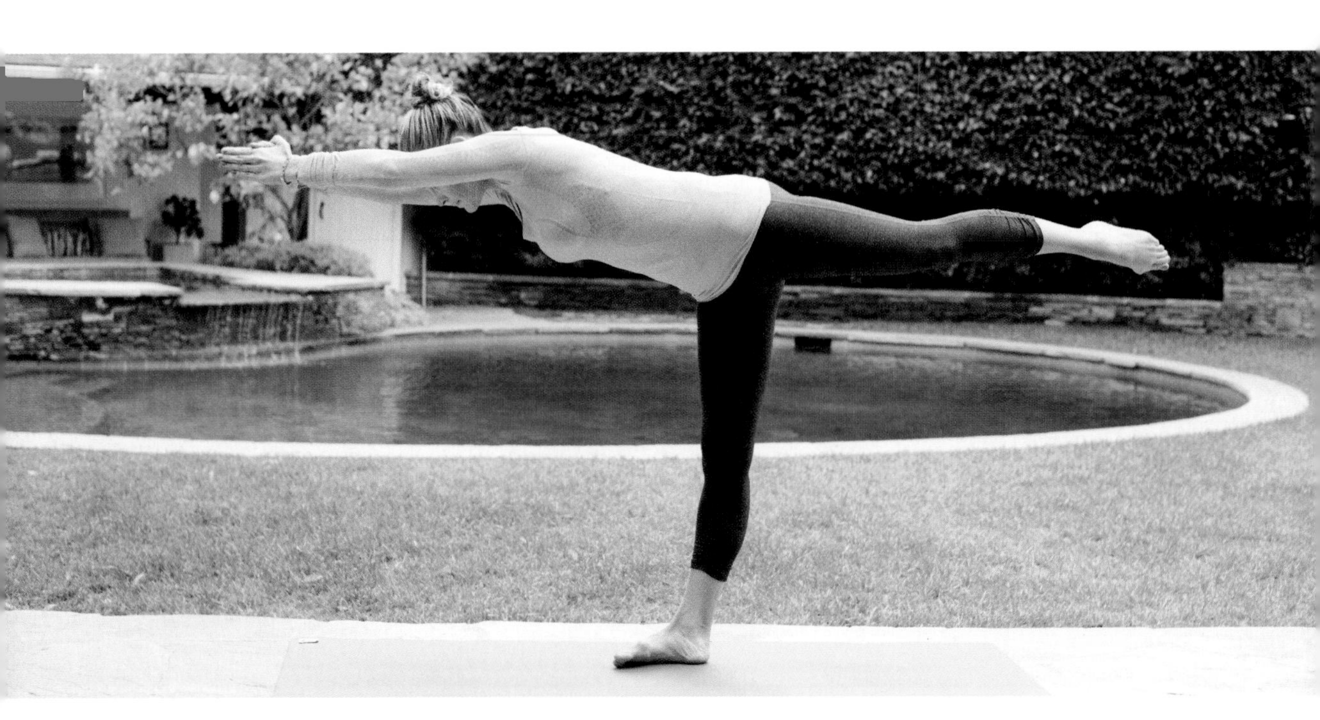

4. warrior

Stretches shoulders and hamstrings, engages abdominals, and helps improves balance and posture.

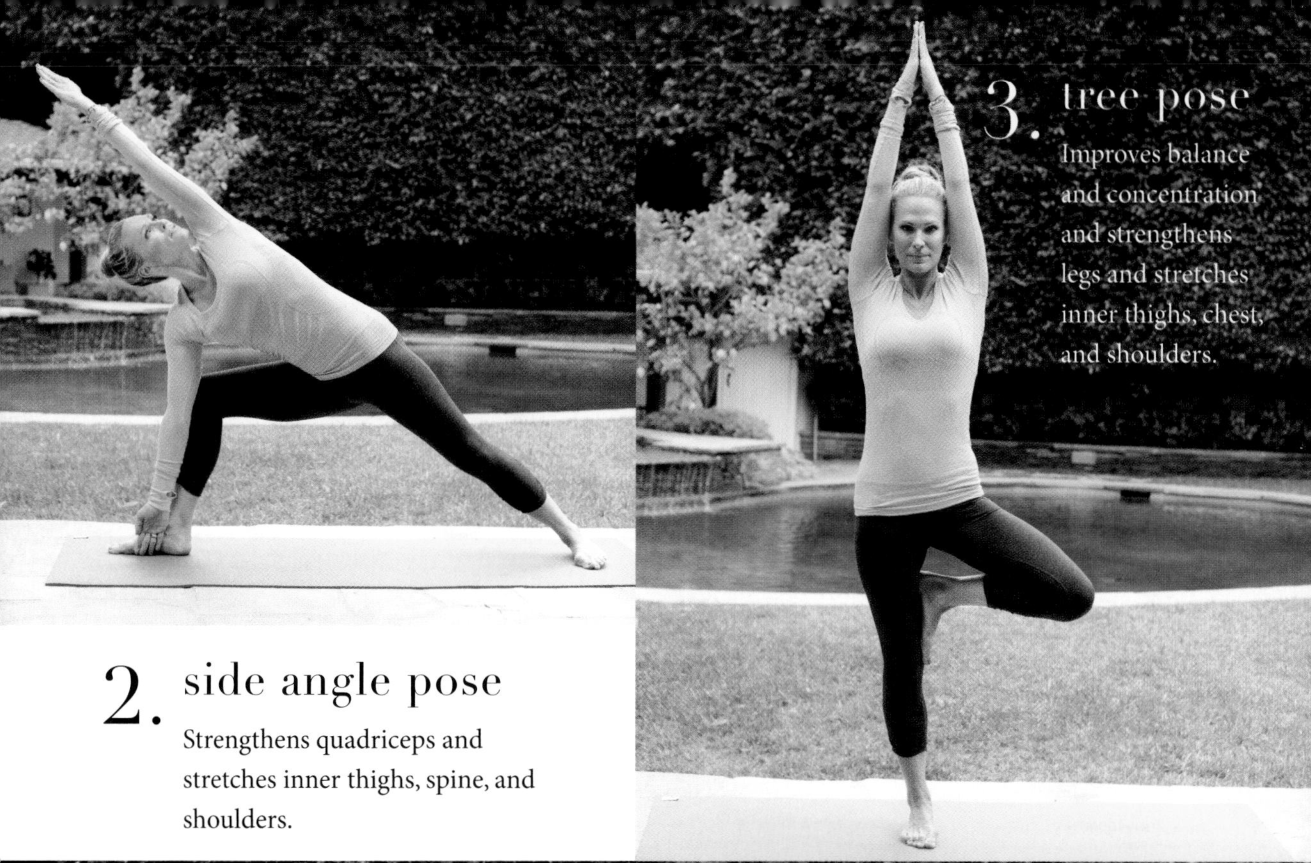

3. tree pose

Improves balance and concentration and strengthens legs and stretches inner thighs, chest, and shoulders.

2. side angle pose

Strengthens quadriceps and stretches inner thighs, spine, and shoulders.

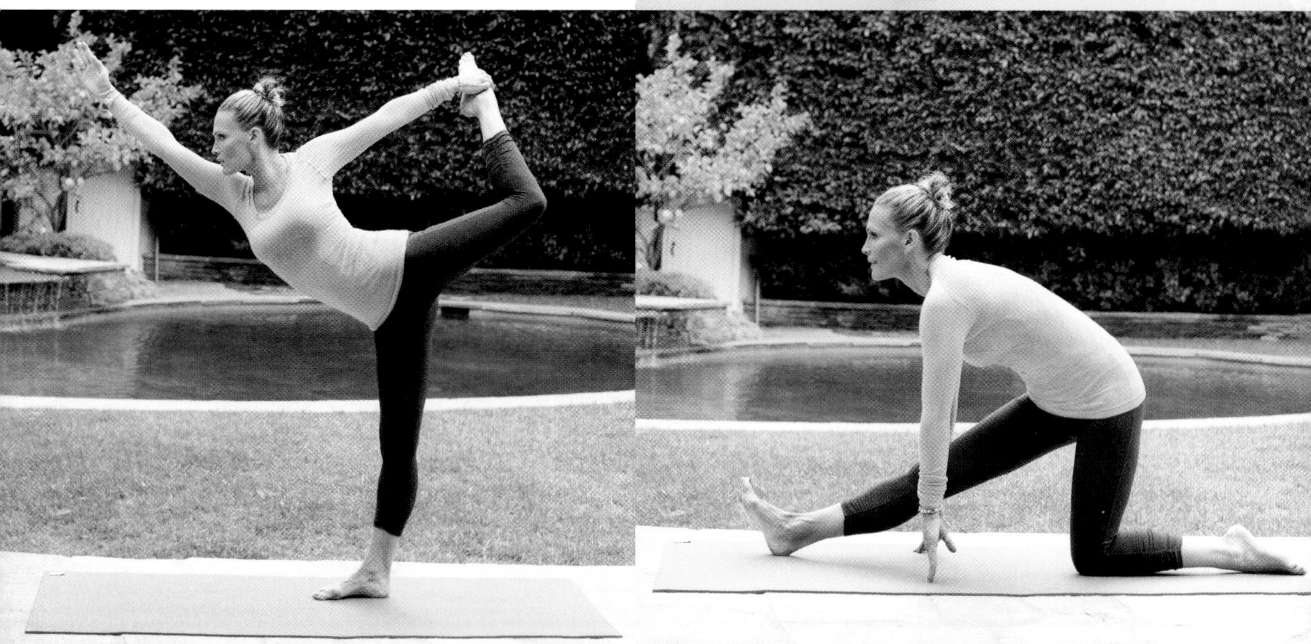

5. dancer

Stretches the shoulders, chest, abdomen, and thighs and improves balance and focus.

6. runner's stretch

Stretches the hamstrings, low back, and spine and stimulates internal organs.

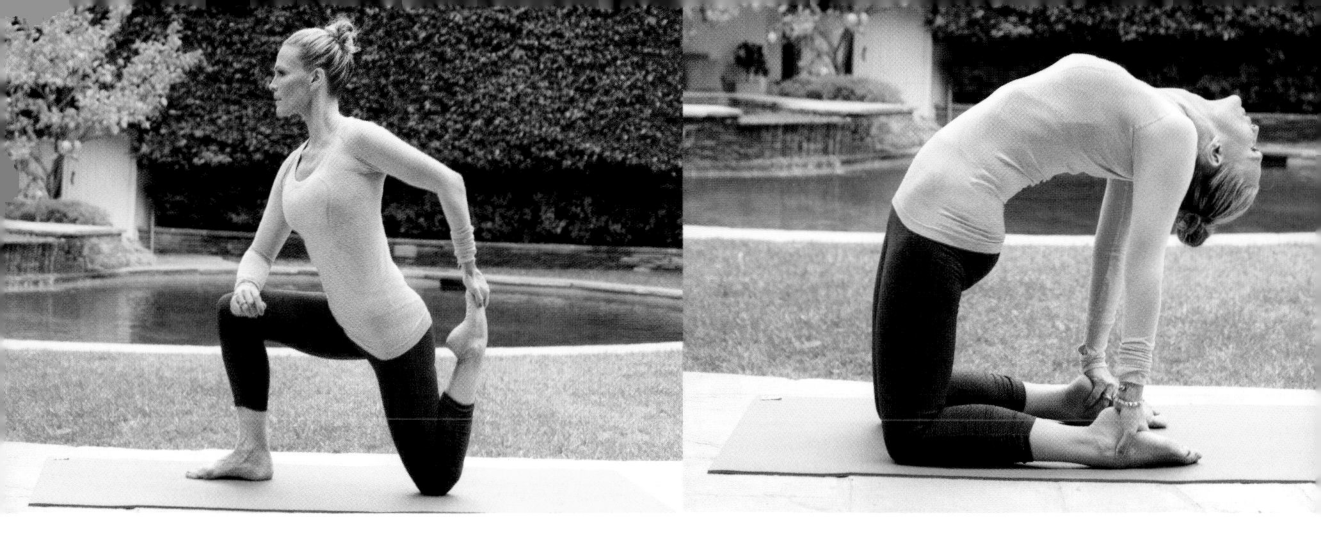

7. low lunge with thigh stretch

Stretches the thighs, psoas (muscle that stabilizes the spine and that allow spine and hips to rotate), groins, chest, and shoulders.

8. camel

Stimulating for the mind and stretches the entire front of the body and strengthens back muscles.

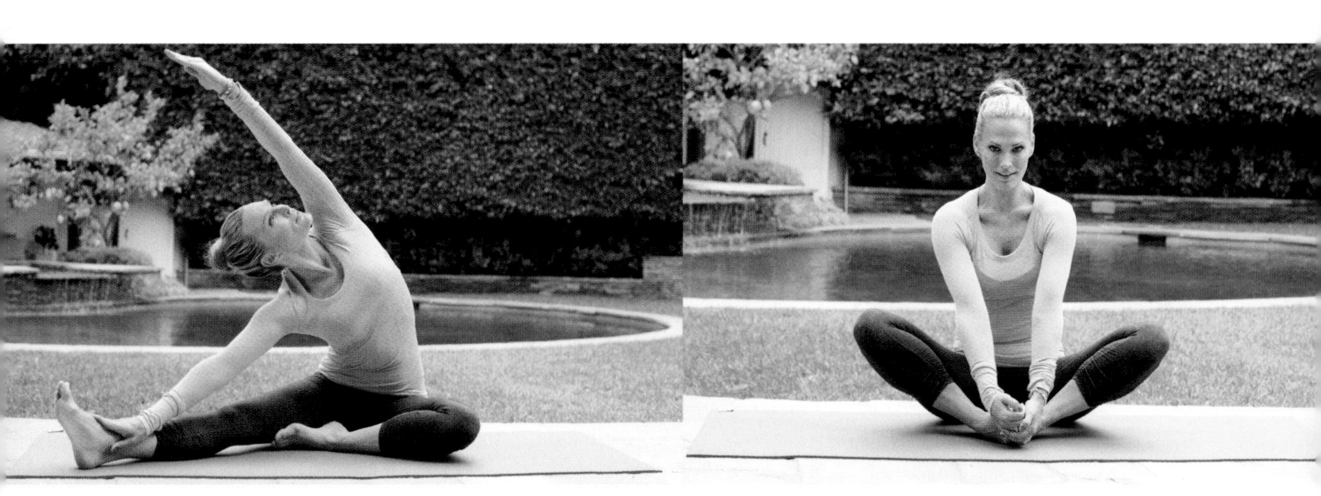

11. revolved head to knee pose

The pose stretches the hamstrings, inner thighs, and spine. It aids in calming the mind and improving digestion.

12. bound angle pose butterfly stretch

The pose stretches the inner thighs, outer hips, and spine. It stimulates internal organs and can help soothe menstrual pain.

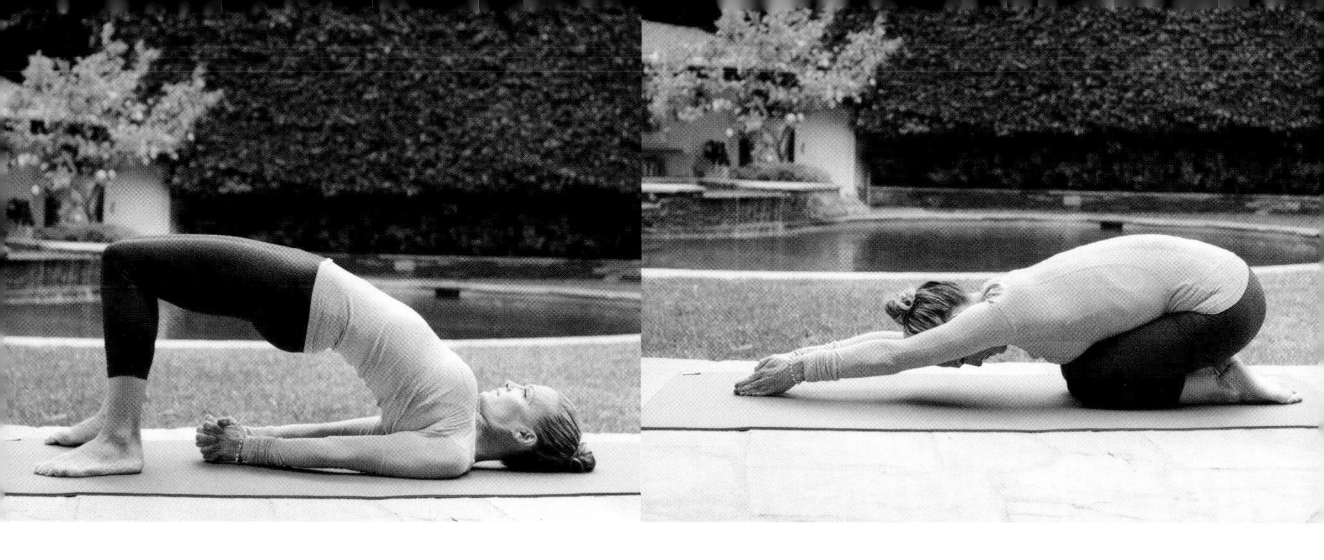

9. bridge pose

Stretches thighs, chest, neck, and spine. Helps calm the mind and expands abdominal muscles and lungs.

10. child's pose

Gently stretches hips, thighs, and ankles. Calms the nervous system and helps relieve stress. Hold for 1 minute if possible. In general, child's pose is a pose you can take at any time in your practice when you need an active break or a transition pose.

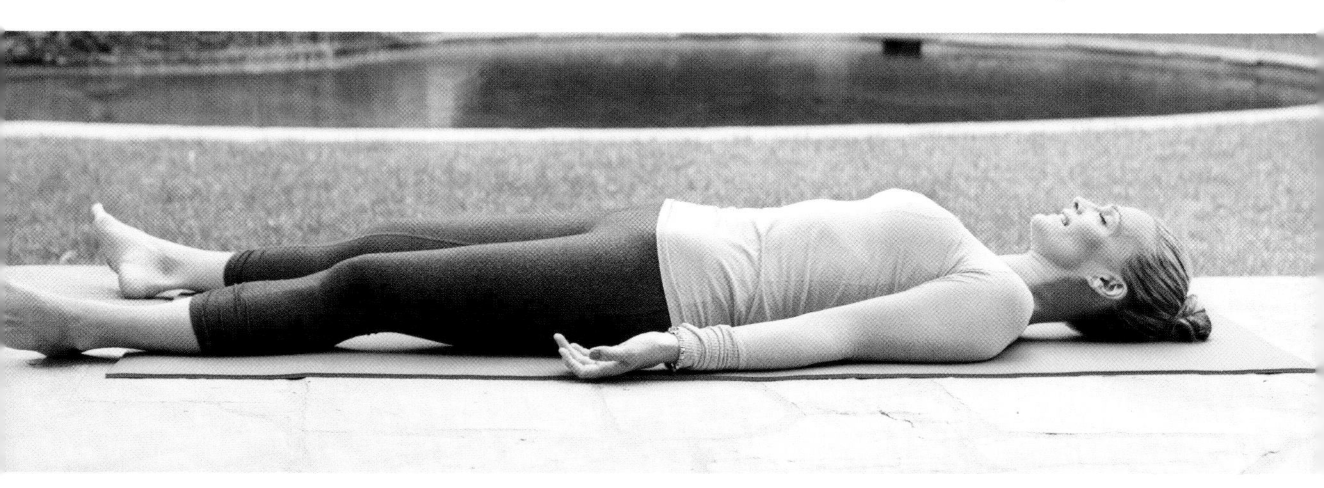

13. corpse pose

Also frequently referred to as *Savasana*. Relaxes the body and calms the mind. Should be held for a least 5 minutes. (Who doesn't love this pose!?)

supermomma beware

The warrior, dancer, and camel poses are not recommended during pregnancy. Keep in mind that twists of any kind can be too much compression as well. Lying on the back and doing poses (asanas) isn't recommended after the first trimester, as it can reduce blood flow to the uterus. Steer clear of poses that stretch the muscles too much like taffy, especially the abs. While pregnant, the uterus and connective tissue are softer due to hormones, so you are more at risk for strains. And let's face it, you might also be feeling nauseated, puffy, and chunky—so no need to add an injury to that!

Everyday Supermodel *yoga Tips*

* Please don't push yourself beyond your limits, and always inform your teacher of any health conditions or injuries before you start.
* Breathe in and out of your nose. It's more calming than in and out of your mouth, and it's proven to slow your heart rate (while breathing in and out of the mouth speeds it up).
* Even when legs are straightened, try to keep a very slight bend in them to avoid hyperextension and knee injury.
* Ask for help to get into difficult poses or use props to assist you: blocks, blankets, bolsters, straps, and pillows are awesome and can keep you injury free. (That sounded kind of kinky—but it's not—when used in yoga, anyway!).

Plank is the perfect postpregnancy pose and an ideal pose for anyone looking to tone the tummy. It's amazing for the core and helps to pull in and tighten the abdominals after they've relaxed and stretched during pregnancy.

—NICOLE HONNIG, yoga instructor

ONLY HAVE 3 minutes?

ONLY NEED 3 moves!

On those days you just don't have a full-on workout within you, do these three moves that engage the whole body—core, glutes, legs, arms. Some might say three minutes of *hell*. Me? I'd say three minutes to *Hello, hot stuff*!

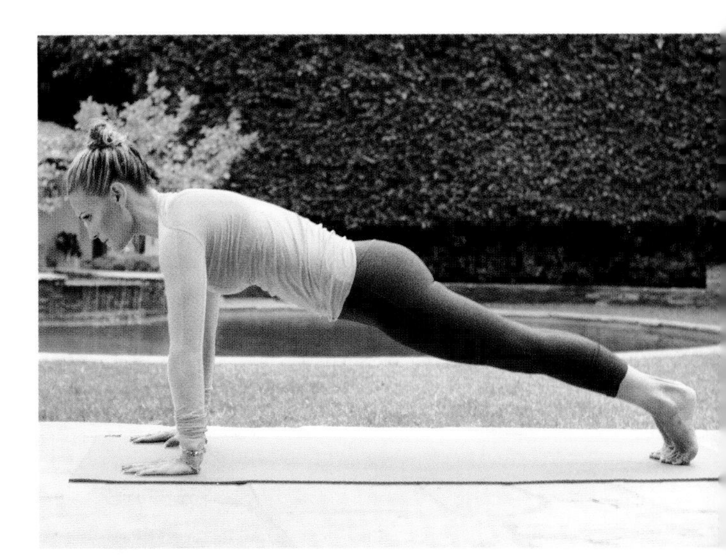

1. forward plank

Hold for one minute.

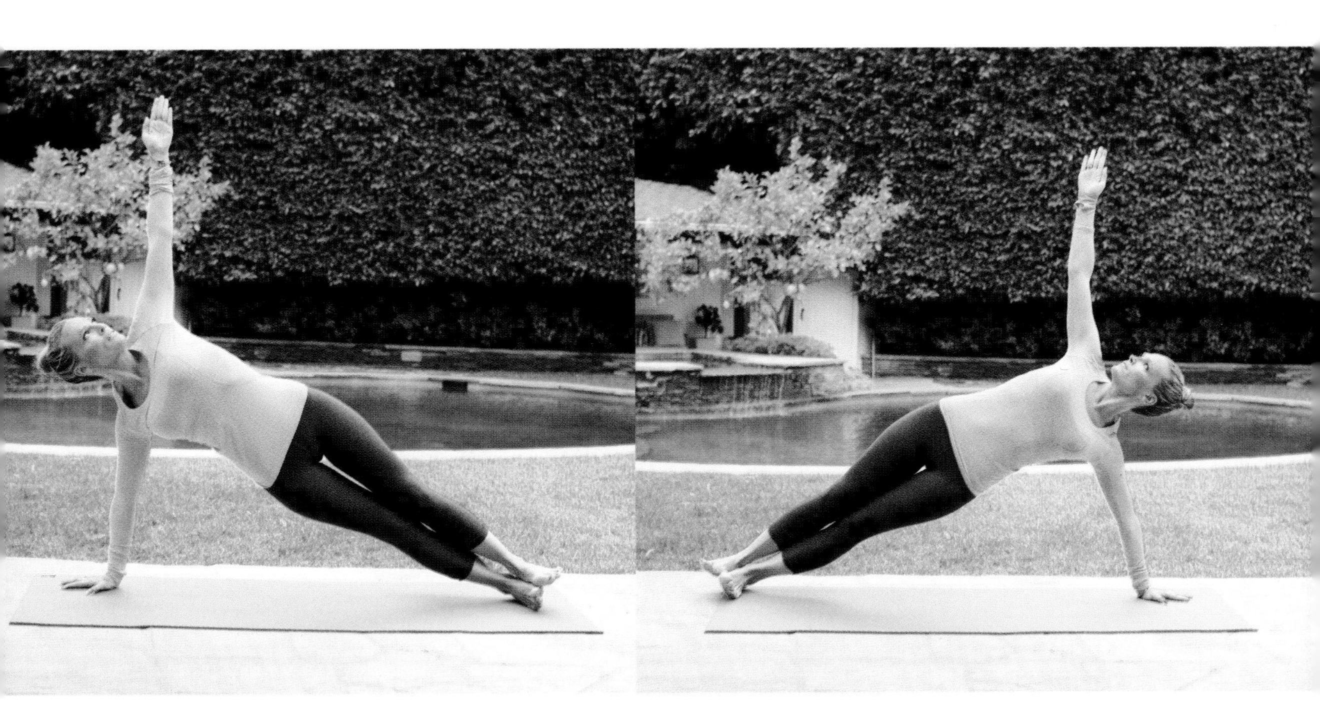

2. right side plank

Hold for one minute.

3. left side plank

Hold for one minute.

supermodel *secret*

Let's talk fitness fashion. Are you wearing bleached-out sweatpants and a sorority rush T-shirt from 1999? Burn those; *do not burn fat in those*. Exercising is not the time to wear items that should be donated to the Salvation Army. Dress to impress yourself. There is nothing worse than looking in the mirror and already wanting to give up. Wear colors you look and feel good in. Get a couple of outfits that tuck and tighten. Find a sports bra that is supportive but doesn't give you uni-boob. Workout wear should be *work-it* wear.

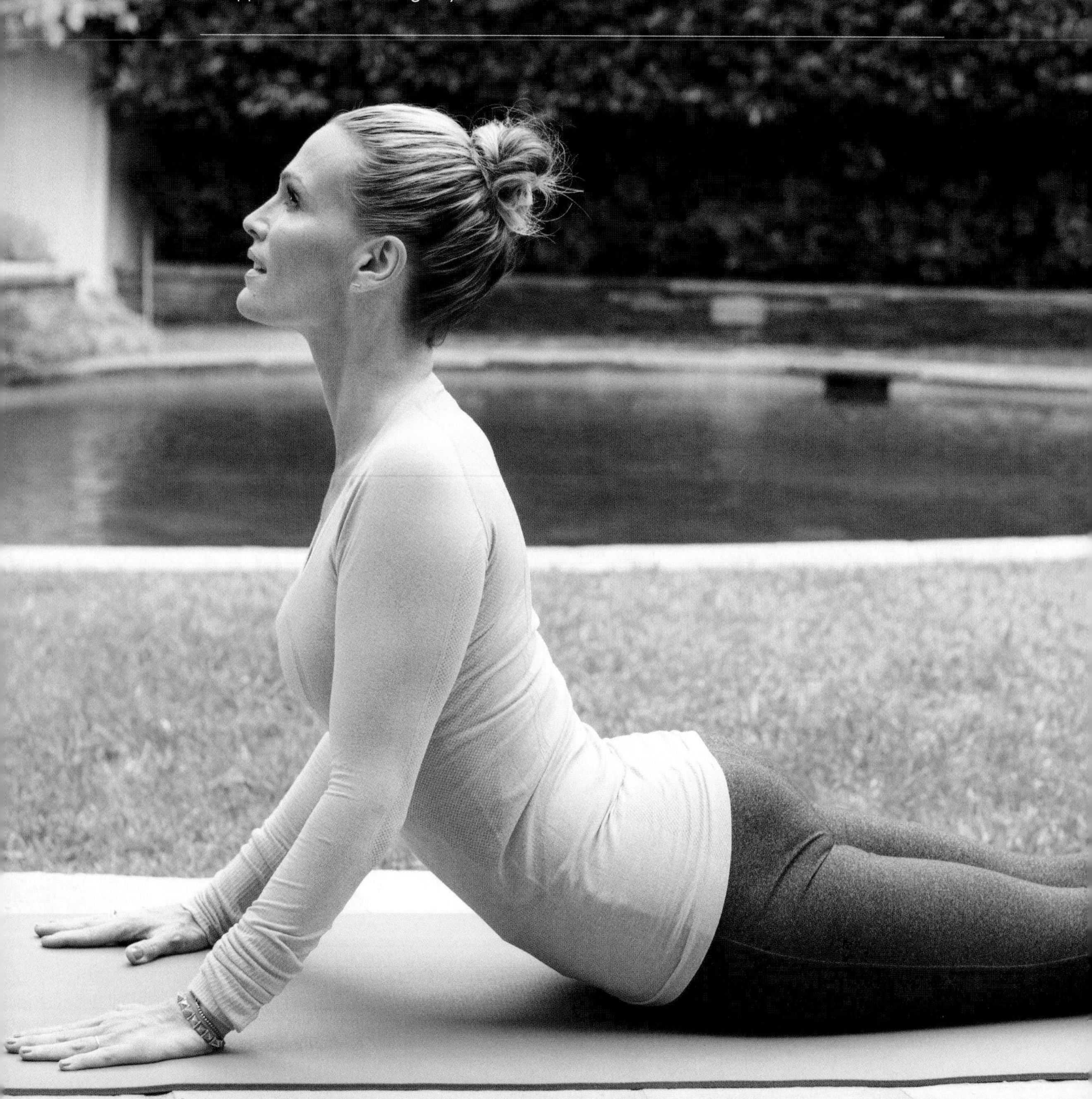

WORKOUT #4: PILATES BODY!

When I was modeling in New York, I started doing Pilates with Alycea Ungaro. All the models were going to her at the time. She still has an incredible studio in lower Manhattan. Alycea designed a specific program for me and my body type and what she did worked. Pilates is still an industry standard for getting a strong, healthy model body.

We have been in a big cardio phase—but studies tell us that resistance and strength training is far superior for overall health and weight loss. Sustained low-grade cardio makes you really hungry. All cardio, all the time, will leave you famished.

—ALYCEA UNGARO, instructor and owner of Real Pilates

The *basics*

* Pilates is tried and true; it has been around since the 1920s. Joseph Pilates was a diver, a gymnast, and a boxer, and he developed this program to train athletes who needed a strong core.
* The foundation of the workout is strength training and resistance using your own body as weight.
* Exercises focus on body conditioning with an emphasis on spinal and pelvic alignment, strong core, coordination, proper breathing—and corrective exercising in order to correct bad habits, retrain muscles, and focus on proper form.
* A typical class is 45 minutes to an hour and may feature a mat workout and weight series or exercises using several pieces of specialty Pilates equipment.
* Specialty equipment includes stability chairs, the Reformer and the Cadillac. The Reformer looks a little like a rowing machine and consists of a platform that moves back and forth along a carriage—and is designed as a resistance device. The Cadillac is a larger piece of equipment that looks a bit like a mini jungle gym but is basically a one-stop exercise shop. It's most often used in private classes because of its size and features leg and arm springs, a trapeze element, a push-through bar for stretching out, and rings or loops for various sequences.

- There are a few kinds of Pilates classes: Mat classes are usually the most affordable because they don't utilize equipment. Reformer classes are generally private or very small group and are more costly. Private instruction classes that feature the Reformer or the Cadillac are the most expensive.
- Pilates is an equal-opportunity workout. It's great for all body types and ages and intensity is easily customized. It's also a program to stay fit, even when you are injured and can't do anything else because the equipment allows for non-weight-bearing or weight-bearing exercises that work many ranges of motion.

The *benefits*

- Almost all devotees witness a shrinking waistline, strong back, flat abs, and lean muscle definition.
- Pilates is ideal for balancing the physique. If you have overdeveloped legs and an underdeveloped upper body, or vice versa, the program will be customized to balance you out.
- It makes you better at everything: tennis, walking with a stroller, whatever day-to-day activities you do.
- Like with yoga, a mat workout can be done anywhere, anytime! No studio needed.
- It doesn't matter what your baseline level of fitness is when you start; the workout is so approachable, user-friendly, and customizeable, it shouldn't be intimidating.
- You will stand taller and have better posture. Also, bad habits will be broken, and injuries you've always had frequently will be corrected.

PILATES FOR THE *EVERYDAY SUPERMODEL*: To replicate the instability and movement of the Pilates Reformer at home, all you need is a towel and a little tenacity! By placing a towel under your feet, hands, or elbows, Pilates can be practiced on your own at home. Amanda Freeman, founder of SLT (Strength Lengthen Tone—a high-intensity Pilates workout in New York City), put together a few Pilates moves for you to try at home.

at-home *moves*

1. Spoon

* Place a towel under your feet and the heels of your hands on the edge of the seat of a chair behind you.
* Using your lower abdominal muscles, pull your torso up while sliding your feet closer to the chair.
* Slowly lower your body while sliding the legs away from the chair.
* Repeat slowly for a minute.

2. Serve the Platter

* Holding light weights, start with hands by your waist and slowly (use a 4-count) lift up to shoulder height.
* Slowly lower down to your waist and repeat for a minute.

3. Newspaper

* Holding light weights, bend your arm at the elbow, like you are holding a newspaper.
* Keeping your upper arms tight to the body, slowly hinge your arms out to the side like you're opening the newspaper.
* Slowly bring your hands together, like you're closing a newspaper.
* Repeat for a minute.

MY FAVE MOVE? THE REVERSE CRUNCH: After doing these, you will never have to do another miserable sit-up again. Just a few of these a day and hello supermodel abs of steel.

* Kneel on the floor with your back in a tabletop position and forearms shoulder-width apart on a towel on the floor.
* Slowly slide your forearms toward your body, rounding your back to activate your lower abdominal muscles.
* Slowly slide your forearms back to the original position so your back returns to a tabletop position.
* Repeat for a minute.

supermodel *secret*

Check out your trainer, the class instructor, and the followers of that method. Do you like what you see? Do you want your body to look like theirs? It's important to do. I take note of what kind of bodies certain programs build. If I like what I see, I'm in. If I don't, it's a good indication it's not right for me.

BRINGING IT ALL TOGETHER

Nike is right about one thing: *Just do it.* We need to approach fitness with a fearless attitude. How do you do that? You make it fun. You try different workouts. But most important, you must take the Olivia Newton John pledge to *get physical.* Remember, we enjoy exercising WAY more than we think we do. When we finish, we feel phenomenal. I stay fitness focused because I enjoy challenging myself and discovering the strategies that work best for me. And for me, that's a blend of cardio and strength training, which includes spin, yoga, and Pilates as a foundation—and then whatever workout is new to the neighborhood that sounds like something I might enjoy. Fitness is key to total health and real hotness, so find a way to make it part of your *everyday supermodel* schedule.

THE SUPERMODEL SWEAT: There's no hard and fast research that tells us that sweating during exercise helps burn more fat and calories. However, I *one-hundred-percent* believe it does and I do whatever it takes to make it rain! Why? It's like a full body flush. And I believe it's essential to banishing bulge and other body woes. I employ every "*bat-sh*t-crazy tactic*" to get myself spouting. Yes, including wearing a giant, black plastic trash bag while I work out. Here are some sweat-your-butt-off benefits:

1. **BLOAT BUSTER:** Sweating reduces bloat. I am the queen of water retention. If I don't sweat for a few days, I look like Puffy the Magic Dragon.
2. **CELLULITE SMOOTHER:** Experts know sweating stimulates circulation and lymphatic detoxification, and some believe it reduces cellulite. Just go to a Bikram hot yoga class and check out the tushes of the regulars. *This alone proves the theory.*
3. **GLOW GIVER:** G'day glow-geous! Sweating opens and unclogs the pores. The improved circulation delivers nutrients vital for healthy skin cells, leaving skin softer, smoother, and yes, "glow-ier" if that's even a word.

How to *turn* Your Workout Space into a Sweat-Cuzzi

1. Heat your workout room or house. I have a small gym and heat the room to about 82 degrees when I'm working out. No fan. No open windows. Just me, my sweat, and I. Simply using a portable heater in a closed room is an easy at-home option.

2. Wear a sh*t ton of clothes: Pile on that Ellie, Lululemon, or Beyond Yoga gear, ladies! Most of the time I wear long sleeves and long everything. Yes, it gets hot. Choose pieces that are fitted and designed for moisture wicking. Or like I said before, wear a trash bag. Yes, you heard me. It's the poor man's sauna suit, but who cares how it looks as long as it works?

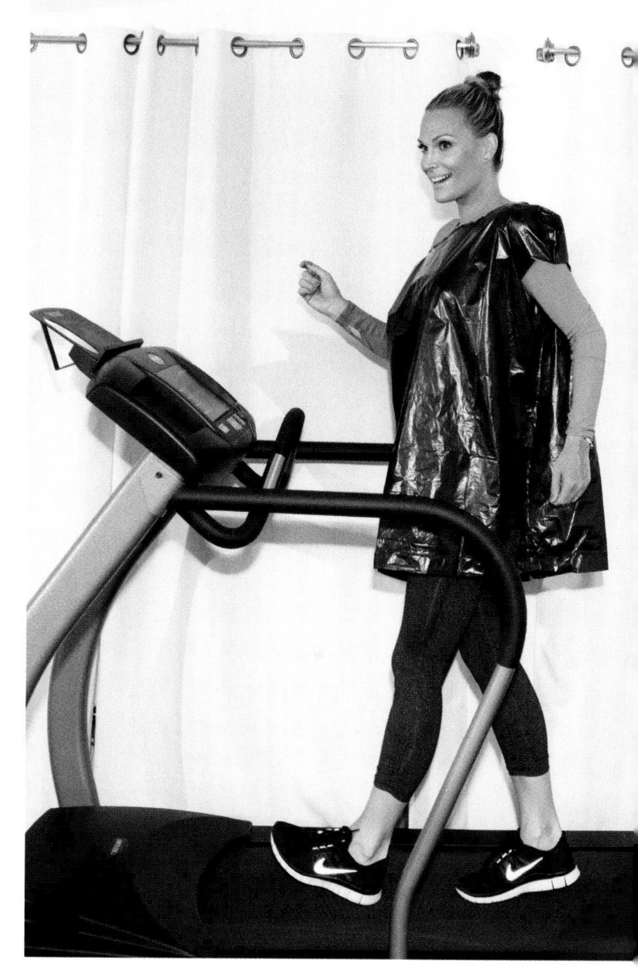

3. Steam or sauna postworkout. Not only is it great for recovery and reducing muscle soreness and stiffness, but it will keep your sweat pumping after your workout.

4. You want to sweat more? Commit. Push yourselves. If you take breaks in class or don't sprint when your spin instructor says to—you are cheating yourself out of serious sweatage and a better workout.

---

supermodel *secret*

Practice heat protection! I really don't want to be picking your sweaty self up off the floor after you've fainted. Please be smart. Hydrate. The more you sweat, the more water you need to drink. The rule: you need to take in more than you sweat out. The more intense the workout, the more water you need to guzzle. Hydrating helps regulate body temperature and increases performance. If working out in a heated room makes you dizzy or lethargic, then it's not the strategy for you.

MIX IT UP TO FIX IT UP: Studies show that changing up your fitness routine helps to constantly challenge new muscles and improves total fitness. Surprise your body by doing different workouts every now and again. Studies also show that when the brain and the body have to work—you get a better workout. Other reasons to rotate your workout?

1. MUSCLES NEED TIME TO HEAL: Different workouts access different muscle groups. When you change it up, you aren't likely to be working the same muscle groups day in and day out. You give them time to repair and rebuild.

2. VARIETY CREATES MUSCLE BALANCE: Doing the same workout over and over can create muscle imbalances in the body. By mixing it up, you help assist in balanced muscle development and will prevent injuries now and later in life.

3. BOREDOM CAN LEAD TO BURNOUT: Same ol' same ol' can lead to boredom, burnout, and eventually . . . abandonment. Uh-oh! When feeling uninspired, don't take the foot off the gas, but rather try something new and different. By keeping your fitness pursuits fresh, you are more likely to have fun and want to stay committed.

HOW TO AVOID a fitness version of *Groundhog Day:*

1. GET OUTSIDE: I live just a few minutes from the Santa Monica Mountains and there are all kinds of nature walks and hikes. The ups and downs, switchbacks, and different terrain makes for a great workout. The fresh air is awesome for clearing out the lungs and the lymphs. Check our your nearest park, trail, beach, or bunny hill for workout inspiration.

2. ANYTHING GOES ATTITUDE: I am ALWAYS open and excited to try something new. I love, love, love to work out with friends, so every now and again I'll find myself in a salsa class across town, a core-fusion class a few minutes away, or in the water on a paddleboard for an ocean adventure. Keep an open mind and you may just find your next exercise obsession.

I believe in living a really active lifestyle, and it has nothing to do with staying in shape, but everything to do with the fact that I think it makes me happier!

—BROOKLYN DECKER, model and actress

---

unmotivated? **SIX TIPS TO GET YOU GOING:** Just like anyone else, there are days I'd rather do anything but work out. So—I rely on a few strategies to keep me motivated and prevent me from falling into a fitness funk.

1. **PREPARE WHAT YOU WEAR:** Kinda like you are in grade school! Lay out your workout clothes in advance. The shoes, the socks, the legwarmers, the iPod. It should all be there within reach so when you wake up in the morning, it's the first thing you see and you can stumble into it without thinking. For me (for whatever reason), neon workout gear really gets me going!

2. **GIVE ME TEN:** Tell yourself: *I'm just going to walk the block for 10 minutes.* Get going and inevitably . . . *you will keep going.* It's getting started that is the hardest part. After a few minutes, your heart is a pumpin' and the endorphins have kicked in, you'll feel so bloody good, *you'll want more.*

3. **PLAN IN ADVANCE:** Sign up for classes online. If it's already on the schedule and in the calendar, working out is much harder to skip out on.

4. **PHONE A FRIEND:** Exercise buddies and activity partners hold you accountable. So when Fergie sends you that text saying, "I am soooo excited for Zumba tonight, *gurrrrl!*" you will not want to let her down.

5. **BLACKMAIL YOUR BOD:** Give yourself realistic goals and a treat for meeting them. Such as: *This week I will work out four days out of seven.* And when you do that, treat yourself to something special.

6. **LAZY-CISES LIST:** Have a go-to list of things you can do when you just don't want to do anything or when time is limited. (See *This for That, Standing Abs,* and *Only Have Three Minutes? Only Need Three Moves* workouts listed earlier. All are a great place to start!)

tip: **COUCH CONDITION!** Prime television time on your couch in your living room can be prime-your-body time. While on the couch, do some leg lifts. Get on the floor and do the plank series while you are watching *Modern Family*. Pledge not to just veg.

this FOR *that*: *Everyday supermodels* . . . get creative! Here are a few ways to sneak in exercise throughout your day. *Micro* workouts all day long can add up to *macro* results.

- **POSTURE PERFECT:** Be conscious of the way you are sitting. If you have a desk job, you can burn up to 400 calories a day just by sitting up straight and constantly readjusting and engaging your core muscles to encourage better posture.
- **HIP HEIST:** Stuck in traffic? Do a few sets of hip raises and butt squeezes and feel the booty burn. Bonus? They work your Kegels. Big Ohh-yeah!
- **WAIT . . . AND LOSE WEIGHT:** How dare you just wait in line! At the bank, the coffee shop, wherever—that's your time to do calf raises, mini leg lifts, and other nonembarrassing moves. Skip the hip thrusts. Those could get you arrested.
- **LUNGE AND RELOCATE:** Why walk when you can lunge? Walking is so 2010. Lunge your way to and from wherever/whenever you can. Ten lunges here and there add up. You WILL be sore the next day. And P.S. there is no longer such thing as an escalator. Take the stairs!
- **WONDER WOMAN IT UP!:** No damsels in distress here. Ditch the cart and carry your groceries. Do a few bicep curls as you go.
- **WORK . . . AND WORK OUT:** Stash a set of light weights under your desk and instead of that five-minute break you take to e-surf and e-shop—pump iron instead.

supermodel *soapbox*

Question—How much do you spend a month on your cable bill?! That's what I thought. So you'll invest in your butt on the couch, but not in your actual butt? And you think hiring a trainer is too expensive. No. You don't need a trainer. But I'm a big believer in trainers for certain people, at certain times, for certain reasons. Not motivated? Plateauing? Really need help losing the weight? Then YOU could benefit from a personal trainer—even if it's just for a few weeks to get the party started. A good trainer has worked with all different ages, body types, fitness levels, and lifestyles. And he or she should be able to help identify what will work best for you. Good trainers also don't chat too much and waste your time—they will push you. Just can't spend the extra cash? YouTube is full of trainers giving daily workout advice. Just check out their credentials—all trainers are not created equal.

SUPERMOMMA BULGE BUSTERS

Losing my baby weight has been a long and winding road for me. It has taken a tremendous amount of effort. Watching what I eat, working out daily, and staying mentally focused have kept me on track. In addition, I've a few more secrets up my supermodel sleeve to keep everyday supermommas fit and fierce.

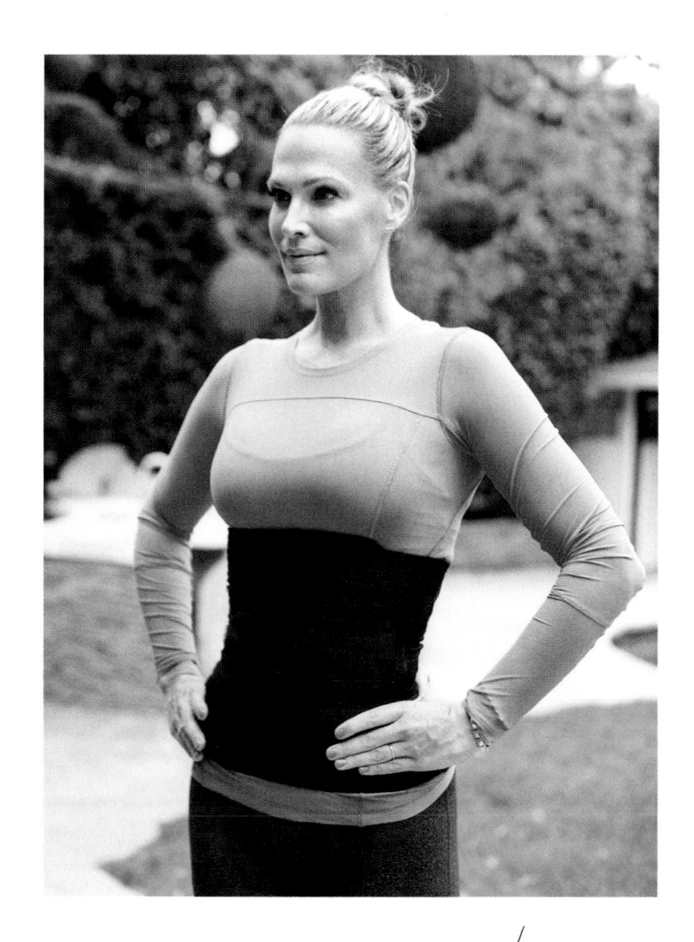

1. **BAND IT TO UNEXPAND IT:** From the day after I delivered (until about nine months post) I wore a belly band *all the time*. Under my clothes day to day and while I was working out. Sometimes, I'll wear Spanx or a corset while I work out. It holds everything in and helps you to concentrate on the ab muscles you really need to tighten. It's great advice even if you haven't had a baby because it makes you extra aware of your core.

2. **AT-HOME HELP:** Those first few months, it's so hard (near impossible) to get out of the house. Not to mention, as a new mom you are on such a tight schedule, you likely need something to come to YOU. Workout DVDs are lifesavers. You can do them in between feedings or whenever you can find the time to squeeze in a few "you" minutes. I still love the classic Tae Bo Billy Blanks DVD—it's a kick!

3. **BABY ON BOARD:** Walk with that child, carry that child, hike with that child. Attach that child to your back and GO! Carrying the baby weight you love will help you to lose the baby weight you *don't*.

4. **MOMMY & ME CLASSES:** There are a variety of supermomma meets exercise meets baby classes where you can bond and fight bulge at the same time. I got involved in classes early on which helped keep me motivated and as an added bonus? I made new friends with babies—so I could ask them lots and lots of questions.

5. **PATIENCE IS A VIRTUE:** Speaking of these classes, I watched a lot of other moms drop weight like it was hot and all I was losing was . . . *my mind*. My body hung on to the baby blubber for the first four or five months. It wasn't until around the sixth month that I even started to see results. So don't give up.

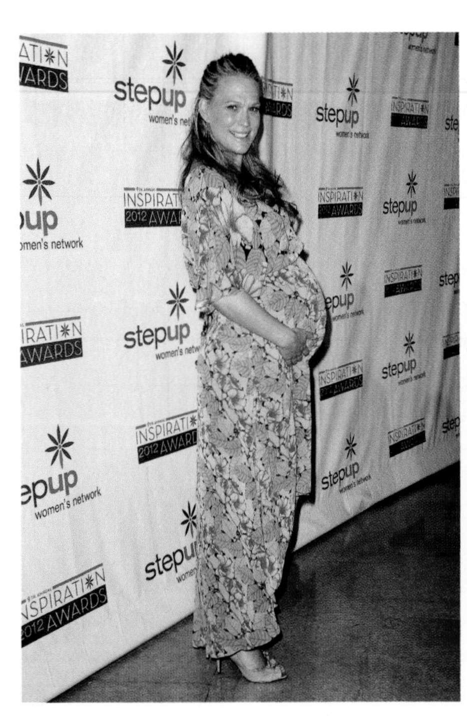

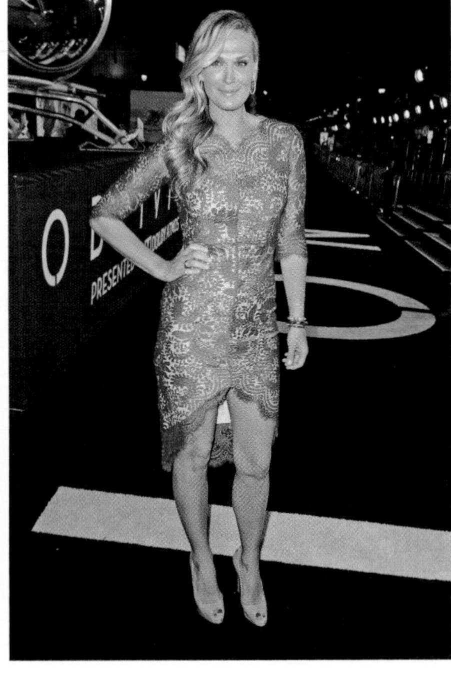

supermomma *secret*

My pregnancy with baby Brooks was pretty easy. I wasn't bed-bound or restricted so I worked out like usual. While I certainly understand pregnancy can pose different challenges for each of us, if you are healthy and feeling good—keep moving. There are a ton of known and unknown benefits to staying active while you are pregnant, including easier delivery and lower rates of gestational diabetes. Just make it known in every class, and with every instructor, that you are knocked up. They can give you alternate moves, adjustments, and positions to keep you comfortable. With any workout plan, do check in with your doc before trying anything new.

GO FOR IT: *Find your inner "fitness version" of Sasha Fierce.* I've read that Beyoncé is shy, so to muster the courage to get onstage, she adopts an alter ego: *Sasha Fierce.* Some of us see ourselves as too old, too overweight, or too "something" to work out. Please don't let any of that nonsense stop you from becoming healthier. Find the alter ego that gets you on your fitness stage. Do not let your mind get in the way of your matter, because YOU MATTER.

Challenge yourself to start. Create a schedule that works for you and that is sustainable. Monday—get out there and walk for forty-five minutes. Tuesday, ride the stationary bike in your garage. Wednesday, sneak in miniworkouts all day long (remember, butt squeezes, calf raises, and office iron-pumping?). Sometimes it's as simple as scheduling weekend recreation that is both physical and fun to reignite the fitness fire. Or maybe it's getting back into something you loved to do when you were younger (my friend Dana got back into tae kwon do after a *twenty-year* hiatus!).

Even if you lose one pound a week, in a few months you'll have lost twenty pounds. Twenty pounds, people! And for those of you who have a friend who is struggling to meet fitness goals, help her out. *Everyday supermodels* need to encourage one another and find ways to strengthen our bonds *and* our bods at the same time. Our bodies were meant to move. It's only recently that we as humans have become less connected to that physical part of ourselves. Let's reconnect! We can all be workout warriors.

I absolutely swear by the Brazilian Butt Lift DVDs. I do them a few times a week at home and I feel the burn even a few days later. They seriously reshaped and defined my behind, especially after the babies.

—KATE HUDSON, actress

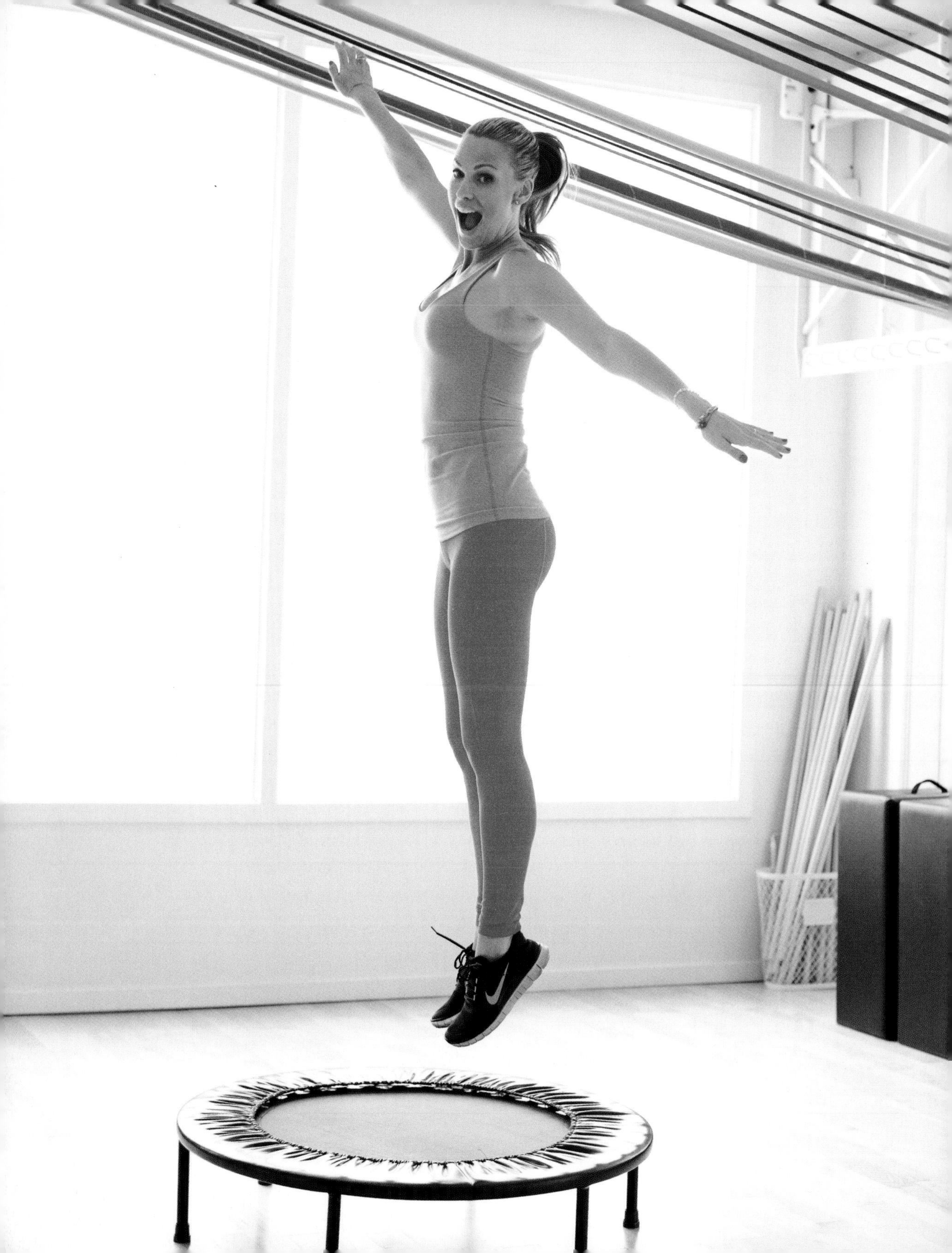

the *everyday* supermodel TOP 10 takeaways

1. Make exercise the rule—not the exception. Take a pledge that you will work out, in some way, every day. That doesn't mean balls-to-the-wall exercise, *but you will do something* active.

2. Look for workouts that feature cardio and strength training for weight loss and toning. And find a workout or combine workouts that will create a balanced, healthy bod.

3. Change it up! Do not get on the elliptical for an hour every day, day in and day out. You have got to surprise and challenge your body. When your mind works harder, so does your body. Change also helps to circumvent the plateau.

4. Sweat it out. Do whatever it takes, but make sure you are a sprinkler system. Your body, skin, soul, and mind will thank you for it.

5. Slow and in control is the name of the game. Do not rush through resistance training. You won't get the same benefits. The slower, the better to strengthen, lengthen, and tone.

6. Hydrate, hydrate, hydrate, and don't forget to add electrolytes for a necessary boost.

7. Sneak in exercises whenever you can. Lunge, don't walk. Bicep curl at work. It all adds up. Leave excuses at the door. If you are traveling, take a jump rope with you.

8. Set specific goals and reward yourself when you reach them. Every pound lost, every week packed with exercise, should be recognized.

9. Find ways to get motivated. Get another *everyday supermodel* on board—you don't have to go it alone.

10. Losing weight and getting fit doesn't have to be a drag. It can be fun. Find a workout you love and start to love the work. After all, you are doing it for YOU.

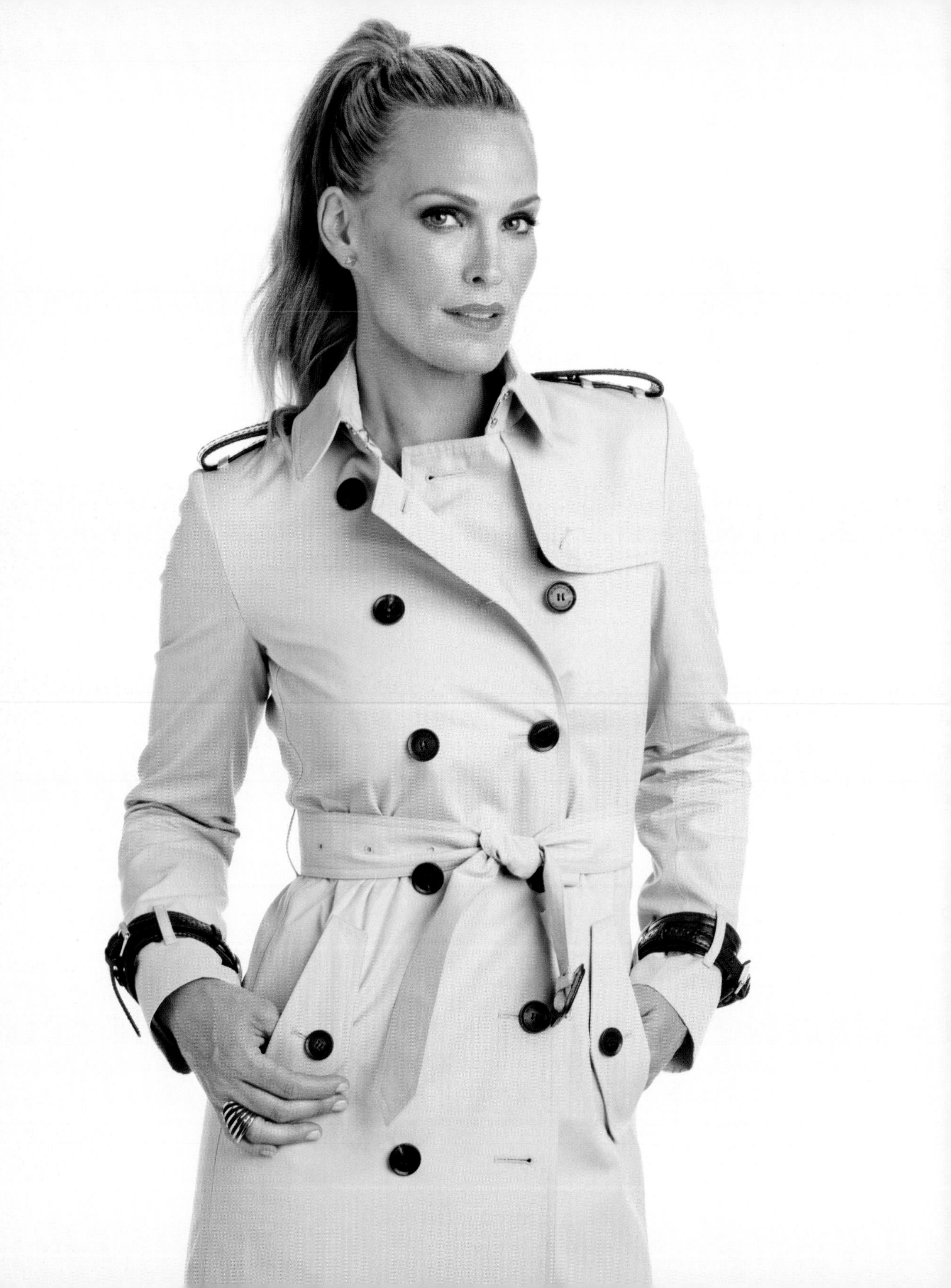

ch/3

fashion institute of mollyology

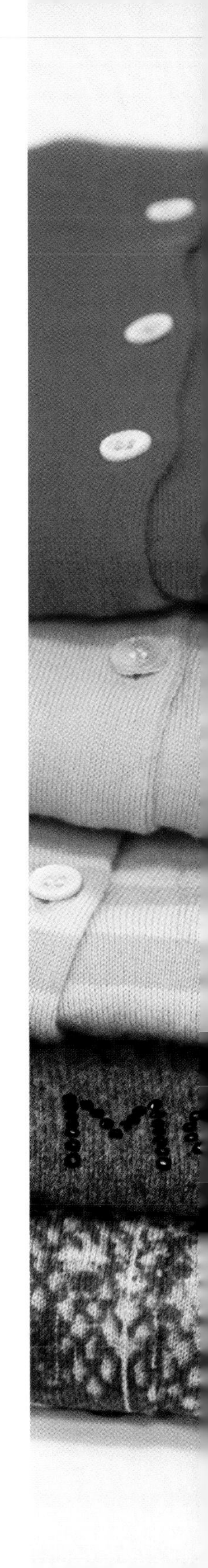

My first lesson in fashion came straight from my momma. My mother was always put together no matter what was happening. Even when she is in the hospital, she has on earrings and lipstick.

Every afternoon after school she'd holler at my brother and me while we were playing in the backyard to "take off our good clothes!" Such is the southern way. My brother, Todd, and I would scurry into our bedrooms and swap our "presentable" clothes for backyard sneakers and "bookstore sweatshirts" from the family business.

Murray, Kentucky, is not the fashion capital of the world, but what I learned there was that *clothes matter* and to *take care of them*. Momma also taught me to read magazines for trends and to save my money. But at twenty years old, I was fresh off the farm and straight outta the Bible Belt and looking the part! Puffy sleeves, Laura Ashley prints, *Little House on the Prairie*–style skirts—I even wore my mom's giant angora sweaters.

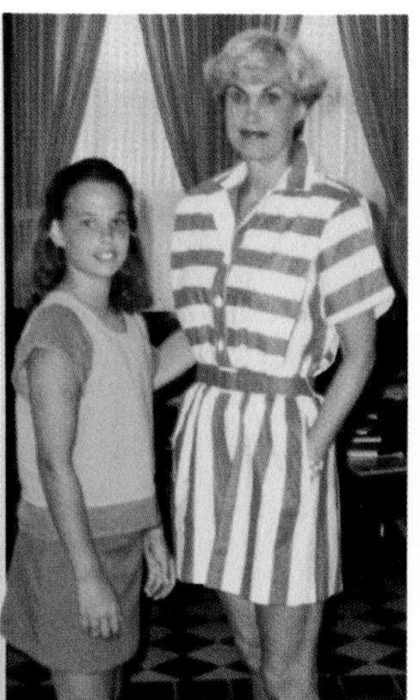

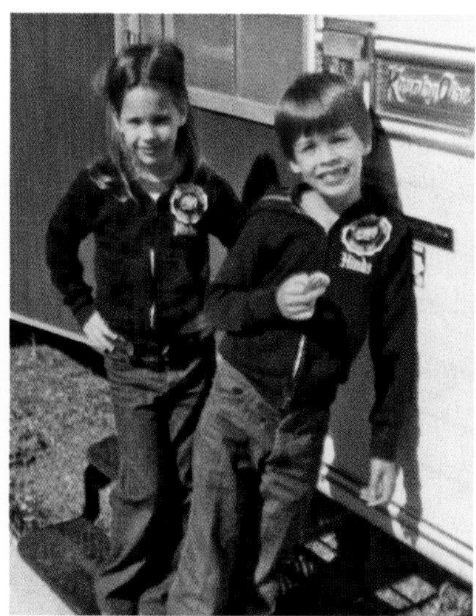

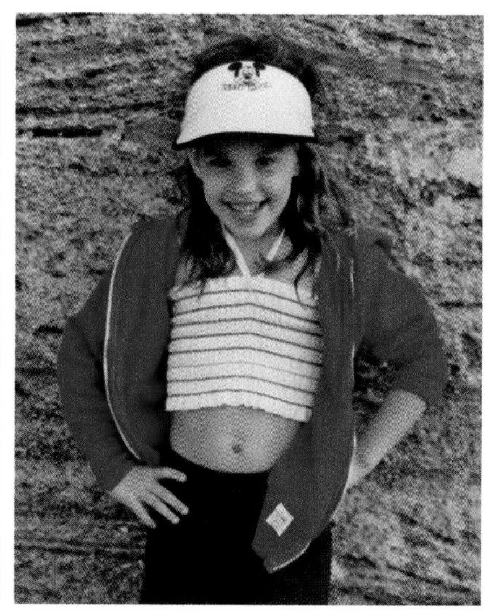

I had to learn quickly to drop-kick my southern ways. I copied all the other models. Fake it until you make it, right? Two models I met, who are still my friends to this day (twin sisters Aimee and Tara Baglietto), were my fashion idols. I worshipped the ground they walked on and facsimiled their looks. I didn't have much cash, but I learned early on the value of investment pieces, and fashion that never goes out of style. Modeling taught me to buy clothes that last, not just to satisfy an impulse, in order to really stretch a wardrobe. After my time in Europe, I could convert ten pieces of clothing into ten thousand outfits, as long as they were high-quality pieces. You can absolutely be stylish without a bulging wallet.

Style comes in every shape and size. It's not about being stick thin. It's about knowing how to build a wardrobe for your figure and lifestyle and how to wear that wardrobe. It's about pulling off easy, edgy elegance—any time/anywhere—rain or shine. When you know how to create a stylish wardrobe and stock your closet with the right must-have pieces—you will look fabulous at every age, at every size. Even at my heaviest, I did not walk around in faded sweats and a muumuu. *I still made the effort. Everyday supermodel* note: Just because you are trying to lose a few pounds does not mean that you throw in the fashion towel until you reach your goal weight. Oh no. Not so fast!

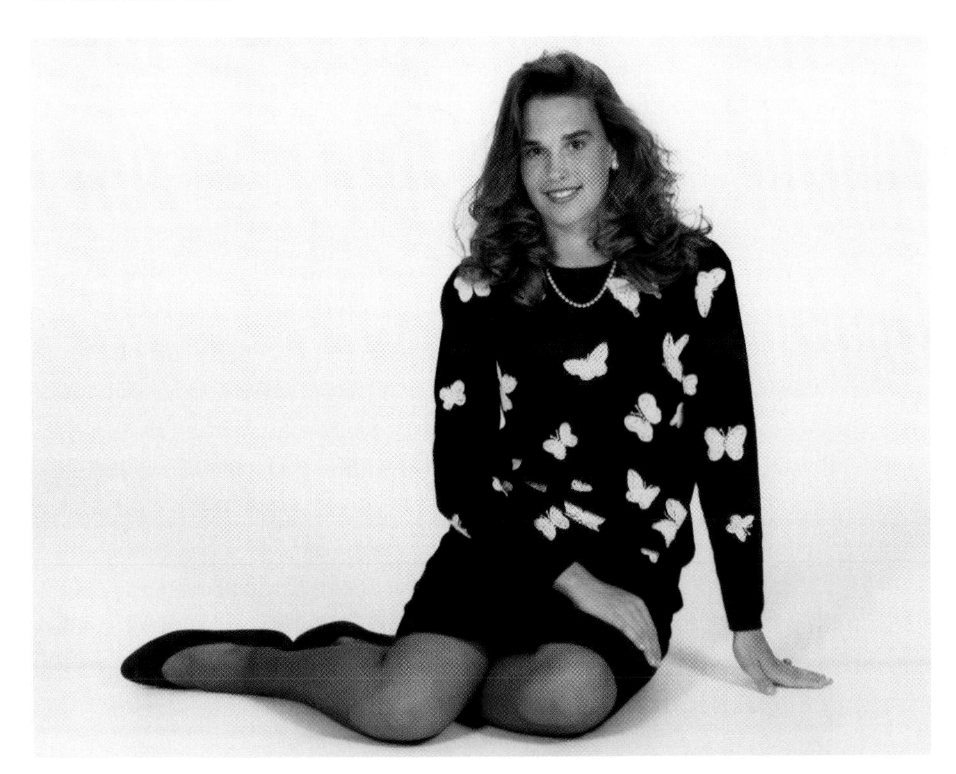

When I was superpregnant, I would wake up in the morning a few minutes earlier and take the time to style myself ten pounds thinner. I made the effort because that meant that I would feel MUCH better about myself *that entire day*. Don't dress down just because you are *feeling* down. In fact—DO THE OPPOSITE. Dress up and you will feel UP. And for those of you who are "X" number of pounds more than you want to be, and you never buy new clothes because you are waiting to lose the weight—*Let's talk*. Go out. Buy a *few* things that make you feel good. Never mind the size on the label (I cut size tags out!). You will lose weight—and guess what? You can ALWAYS have them tailored when you do. I don't care what size you are. You deserve to feel and look good at every single stage.

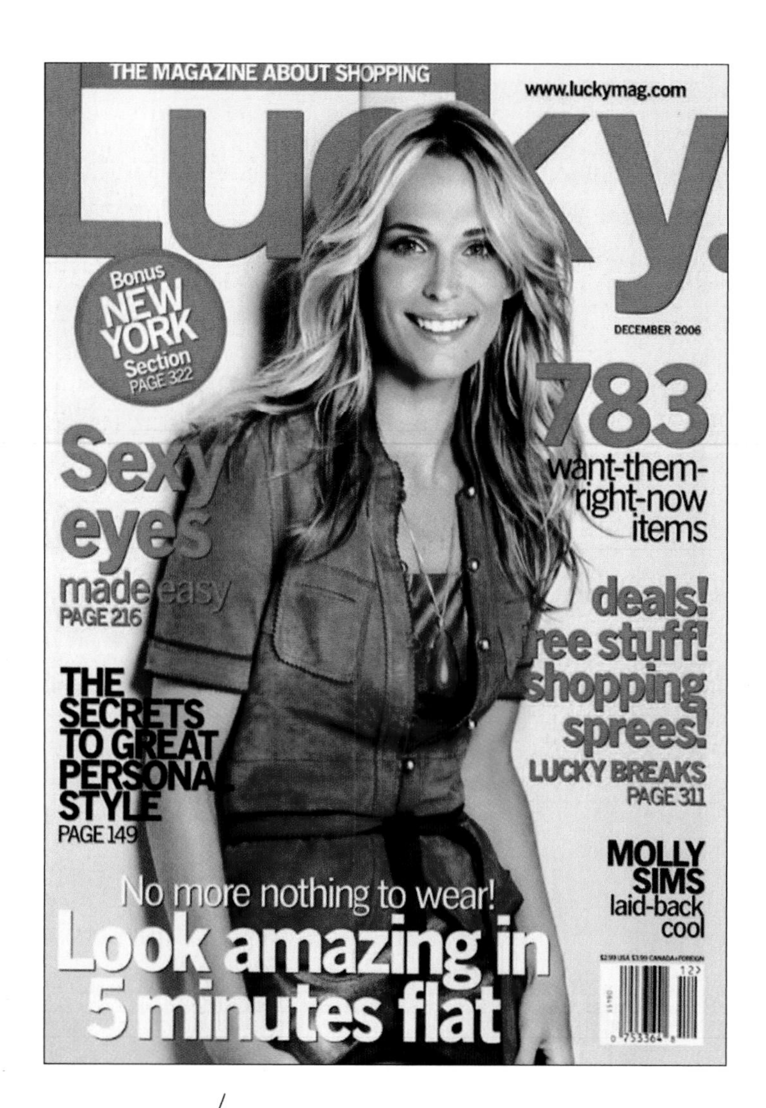

In this chapter, I have recruited a professional team of fashionistas, including Beckie Klein and Martina Gordon (aka The Re-Stylists), models-turned-image-consultants, to help you build and rock an *everyday supermodel* wardrobe. Some people flip houses; we are here to flip closets! Your closet. In the following pages, you will learn how to develop a core wardrobe of classic pieces, trend-driven additions, and essential accessories. And then you'll learn—what to do with it all! Because knowing *what to wear* and *how to wear it* can transform the everyday woman into an *everyday supermodel*. The right fashion choices and styling can take all of us from ordinary to . . . extraordinary. I know this because I've watched it work for many women in my business, including ME. Regardless of what you've got going on (long legs, superstar shoulders, curves and cushion)—let's supermodel you up! After reading and using the advice in this chapter, I *promise* you will never again utter the words *I have nothing to wear!*

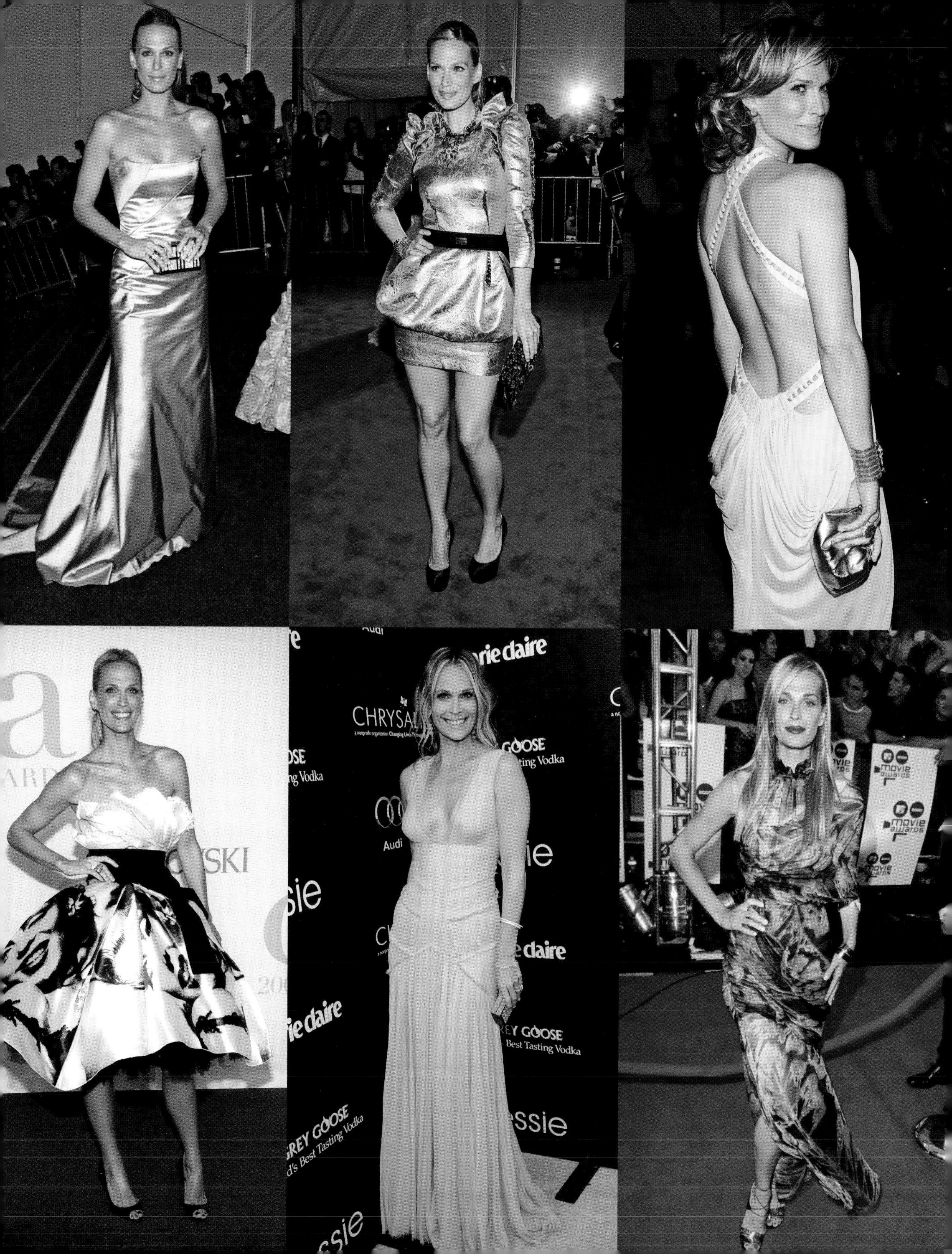

Audi
Best Tasting Vodka
movie awards

My Style *squadron*

- **THE RE-STYLISTS: BECKIE KLEIN AND MARTINA GORDON:** They've walked runways, been in countless fashion mags, and today they style for television and real people. Beckie and Martina turn lawyers, doctors, and momma bears into the *everyday supermodel* versions of themselves. You're next.

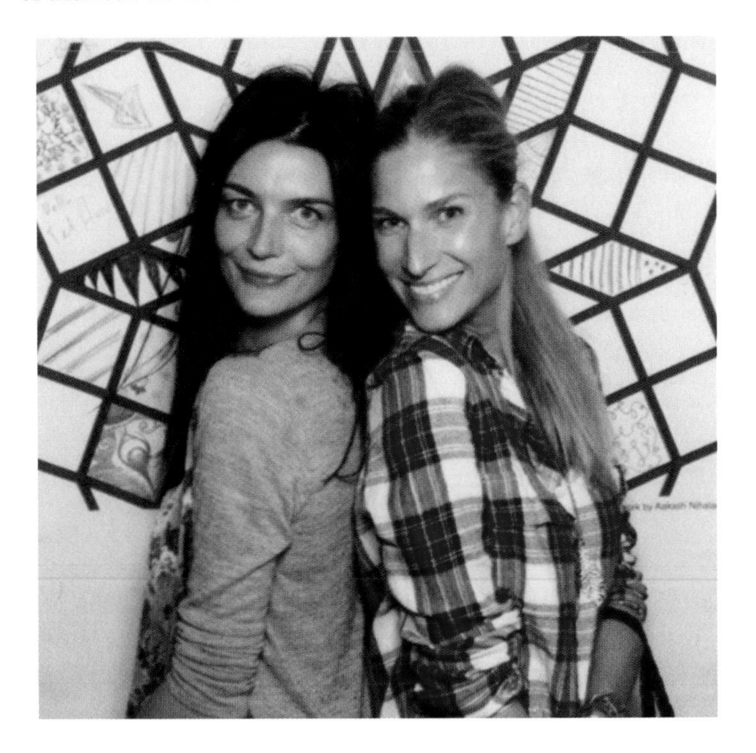

- **RACHEL ZOE:** I've known Rachel for a decade. She has styled me for more red carpets than I can count. Bottom line: Rachel has taught me to take risks and *I trust her with my fashion life*. When we work together, I always love the way I look.
- **MIMI BROWN:** fashion stylist and closet consigliere. She will help you transform your closet into an MTV crib's worthy space—functional and fierce.
- **MICHELLE VICK AND ERIN BUNCH:** Creators of the Broke Girl's Guide website (www.brokegirlsguide.com), they are experts on how to be frugal fashionistas. You don't have to always flash labels to look luxe. Amen wallet warriors.

supermodel *secret*

When it comes to style, I am not special. I definitely didn't win "Best Dressed" in high school. (You've seen the photos, and I think you'll agree.) That said, fashion can be studied, learned, and applied—*and that's exactly what I did.* Like beauty, it can be bullied out of you. If I can go from this—to THIS—so can you. Consider this chapter a how-to on style. And then look all around you. Read the blogs. Pay attention to what you like on people in magazines and on TV. TRUST ME, they didn't always look that stylish. Everyone can do it.

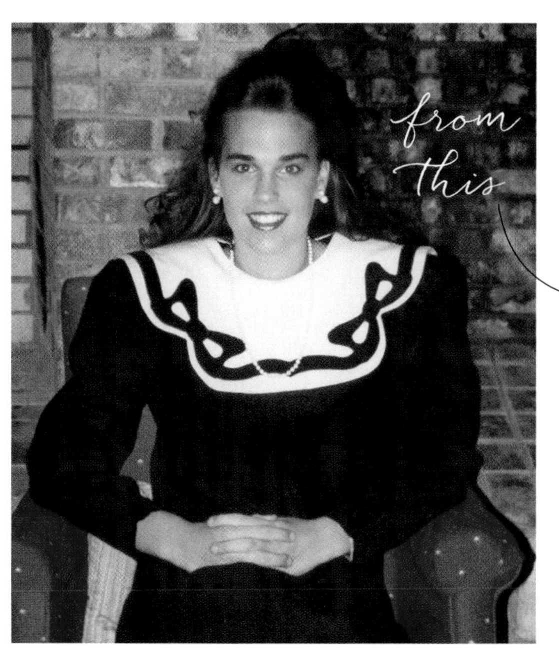

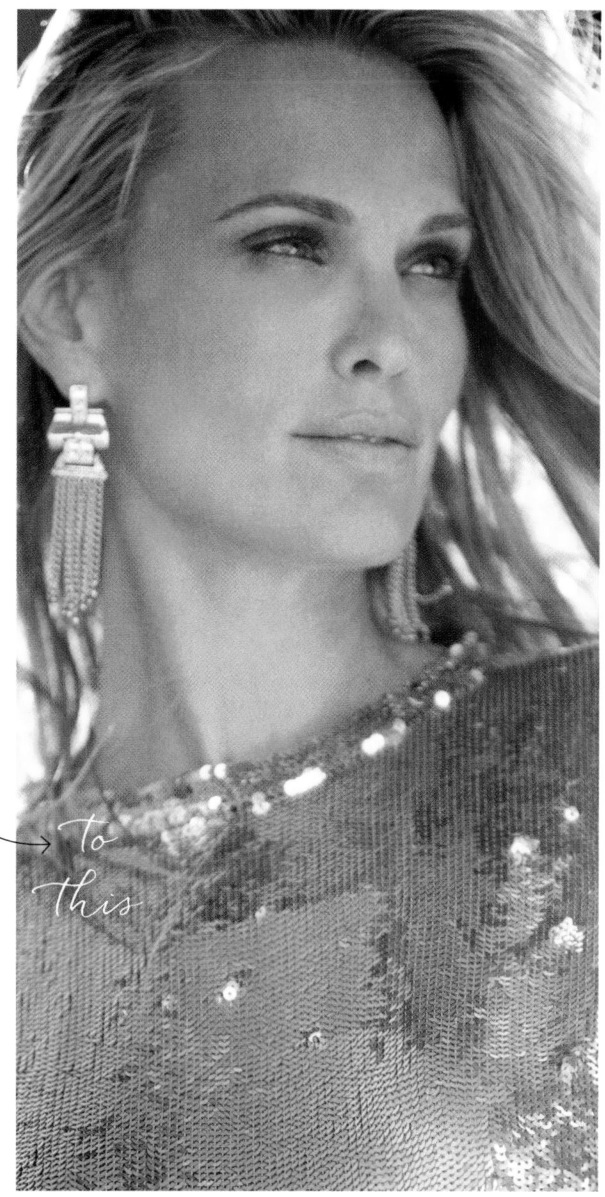

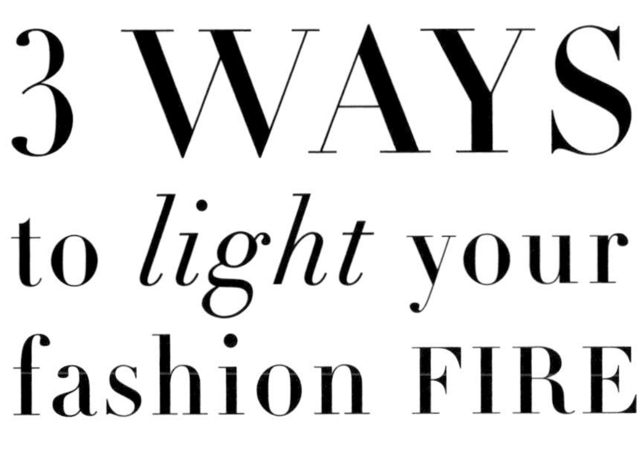

3 WAYS to *light* your fashion FIRE

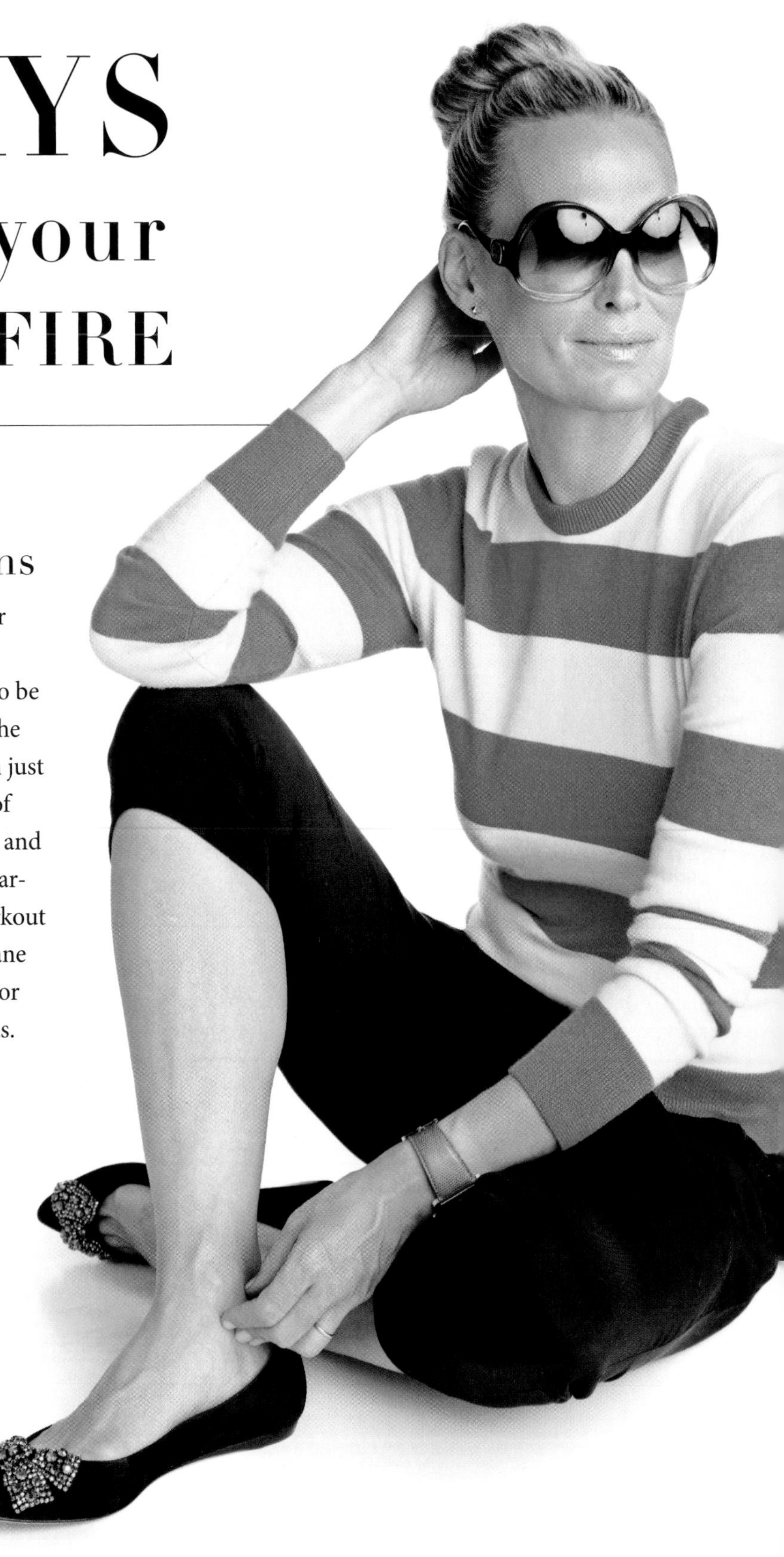

1. study the icons

Study style icons and their signature looks. Running errands? It's your choice to be fashionable or frumpy—the effort is the same. You can just as easily throw on a pair of pedal pushers, ballet flats, and striped tee (à la Brigitte Bardot!) as you can tired workout wear. Channel Jackie O, Jane Birkin, Audrey Hepburn, or contemporary fashionistas.

supermodel *secret*

Speaking of style stalking, I was at a baby shower and one of the hostesses was wearing this chic (and comfortable!) Alice and Olivia maxi dress with a black leather motorcycle jacket. She was pregnant and managed to look fantastic. I didn't waste any time asking her where she got the dress and immediately ordered it online. The following week I cohosted *The Talk* on NBC and wore her exact ensemble.

2. sidewalk stalk

You like that girl's shoes? Stop her on the street and don't be afraid to ask where she got them. Look at body types like yours and note what looks good on them—*and what doesn't.* Whenever out and about, pay attention and take fashion notes.

3. go global

Globe-trotting will awaken your inner fashion guru. In France, I learned that adding a scarf to any outfit ups the ante and oozes chic. The Parisian woman is the definition of effortless sophistication, confidence, and sensuality all at once. If you truly want to understand style—get yourself to Paris, people! Or even easier . . . check out the book *Parisian Chic* by Inès de la Fressange. In London I learned to mix and match vintage with contemporary fashion. Don't get out much? No worries. Style bloggers have got you covered. Fly Air Google and you can be on the fashionable streets of Stockholm, New York, or Milan in minutes. Pinterest is also a useful way to collect (and then copy!) outfits and looks you love.

supermodel *secret*

I am constantly reading magazines. British, French, and American *Vogue; Harper's Bazaar; Elle; Marie Claire; People Style Watch.* I even flip through every J.Crew catalog (Jenna Lyons, the creative director, is a genius!) because I'm inspired not only by the clothing and the color, but also by the way the clothes are styled on the models. Some sites I visit are Polyvore.com (love their collaging), Style.com (for trends), and whowhatwear.com (for all the above).

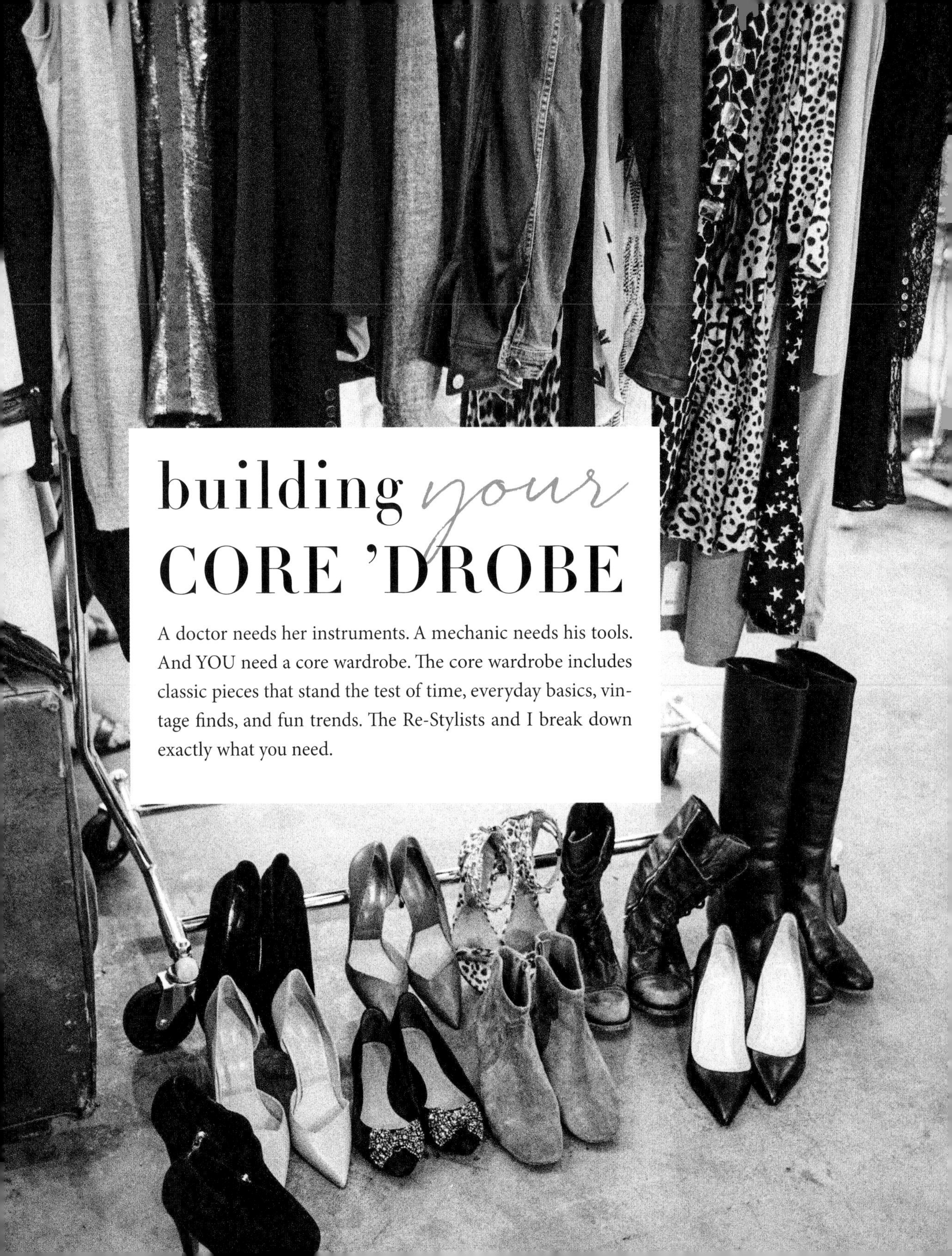

building *your* CORE 'DROBE

A doctor needs her instruments. A mechanic needs his tools. And YOU need a core wardrobe. The core wardrobe includes classic pieces that stand the test of time, everyday basics, vintage finds, and fun trends. The Re-Stylists and I break down exactly what you need.

CORE clothing

These are the foundation pieces every complete wardrobe needs—and we could not live without.

1. tailored black blazer

2. white collared shirt or blouse

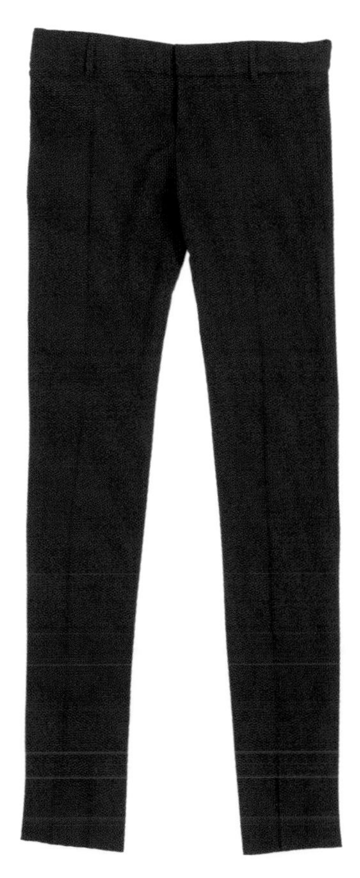

3. pencil skirt

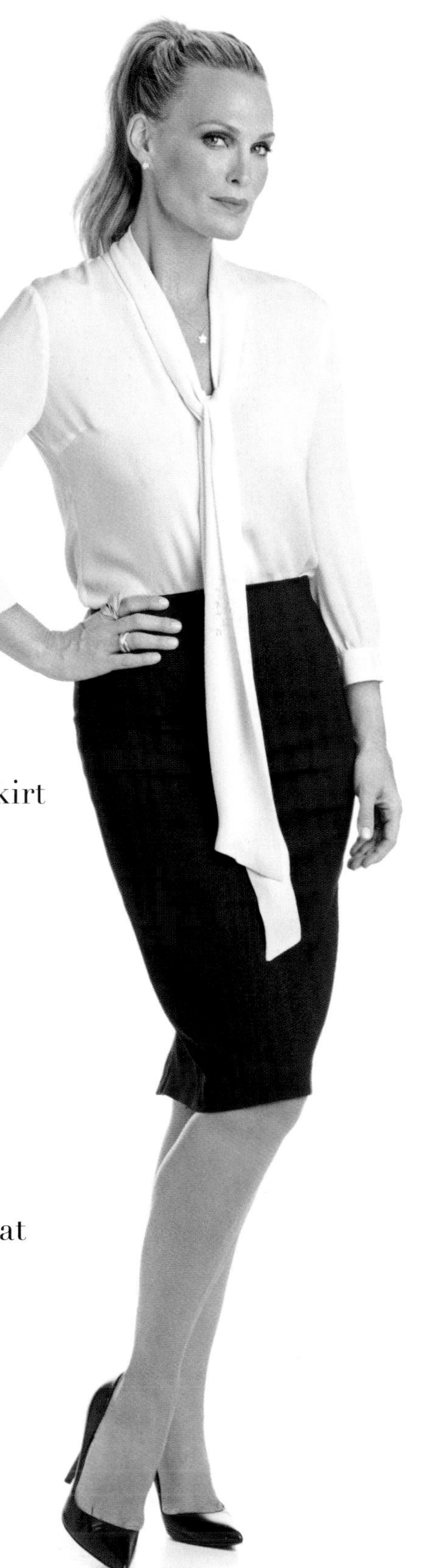

4. tailored black dress pants

5. little black dress

6. classic trench coat

7. black leather jacket

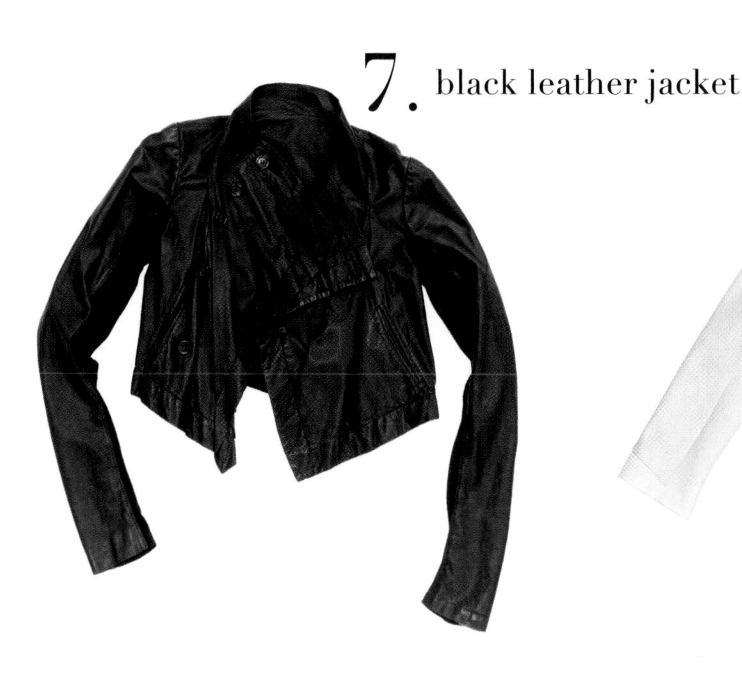

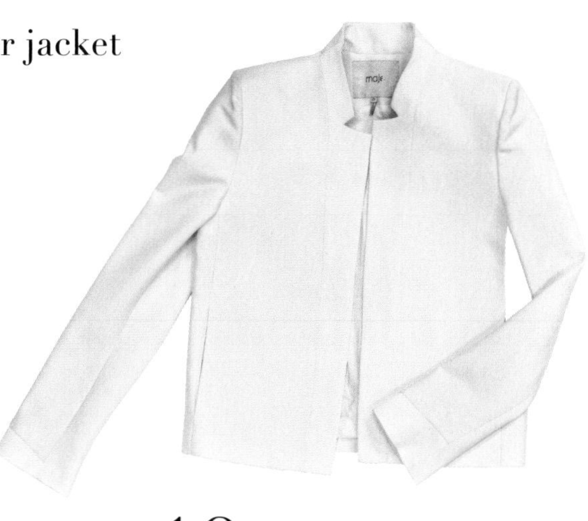

10. White jacket or blazer

11. summer pant in white or neutral

12. cashmere pullover knit sweater

13. long, layering tanks and tees (in neutrals)

14. jeans:

- a skinny (dark denim)
- a boyfriend jean (washed-look)
- a flare leg

15. cardigans: long, short, and one in between

16. boho/long flowy skirt

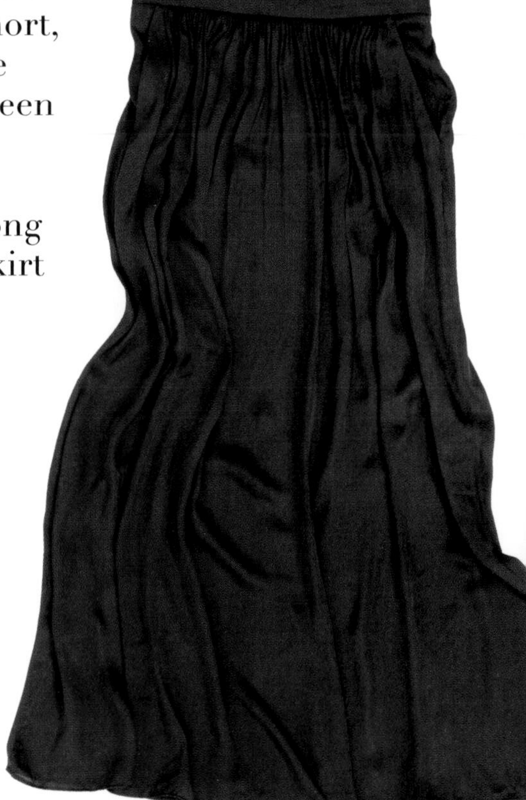

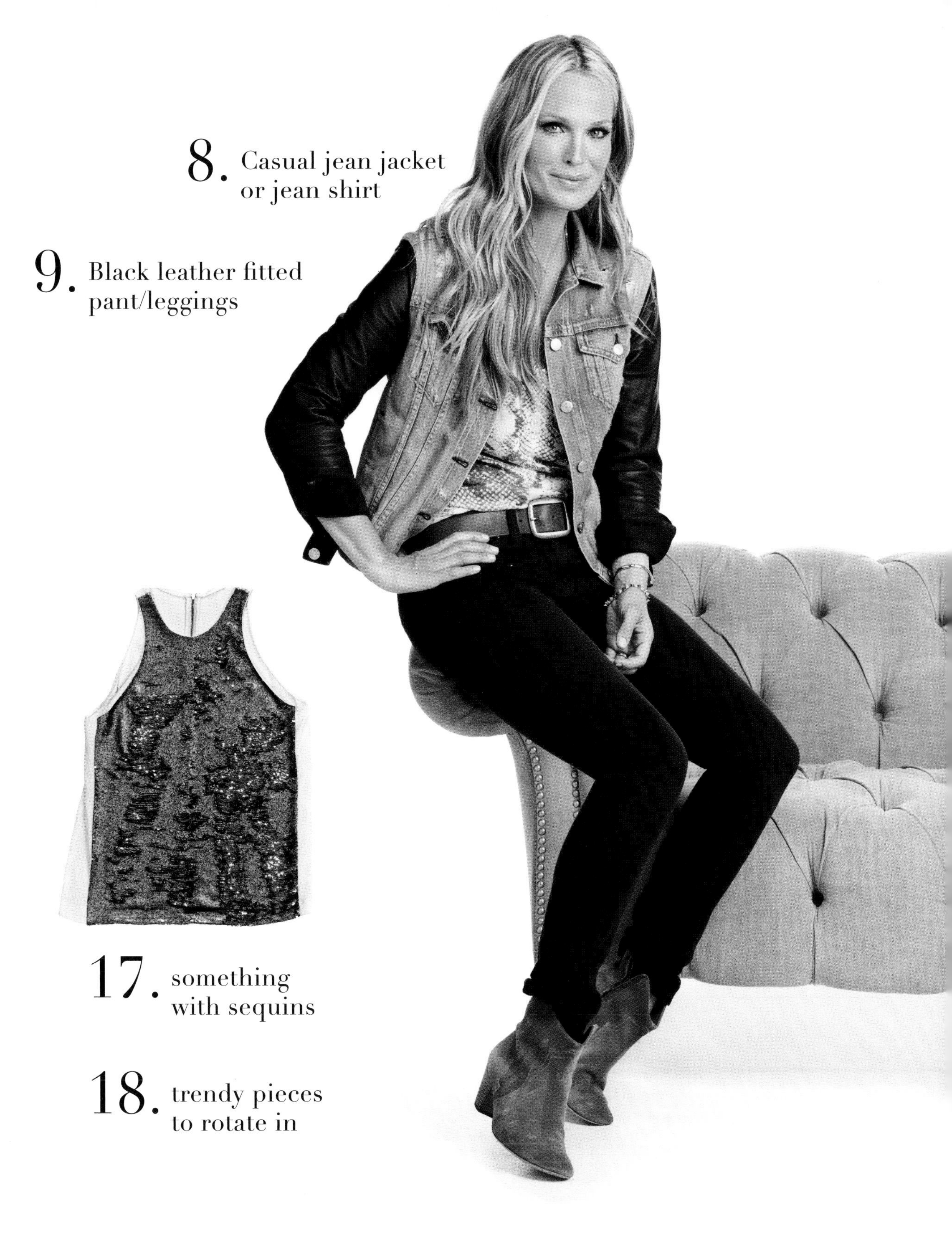

8. Casual jean jacket or jean shirt

9. Black leather fitted pant/leggings

17. something with sequins

18. trendy pieces to rotate in

invest **WHERE YOU CAN:** When building your core wardrobe, invest in *what* you can, *where* you can, *when* you can. If you have the cash, by all means go out and check everything off the list. But we all are working with different budgets. What you spend on your investment pieces and what someone else does will be different. Most of us invest slowly in the most important pieces and acquire them over time. If I can find a high-quality, classic black blazer from H&M or Zara (and I don't have to spend a ton of money on it) = SCORE! Today you can find well-made pieces at *affordable* prices. Without a doubt, absolutely invest the most money in the items you *will wear the most*. That definitely includes investing in the nicest-quality handbag your budget will allow.

MY FAVORITE DESIGNERS FOR "INVESTMENT" PIECES: Fashion is not about label lusting. However, there are designers that just do it right. I will invest hard-earned cash in select pieces from certain collections, luxury designers, or high-end stores (but more often, I look for lower-priced labels that imitate my favorite designer pieces). You'll have a well-designed classic forever. Below are a few of my Designer Crushes and Luxe for Less Labels.

Designer *crushes*

1. **ISABEL MARANT:** Relaxed, BoHo clothing with a slightly androgynous attitude.
2. **LANVIN:** Models are obsessed with Lanvin. Amazing evening gowns and outerwear, gorgeous feminine fabrics, lots of draping, some edge—and chunky jewelry.
3. **STELLA MCCARTNEY:** Unrivaled tailoring, vegan friendly, and classy.
4. **ALEXANDER WANG:** Clean, simple, masculine. The T-shirt and blazer master.
5. **MICHAEL KORS:** Uptown and elegant, with sex appeal—clothes made for real women.
6. **CHLOÉ:** Cool, Parisian sophistication. Refined classics, with a bit of hip edge.
7. **DOLCE AND GABBANA:** This Italian powerhouse stands for luxury, decadence, and sex. I never met a body-hugging lace dress from them I didn't like.
8. **JASON WU:** Park Avenue chic meets soft, fresh fabrics. If Mrs. Obama loves him, I do too.

luxe for *less* Labels

1. **J.CREW:** My go-to store for basics, color, and wearable trends.

2. **RAG AND BONE:** These are cool clothes you can wear every day. Their men's line is so good too!

3. **ZARA:** They knock off pretty much everything and do it very well. Great for the office.

4. **TOP SHOP:** Always on trend—I never, ever leave there empty-handed—lots of off-duty supermodel looks.

5. **H&M:** Two words = designer collaborations! You get pop-up access to big-ticket designers (think Isabel Marant and Lanvin) at fast-fashion prices. Everything always sells out, so you've got to be in the know and arrive early.

6. **ASOS.COM:** One of the ONLY online stores with a diversity of chic, cool clothes from low to high prices.

7. **TARGET:** Designer collaborations, cheap and cheerful workout gear—and stylish swimsuits.

8. **T. J. MAXX:** You can always score luxe labels here, but at a discount.

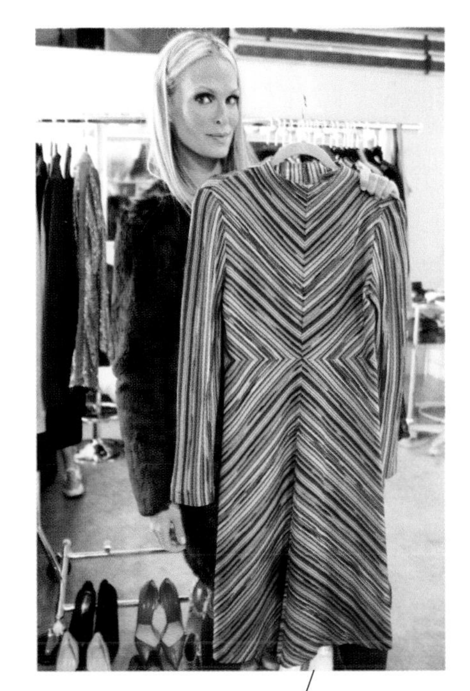

supermodel *secret*

I still have the first designer piece I ever purchased. I had saved up a little modeling money and bought a Missoni dress. At the time, it was a small fortune. But Missoni is timeless—and guess what? I still wear it. (Yes, it's a little tight—but the point is—it still *almost* fits!)

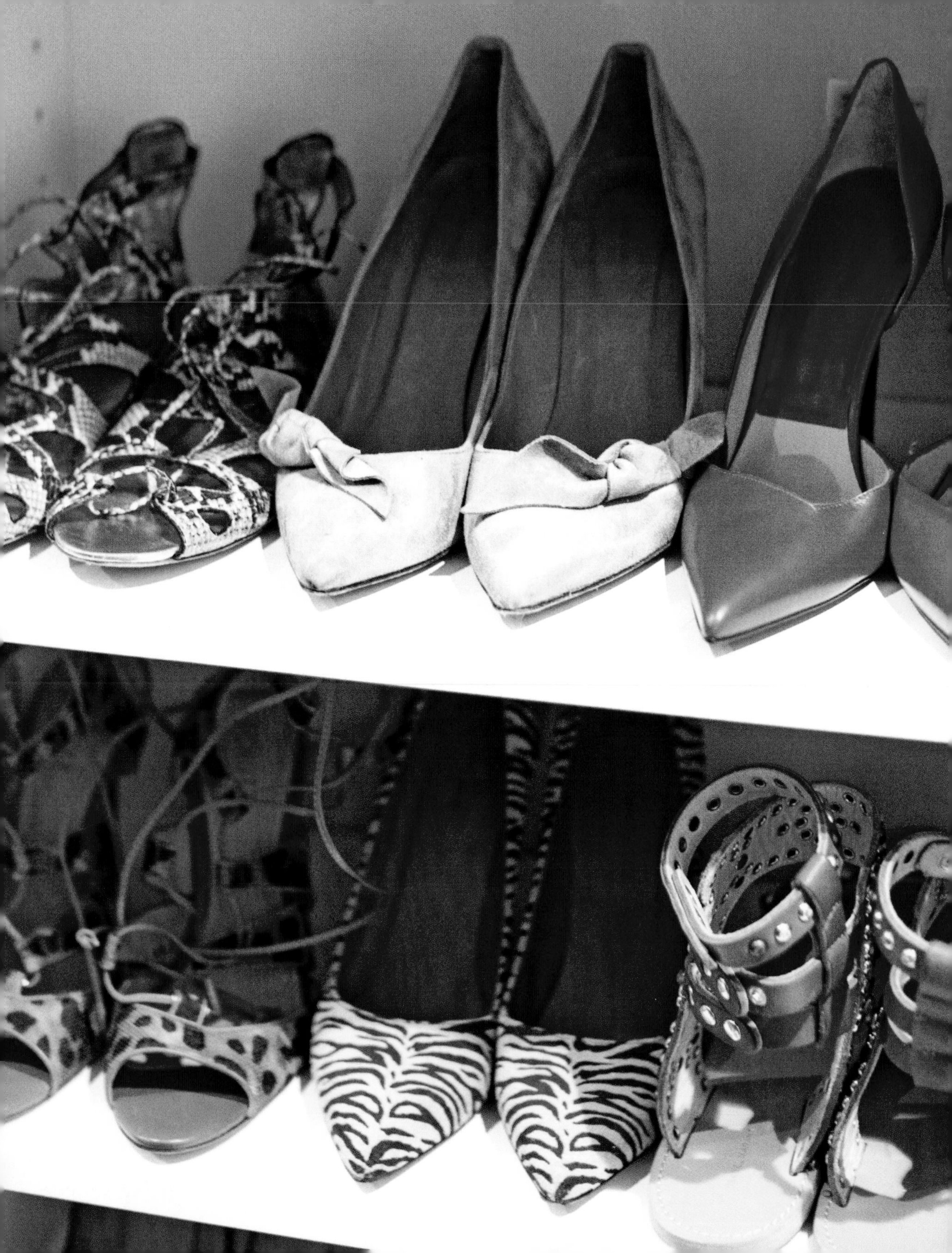

CORE shoes

While most women have a bit of a Carrie Bradshaw/Imelda Marcos mentality when it comes to foot fashion, the truth is— more is not always more. We've identified the seven (maybe eight) shoe styles that will get you through any event in style. If you have these, you have everything!

1. NUDE PUMPS: These are a nonnegotiable. You must own a classic pair that can be worn winter, spring, summer, and fall. When choosing a nude, choose a shade that complements your skin tone and extends your leg (that is truly different for everyone). Nothing lengthens the leg like a nude heel! Pointy or flat? The Re-Stylists and I thought long and hard about this. The verdict? When investing in a heel you'll have forever—always go with a classic point. It stands the test of time . . . and elongates the gams, ladies.

2. BALLET FLATS: Loooooove Lanvin ballet flats—I could go broke collecting them. They are comfortable, stylish, and feminine. I've had mine for six years and have had them resoled three times. And for the heel averse, they can be paired with a dressy look. Even more . . . you can slip 'em in a tote for on-the-go comfort or chase after toddlers wearing them and still look fabulous! There are several great brands out there. D'Orsay flats are comfortable, stylish, and versatile too, and even more flattering for those with shorter legs.

3. TALL BLACK BOOTS: Now if you live in the tropics, maybe you can skip these, but for everyone else—pay attention! Invest in quality leather or leather look-alike (it shouldn't look like plastic). Go with a classic heel that isn't too high. If you tend to be more casual, you can go with a sleek, riding boot with a round toe and box heel. If you are have more nights *out* than *in*, buy a foxier pair with a narrow heel and a pointy toe.

4. NEUTRAL CASUAL BOOTIE/ANKLE BOOT: Isabel Marant makes the best suede ones, but Rag and Bone's are good too, and good knockoffs abound (think Aldo and Steve Madden). Buy them it in any neutral color and pair them with almost everything. Skinny jeans, short-shorts, floral dresses, or leggings and a chunky knit. Wear them with bare legs, tall socks, or tights. Dressy versions work too if that's more up your alley. You can't go wrong with this style.

5. **BLACK HEELS:** You all have these, but do you have the right ones? This is a hands-down investment piece . . . so let's talk. If you choose to smartly invest in these, and maybe even splurge on a designer pair, how do you know which pair to purchase? *Which will stand the test of time?* Here's our advice: Again, pointy toe—not round. A heel with a platform is fine, but choose a design with a hidden platform. Go with leather—not patent leather or suede—and select a feminine, narrow heel (not chunky) at whatever heel height you are most comfortable in.

6. **MOTORCYCLE BOOT:** My weekend wear is all about the motorcycle boot. I'll wear moto boots with a casual dress or a white tee and boyfriend jeans. The longer you have the boots, the better they look. If yours look brand-new, scuff them up a bit. A little Harley-Davidson on your heel is hot *and* supermodel cool. Vrooom, Vroooom!

7. **CHIC SANDAL:** Preferably a flat, but a small kitten heel also works if you like height. Nude will go with everything, black is a close second. A modern, leather, strappy something with a touch of glamour (think a simple jeweled or metal detail) will take you far. The right sandal can be dressed up or down and will pair perfectly with a casual tee and shorts or a dress at a spring wedding.

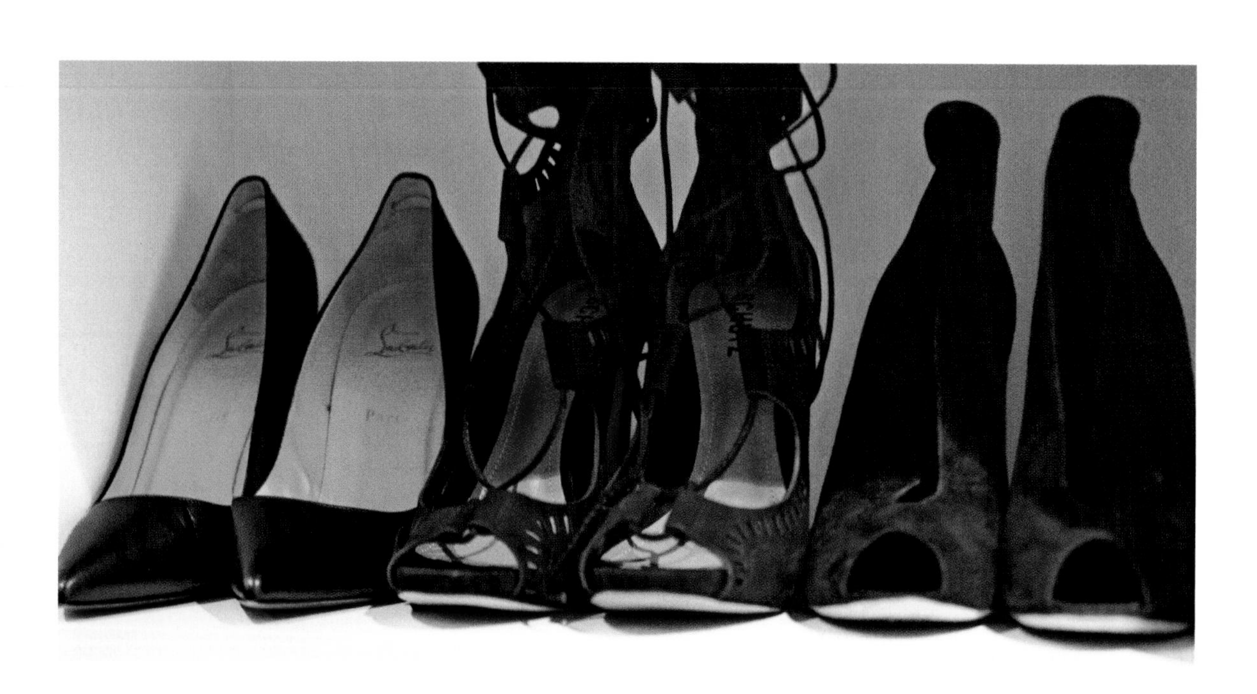

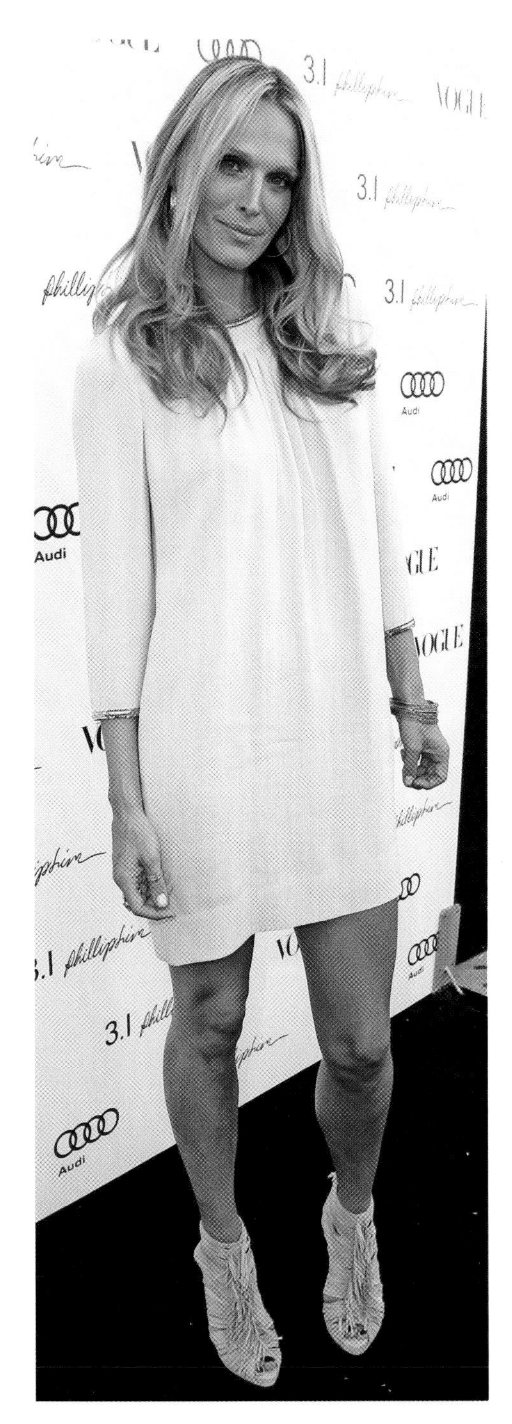

supermodel *secret*

THE STATEMENT SHOE.

Possibly #8 on the list. Every woman should have a shoe that steals the show. You wear it with something extremely simple. It makes the outfit and gives you the *everyday supermodel* edge. Think a bright red pump, studded high heel, something with embellishment, diamonds, or fringe. It's a shoe that says and does it all *so you don't have to do anything else*. Fashion truth-be-told: It's so easy, it's almost cheating. Busy babes: pay attention. The statement shoe is a guaranteed way to look stylish without doing a *damn thing*. Prepare to be complimented.

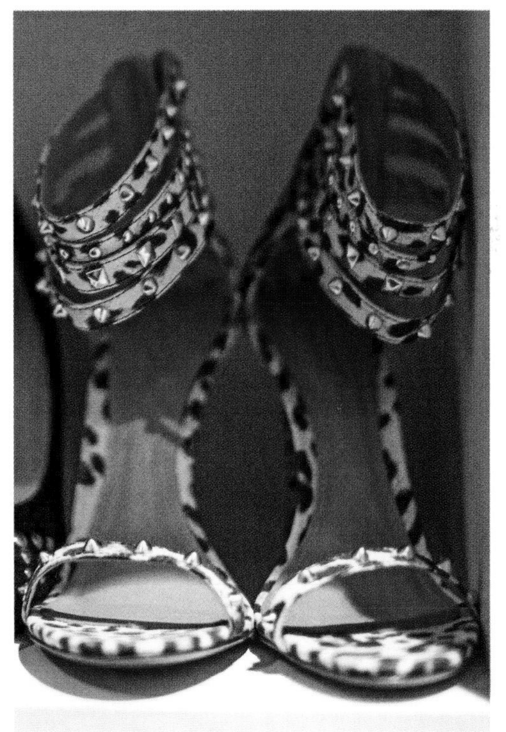

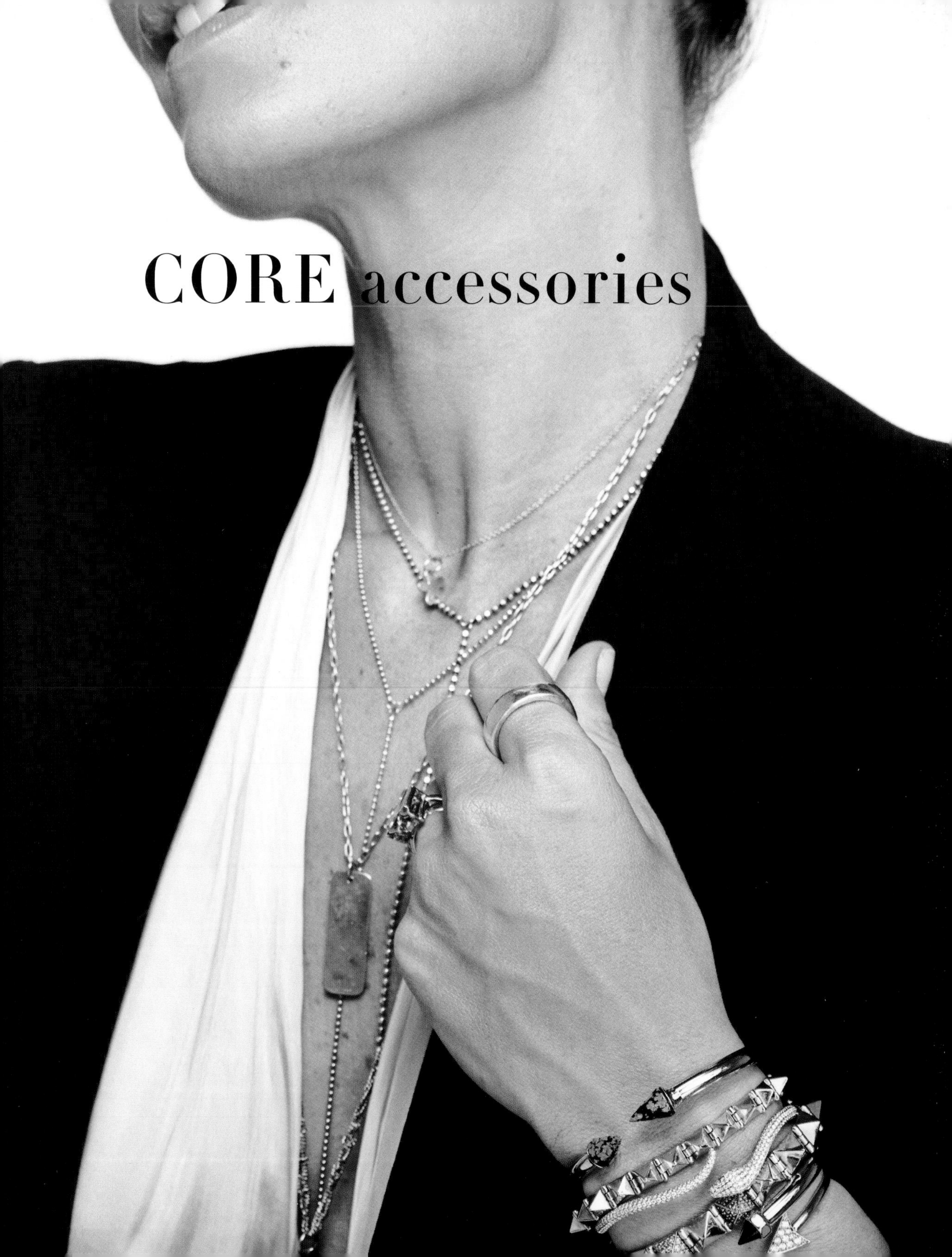

CORE accessories

1. shades

Nothing says *everyday supermodel* more than a pair of superchic sunnies. You will never go wrong with classic Ray-Ban aviators (um, the Jolie-Pitt's—hello?) or an oversized pair of black (or tortoiseshell) Jackie-O style shades.

2. scarves

No closet is complete without them. You need a neutral color for layering and versatility and a fun/bold color or stylish print for pop. When it comes to fabric, think wool/cashmere scarves for fall and winter and cotton/linen blends for spring and summer. Theodora and Callum prints top my list of faves. I don't lie on a beach or by a pool without one.

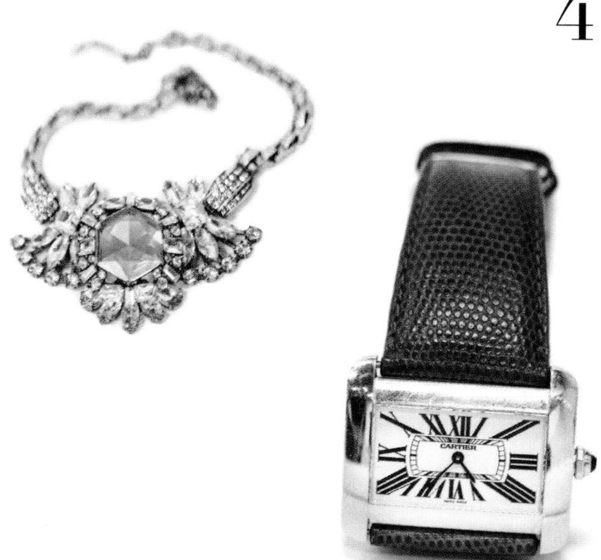

3. jewels

For earrings, every woman needs a pair of diamond studs or look-alikes, gold hoops in a medium size, and the wild card—something sparkly/shoulder sweeping! For rings and bracelets: do stackable pieces in a variety of metals. And you can never go wrong with a solid, modern, metal cuff. For necklaces, you need one versatile "statement piece" that will transform an ordinary outfit or little black dress into an *everyday supermodel* look. Finally, a long chain necklace or necklaces you can layer. Designers I wear include Anita Ko, Jennifer Fisher, and Stella and Dot. Zara and H&M have good trendy pieces. J.Crew makes luxe-looking statement necklaces.

4. watches

Nothing says I'm classy (oh, and responsible!) more than a timeless timepiece. The most classic version is simple and not flashy. It isn't covered in diamonds or Swarovski crystals. It can have a metal band or a leather band, but the design should be traditional and embody understated elegance. Certain labels, like Rolex and Cartier, generally do not lose value and will even gain value, making them *actual investments*. Michael Kors designs chic, more affordable versions.

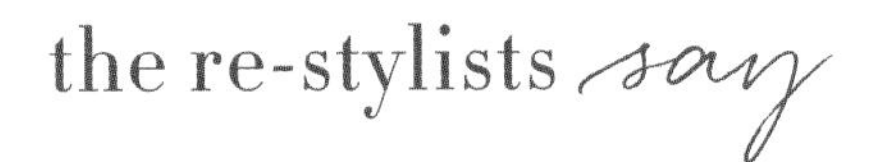

the re-stylists *say*

Mix it up, baby! You *can* wear silver with gold. The goal is to create texture and dimension. When wearing necklaces, have an anchor piece (the main event piece) and then add/layer on top—different lengths, different colors, different textures, and different weights. Yes, combine rose gold with yellow with white. That is true supermodel chic.

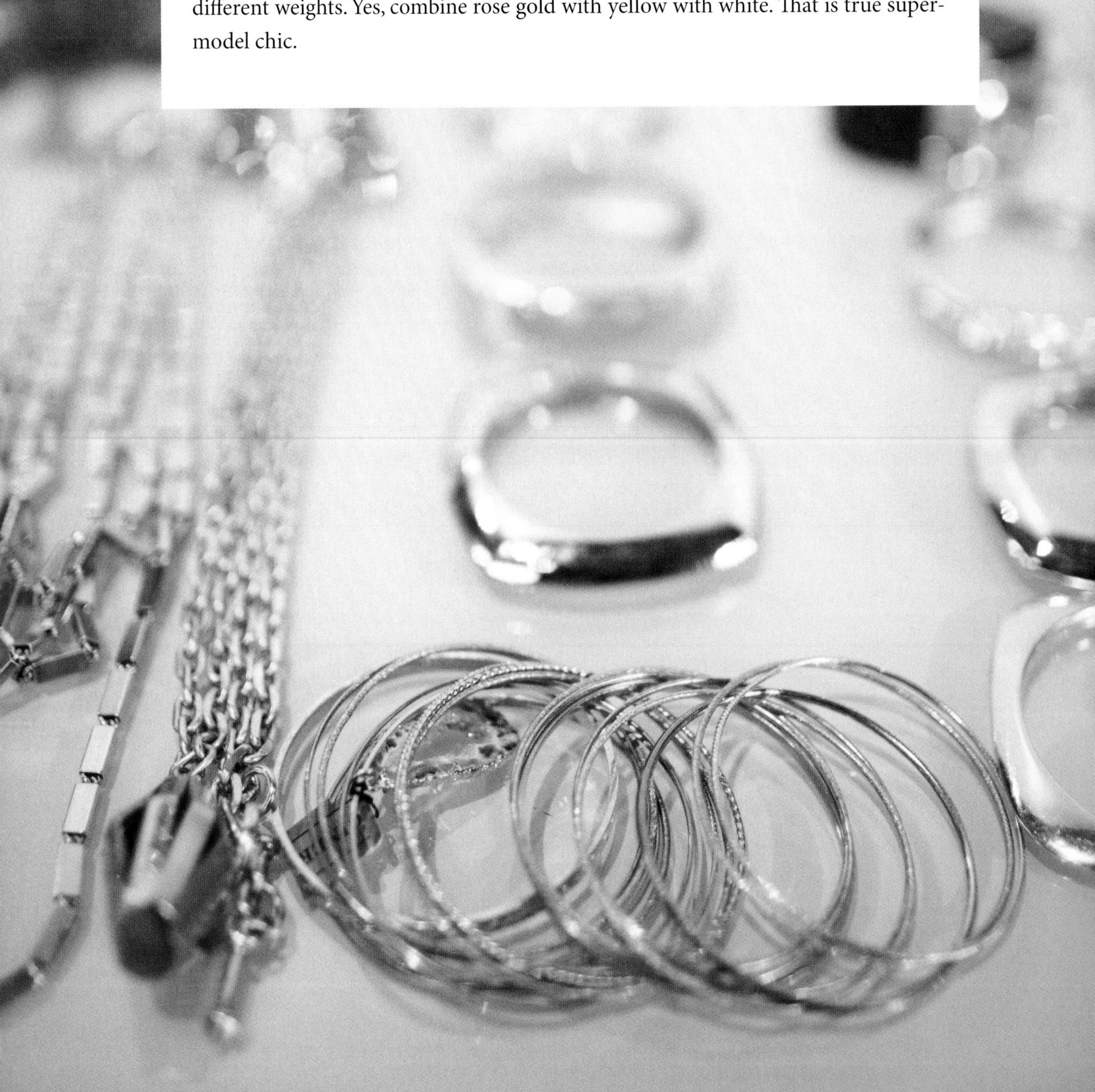

jewelry *travel tip*

Bring extra backings! Also, thread your chain necklaces through one end of a straw, latch the clasp, and place in a zippered pouch. This will keep chains from dreaded tangling. Also, always double-check the backings of expensive earrings—confirm they lock securely. If they don't, get new backings. —MIMI BROWN, stylist

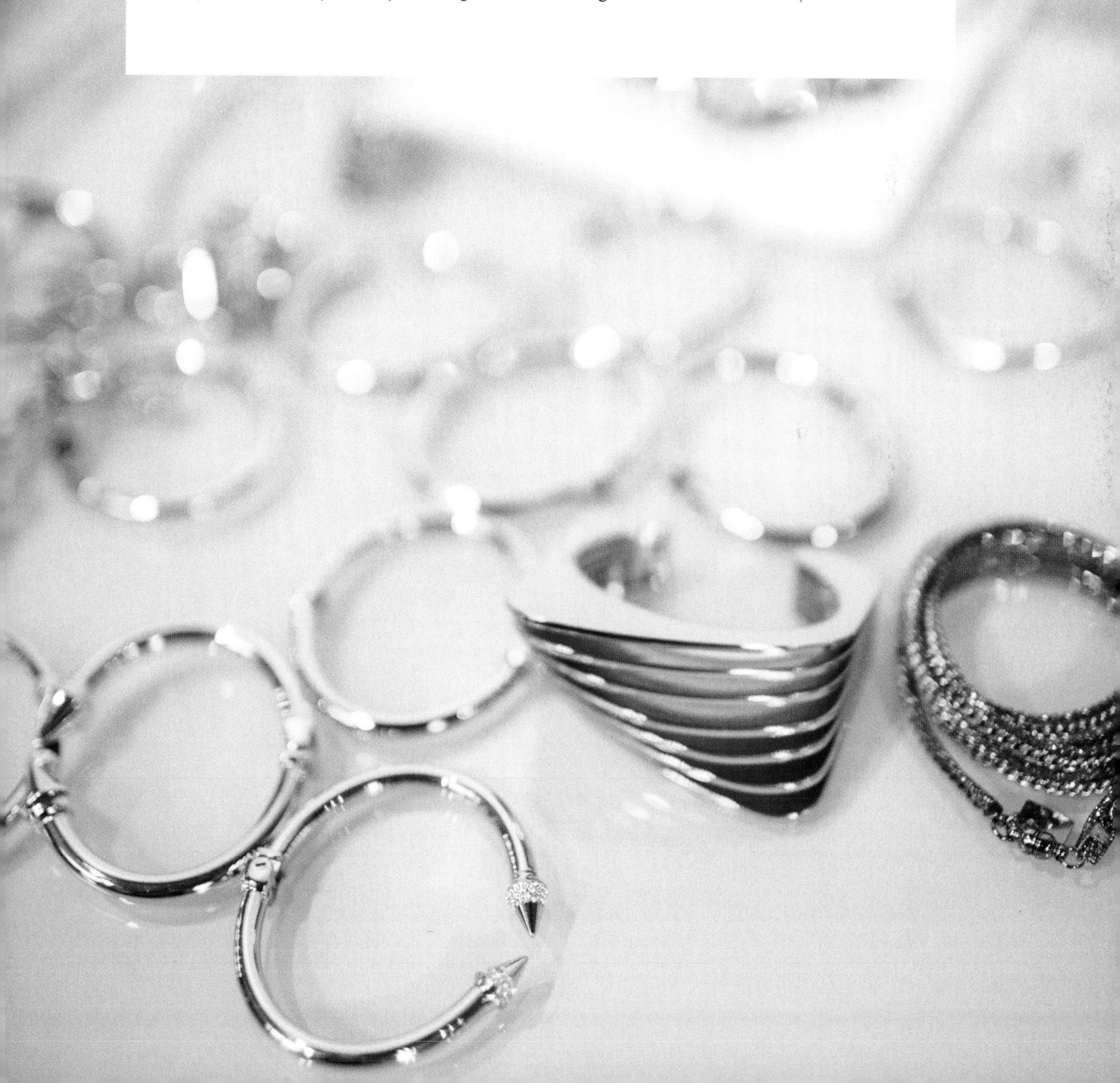

CORE handbags

Building your handbag collection is key. You have got to have the right ones that will last, look good, and function well for your lifestyle. Below, we identify the four styles of handbag that will serve you well and round out your core 'drobe.

1. professional handbag

Choose a classic boxy or bucket shape, slightly oversized to fit a notebook, folders, a pair of flats, and a small makeup bag. It must have a zipper or snap closure and interior compartments for *life necessities* and to help organize. It should be large enough to get you through a workday, but small enough to transition into night. It should be stylish enough for lunch with friends, but conservative and classy enough for a business dinner or something more somber.

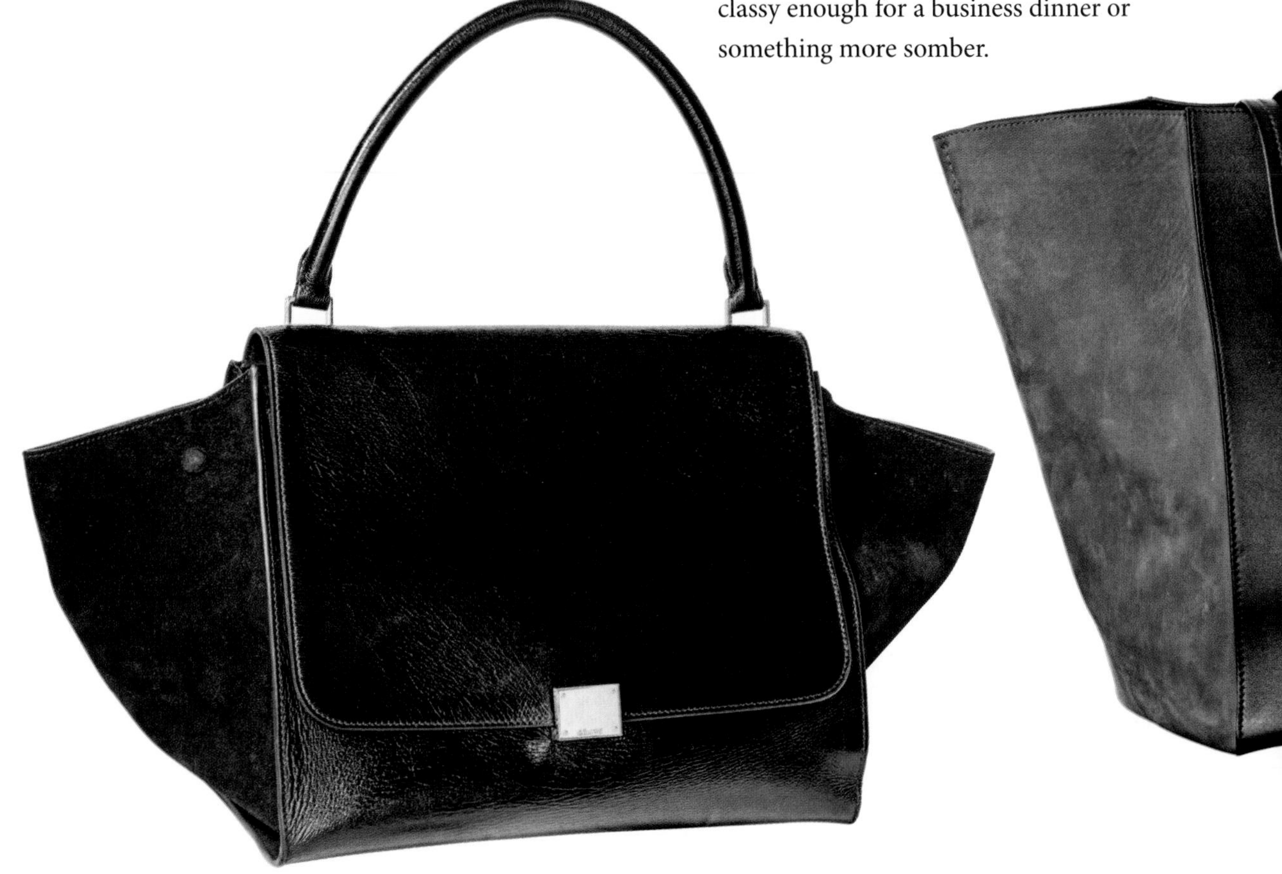

2. carryall tote

A do-it-all! This can go to the office, the gym, the beach, a birthday party with the kids, a shopping spree, or on the plane! A tote can be a black hole, so simplify the "shuffle" when using one by having smaller bags inside to organize items. (I'm thinking about my son's little race cars as I write this. I put them all in a separate, Ziploc baggie so I'm not digging like a gopher for his red mustang.)

3. crossbody bag

I cannot live without this bag and have single-handedly convinced every last one of my friends to get one. It's functional and understated, but is an absolute must for on-the-go. Yours should be just big enough to fit the absolute essentials. Best part of all, it's lightweight and hands free—and can go with you to anything/anytime.

4. the clutch

This is your go to evening bag. Black. Nude. Or something sparkly. Wear to weddings, anniversaries, New Year's Eve parties, red carpets, or special events. A superchic clutch also spices up a pair of jeans and heels on a casual night out. Clutches can be so annoying to hold, so try to find something that's comfortable.

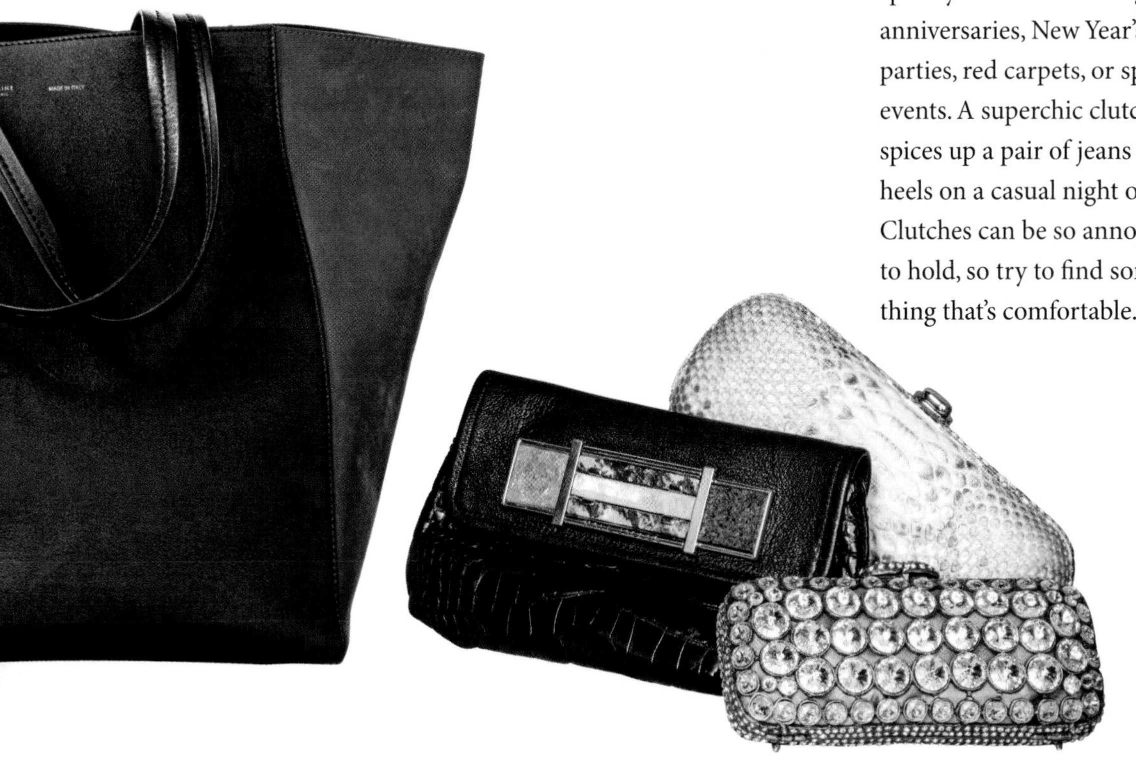

the re-stylists *say*

HOW TO IDENTIFY A CORE CLASSIC HANDBAG

Certain designer labels are known for their haute handbags. I wear mine with pride and take care of them like they are my children. But the truth is, you do not have to spend thousands of dollars on a luxury label. You do however need to know *what key features to look for in a classic handbag*. Pay attention to these hallmarks of a high-quality and invest wisely. You will want to invest as much as your budget will allow. Think about it—when it comes to cost per use, a handbag is always a good return on investment.

- **LEATHER ALERT:** Know the difference between leather that looks cheap and luxe. Look for leather that is slightly pebbled, with a soft matte finish. Not too shiny! Choose a leather that has some texture and weight. If you prefer vegan options, there is a difference between rubbery, cheap-looking faux leather and buttery, near replica.
- **HONE IN ON THE HARDWARE:** If the bag has hardware, look for sturdy pieces with weight, nothing chintzy, that will rub or break off. If the bag features a detail, such as a stone or something special, it should be a quality detail and secured well. If there is metal anywhere on the bag, make sure it's a neutral color metal that you wear the most. If you aren't sure, look for a bag with minimal to no metal accents. Note: crap hardware and fake, plasticky metal is a dead giveaway your bag is CHEAP.
- **IN STITCHES:** Pay attention to the stitching. It should be elegantly executed and match your bag's leather. It goes without saying, there should not be fraying, weird double stitching, or loose stiches.

* **PARK IT IN NEUTRAL:** If you are investing in only one bag, invest in a versatile neutral. Black, gray, taupe, tan, and brown all work. But keep in mind, lighter neutrals tend to get dingy with lots of wear. If you are hard on your bags or have kids, a dark neutral is the only way to go! Consult your wardrobe. What neutral colors do you wear most? Use that as a decision-making guide.
* **AVOID GAUDY DETAILS:** It does not matter if it's the most exclusive label. If there is a trendy detail, like a giant oversized metal lock or a graphic image, please do not buy it. It will date you. A classic bag that lasts years and even decades is almost always simple and sleek.
* **SIGNATURE DESIGN:** Certain designer labels feature signature monogrammed designs (Louis Vuitton, Gucci). Generally speaking, those bags are classic no-brainers. But! *Everyday supermodels,* be wise: spending a lot of money on a designer handbag does not guarantee that it's a classic. If you don't pay attention to the aforementioned guide, you might woefully invest hard-earned cash into something that is actually a trend. In a year's time, you'll be left with a hole in your wallet . . . carrying a pocketbook that's passé. Double ouch! When buying designer, all the above rules still apply.

---

supermodel secret

Knowing your body and dressing to accentuate it is a big one. Acknowledge your assets. For example, I have really broad shoulders and athletic arms. Cap sleeves make me look like a Green Bay Packer so I never, *ever* wear them. Instead, play up your strengths. What pieces or outfits make you appear leaner or more balanced and proportioned? Compare pictures of yourself in different outfits and you'll be able to tell in an instant. Try snapping a picture of yourself in the mirror wearing two different jackets with the same outfit—one longer/one shorter. Compare the pix: does one look better? Take note!

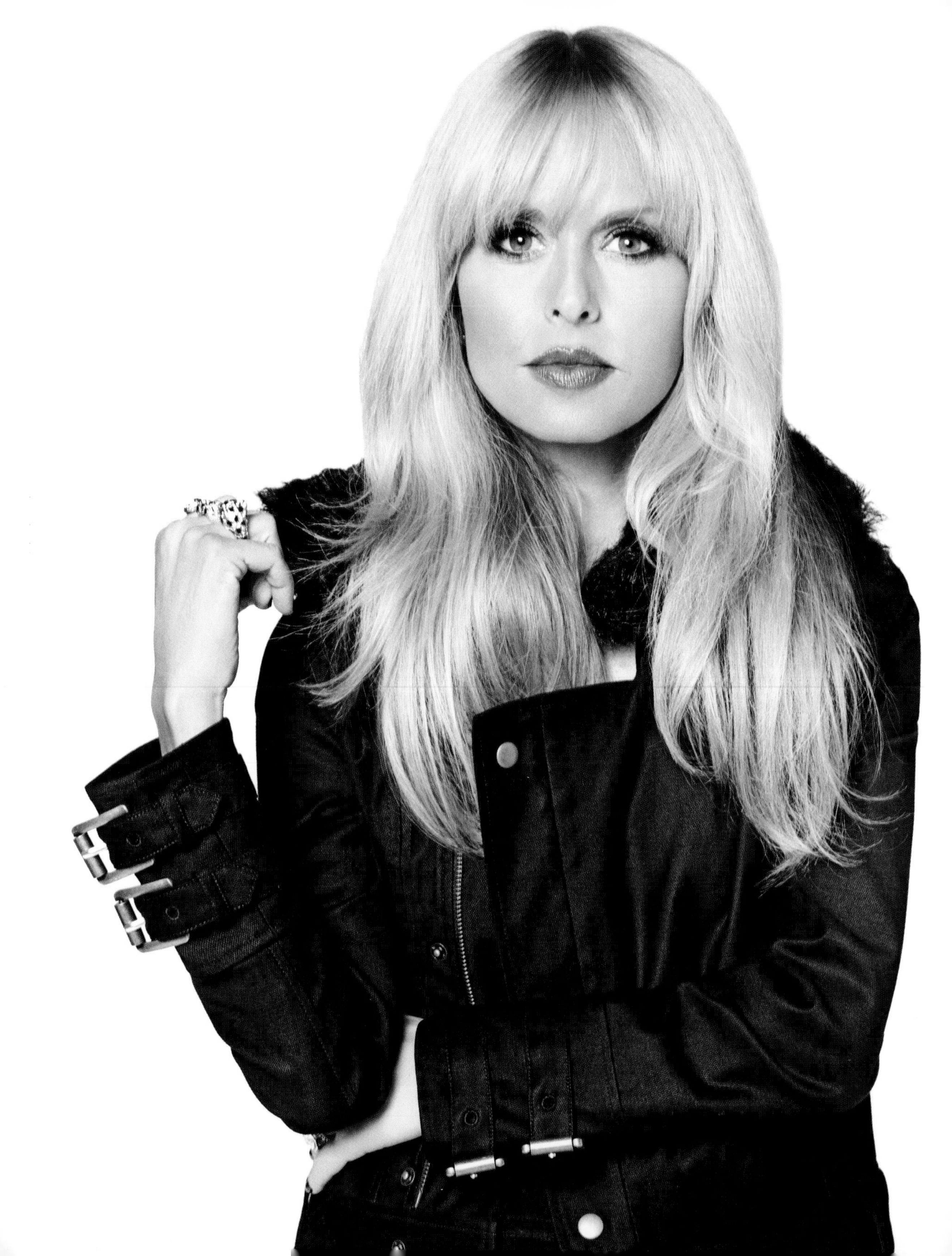

convo with *the zoe*

Rachel is a genius. As a stylist, she revolutionized fashion in Hollywood. Her innovative styling has helped actresses build careers and even become household names. Rachel combines classic glamour and '70s flair, with a little creative risk.

She also makes serious fashion accessible for everyone. Her clothing collections are sometimes bold, but always wearable. Rachel has been my stylist for years. I trust her and she gives good advice.

1. Your top three tips to looking GREAT?

   ATTITUDE IS EVERYTHING. No matter what you are wearing, *wear it confidently.*
   LESS IS ALWAYS MORE. Like Coco Chanel always said, "Before you leave the house, look in the mirror and remove one accessory."
   MY MOM TAUGHT ME to never leave the house without lipstick . . . and she is the most glamorous!

2. What is an ABSOLUTE fashion no-no?

   I THINK TOO MUCH OF ONE TREND is never a good thing. With "of the moment" statements, moderation is key.

3. What is your most favorite piece you own?

   THAT IS THE HARDEST QUESTION I GET ASKED! My dear friend William Banks-Blaney, of William Vintage, recently gave me the most insane Jean Patou vintage dress. It is incredible and I am beyond obsessed—it is literally covered in crystals from shoulder to hemline. One of a kind.

undercover agents and *hidden* helpers

Rachel Zoe herself will tell you that when she and her team style a celeb, looking poised and polished is often as much about what's *under* the clothes as the clothes themselves. I have worn it all when it comes to figure fixers. Belly jelly anyone? Bra-induced back fat? After baby, I'm all too familiar! Trust me, there isn't a girl on the red carpet today that isn't getting undercover help from a tummy tamer or a behind binder—or who knows—maybe even duct tape! Stylist Mimi Brown and I outline a few ways to tame your fuller frame.

- Stock up on control/support items: shorts, tummy control tights, and body suits. Waist cinchers are always helpful under tight or clingy tops and dresses. Some of these wardrobe warriors are so commonplace you can even find them in drugstores, like Walgreens.
- Buy your favorite strapless and T-shirt bra in nude and black—most come with a variety of straps you can rig different ways to accommodate different necklines. Make sure you own at least one bra that does not have any wire or boning around the base; that's what creates the bra bulge in the back. If that's not enough support for you, add foam inserts or "chicken cutlets" to the inside of your favorite nonpadded bra or no underwire bra for more lift. Tanks that tighten and smooth bra bulge are lifesavers too!
- Breast petals and breast tape are great if you need to go totally braless. Double up on the breast tape and apply under each breast in a half moon and jerry-rig up on each side to mimic the lift underwire would normally provide. (Duct tape will work in a pinch!) Then, top off with a breast petal to cover the nips. A lot of work—but it does do the job.
- A variety of briefs and thongs in nude for light-colored bottoms and skirts. Truth be told, when necessary, commando is best—no lines under tighter clothing. Just say no to grandma panties, unless it's that time of the month, or you are pregnant (then you are off the hook).
- It doesn't have to be uncomfortable, but some lacy and sweet lingerie can make you feel like a femme fatale. A nude and a black lace bra/panty set should do the trick. For lingerie that's *everyday supermodel* sexy our picks include Elle Macpherson, La Perla, Eberjay, Cosabella, Eres, Hanky Panky, and Maje/Sandro.

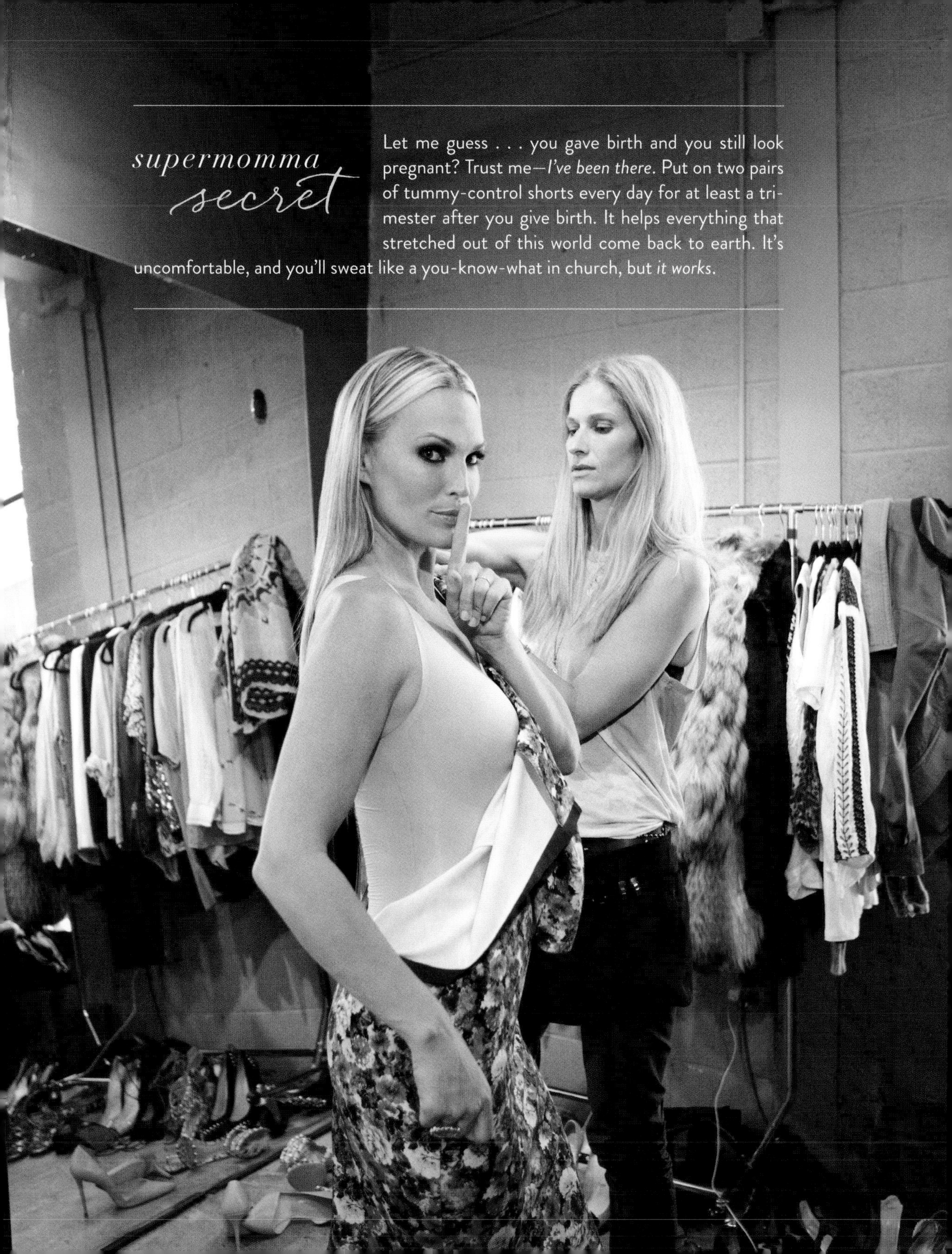

supermomma secret

Let me guess . . . you gave birth and you still look pregnant? Trust me—*I've been there*. Put on two pairs of tummy-control shorts every day for at least a trimester after you give birth. It helps everything that stretched out of this world come back to earth. It's uncomfortable, and you'll sweat like a you-know-what in church, but *it works*.

I love how she can look effortlessly chic no matter what she wears, how she can mix something worth $5 with a $5,000 item. So with her, it's as much about her image as it is her attitude and approach to fashion. Some of the most stylish glamazons are living it up on a dime. They just know how to reinvent a look with a belt or by wearing their hair another way."

—RACHEL ZOE ON KATE MOSS

THE *signature* SUPERMODEL PIECE

Your *everyday supermodel* piece is your signature piece. Every core wardrobe should have one. It's a little bit like a statement piece, but it doesn't have to be flashy. Simply put, it's a beloved item that has you all over it. Maybe it's a jet-black fedora you wear all the time that looks extrachic on you. Perhaps it's an heirloom necklace (like it is for me) you layer on with everything. When people think of you . . . they might even think of *it*. To me, that is style.

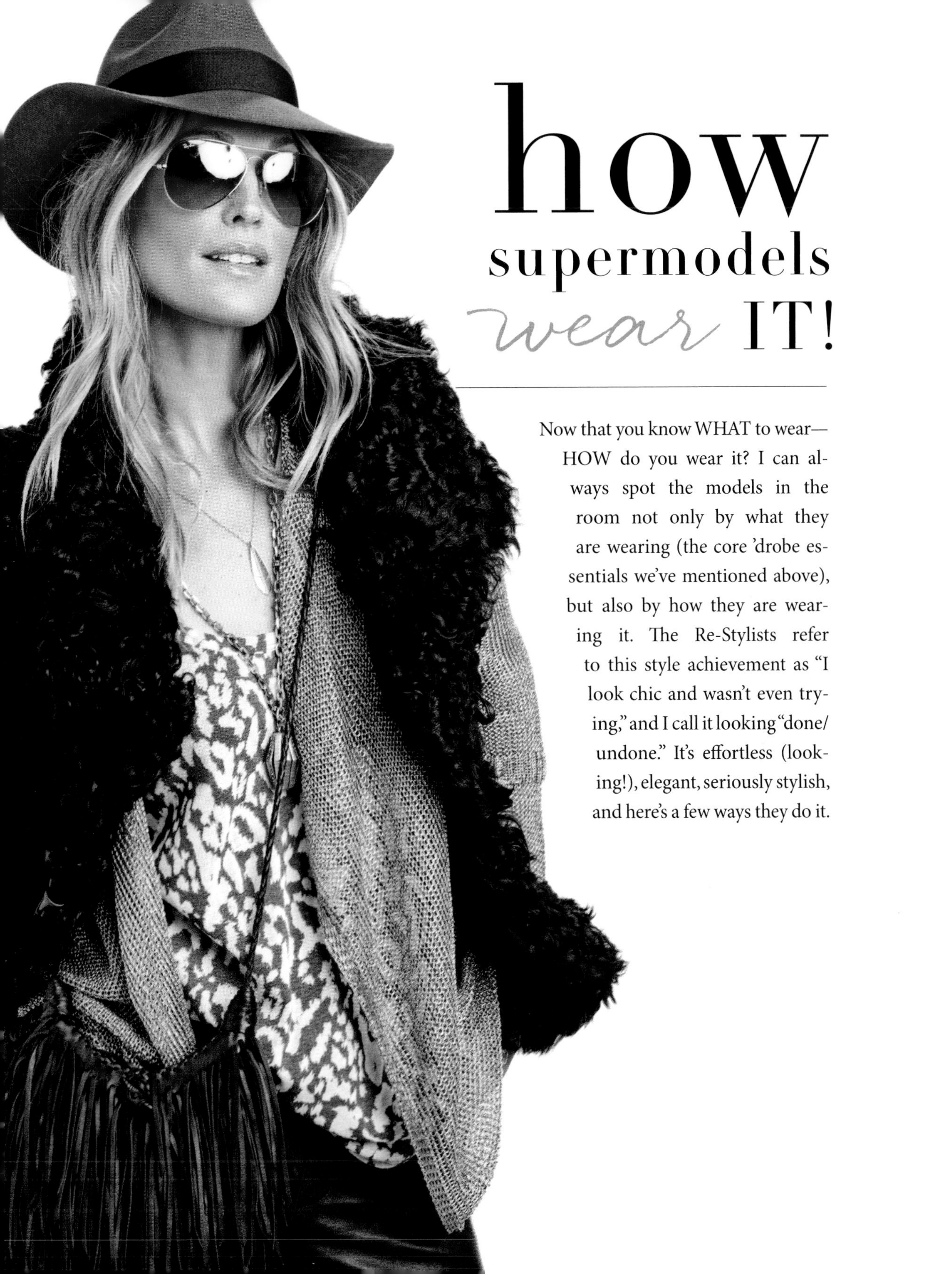

how supermodels *wear* IT!

Now that you know WHAT to wear—HOW do you wear it? I can always spot the models in the room not only by what they are wearing (the core 'drobe essentials we've mentioned above), but also by how they are wearing it. The Re-Stylists refer to this style achievement as "I look chic and wasn't even trying," and I call it looking "done/undone." It's effortless (looking!), elegant, seriously stylish, and here's a few ways they do it.

8 *signature* model moves

1. buy a size up (almost always)

Models almost never wear clothes that are tight (there are of course exceptions to every rule). As an example, while most girls at a club will be dressed in skintight minidresses, the models will likely be wearing something loose and edgy. This goes for everyday clothes too. Most of us try to squeeze into the smaller size because the smaller number somehow makes us feel better. But please don't—who cares? (Remember . . . cut the tag out!). When things are too tight, fabric often pulls, looks funny in places, and worst of all, *looks cheap and will make YOU look cheap*. The slightly bigger size almost always lays better, drapes better—and honestly, will make you look thinner and taller.

YES. I said it. When you try to squeeze into something, a lot of times you get sausage arm or leg or butt or back. No woman wants to channel Chris Farley in *Tommy Boy* . . . "Fat guy, little coat." You get the picture. The added benefit to buying bigger, you can always tailor something for better fit.

And finally . . . ALWAYS BUY BIGGER IF THE ITEM IS CHEAP. The fabric usually isn't as refined, so the fit and tailoring won't be as precise. When there is a little more play in the fabric, the piece will almost always present better.

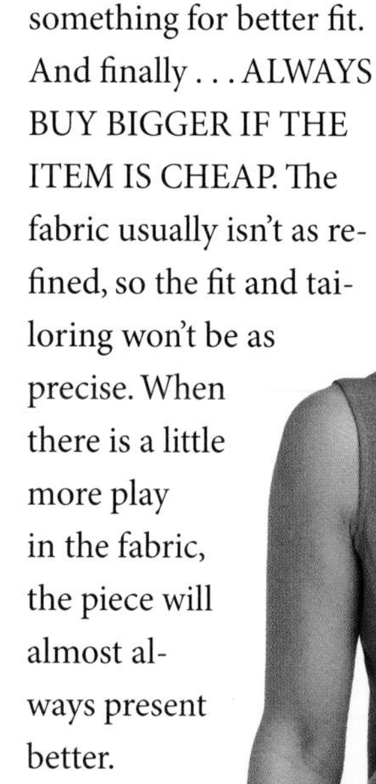

my "size" but way too tight

a size bigger but much better

2. tailor made

It might sound like a splurge, but models are so into fit, that some will even have their T-shirts tailored. I know a young model who buys vintage men's tees at secondhand stores and has them redone by her tailor to fit her body. This rule goes for everything. Suits, dresses, pants . . . models have their tailors on speed dial. And while it can be, tailoring doesn't always have to be expensive and doesn't always mean a complete overhaul of the item. Some department stores do basic tailoring for free. Tailoring can also be as basic as adding snaps to a button down blouse so it doesn't gap. It might mean making the slightest adjustment so it's most flattering. For expensive clothes and big fixes, research a well-respected, tried-and-true tailor in your area. For smaller jobs, most any local dry cleaner will do.

3. mixing high & low

Pairing designer pieces with affordable fashion is where everyday supermodel style is right now. No model wears head-to-toe designer anymore unless it's for a photo shoot. The everyday supermodel has shopping savvy—knowing when to splurge (on something you will wear a lot or that you'll have forever) and when to save. Every day you see fashion femme fatales on red carpets and city streets wearing $50 dresses or ensembles from Top Shop or an H&M/Target designer collaboration. They'll complete the look with a Chloé handbag, Saint Laurent boots, or Marni sunglasses. The entire ensemble will look expensive, even if only one item is.

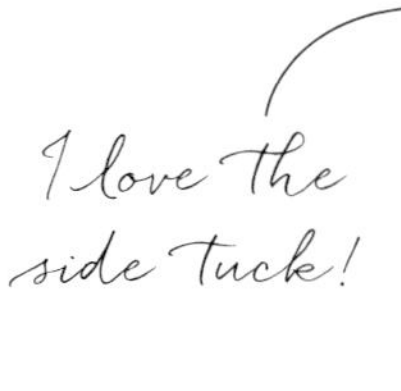

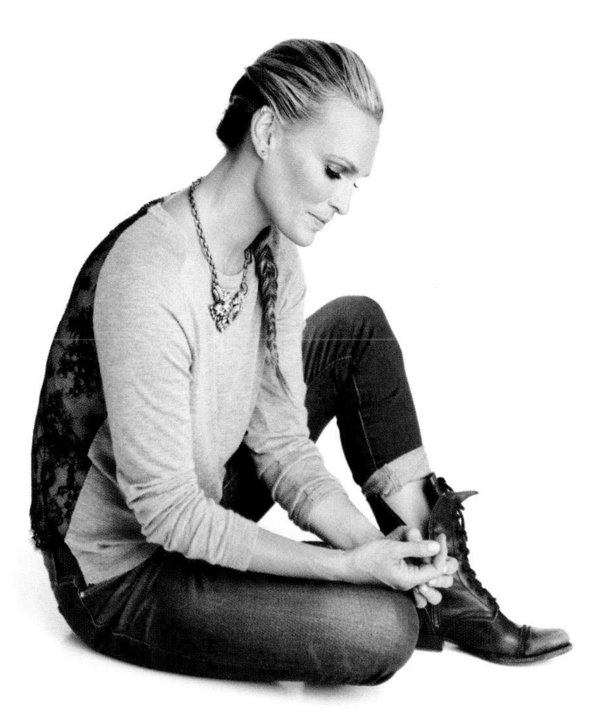

4. combining casual & dressy

Who can forget Sharon Stone and the infamous black Gap tee with the Valentino trumpet skirt? Models have been working this kind of thing for years. It's a bit like pairing a casually chic hairstyle, a bit loose, a bit disheveled—with an evening gown. You don't always have to go for the formal updo. Pairing clothes is the same. Just step out of the box and get creative. What's great about a look that combines both casual and dressy—it's so versatile. With just the switch of a shoe (a flat to a heel, or a sneaker to a stiletto)—you easily go from day to night, without changing clothes, and look both appropriate and AMAZING!

5. contrast

Models mix fabrics and textures. Models rarely ever go all shiny or all matte head to toe. If you have a wool suit you wear to work, try a silky blouse underneath with a little sheen or a lurex tank with subtle sparkle. Also, contrasting styles is unexpected and supermodely. Think mixing masculine and feminine pieces. A feminine sweater, with a boyfriend jean, studded earrings, and motorcycle boots can be really interesting. A minimalist dress, chic and simple, with decadent, glamorous costume jewelry. Contrast is surprising and sexy.

6. think outside the box

Models get creative and know when to break rules. Including any we list in this book! They may even wander into the men's section of their favorite store and buy a sweater. (FYI, men's sweaters are cut longer and often drape nicely.) Same goes for men's collared work shirts (and they make for a sexy beach cover-up). A model might wear a top or a dress backwards—and the front V-neck is now a plunging V in the back!

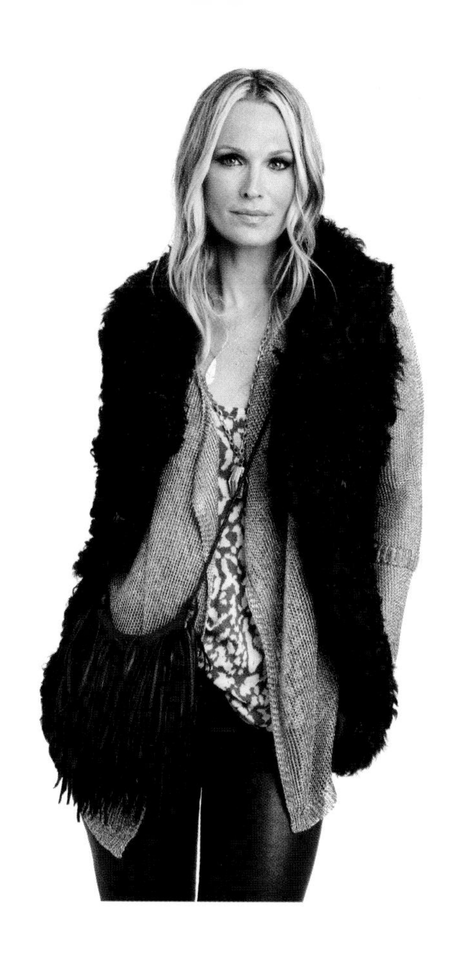

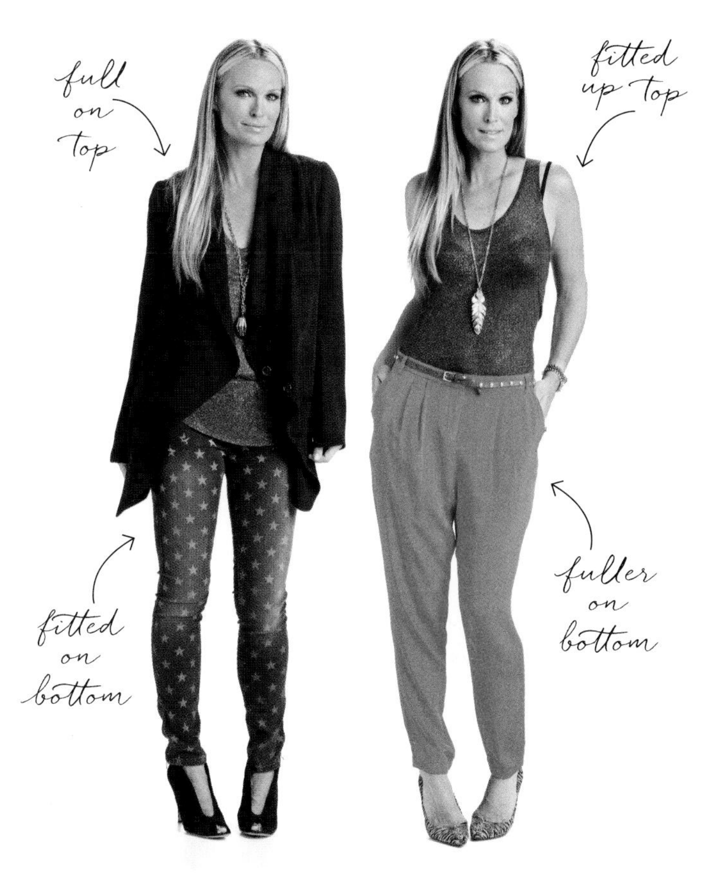

7. layer player

Rachel Zoe and Jessica Alba do this best. You will never see either of them in just jeans and a tank top. They create dimension and supermodel style by layering pieces and building up a look. A long tank, a cardigan, then maybe add a fun fur vest (faux if you like!) or a scarf—that's layering. Don't forget about accessories—you can almost always top off with some sunnies or a hat for an extracool factor. Copy style mavens featured in the media to get it right (I do!).

8. balance scheme

Follow the principle of proportion. If something is tight on top, go looser on the bottom. If you have a tight jean on bottom, reverse it, go fuller on top. All tight or all balloon-ish generally doesn't look as chic. It also creates better balance and gives the impression of an hourglass figure.

jessica alba's style *secrets*

WE ASKED, SHE ANSWERED

The top three accessories every girl should have in her closet:

1. Great bag
2. Stylish pump
3. Leather moto jacket

These staples dress up any outfit—from jeans and a T-shirt to a slip dress. And don't be shy with your style. Try a bold take on a classic: a white pump, a metallic cross-body bag, or a studded leather jacket are all cool reinventions of classic, fashion must-haves.

ON LAYERING: Molly said it. I do love to layer. To layer right, there are a few things you need to consider. Foundation pieces need to be thin and cut at different lengths and proportions for versatility. The top layer can be heavier, like a chunky knit or a leather vest, but the bottom layers always have to be lightweight. When layering, the key is to make sure you're getting an elongated silhouette.

MY STYLE MOTTO: Really get to know your body and dress to accentuate it. If you only wear silhouettes flattering to your figure, you can't really go wrong. That way, you can be daring with trends or stick with classics, but as long as you are dressing to enhance your shape, you will look and feel great—and that's what matters most. It all works if it looks great.

FASHIONABLE FINISH: To complete a look, I love to add a statement-making pair of sunglasses. I have lots of different colors and styles. I mix it up. Some days I go with a chunky frame, other days metal—depending on my outfit.

supermodel *it up*

The same outfit/pieces can go from ho-hum to hot-to-trot—just by adding a few styling touches. Check out how subtle tweaks by the Re-Stylists took this look from blah to *everyday supermodely.*

It's *all* in the Styling.

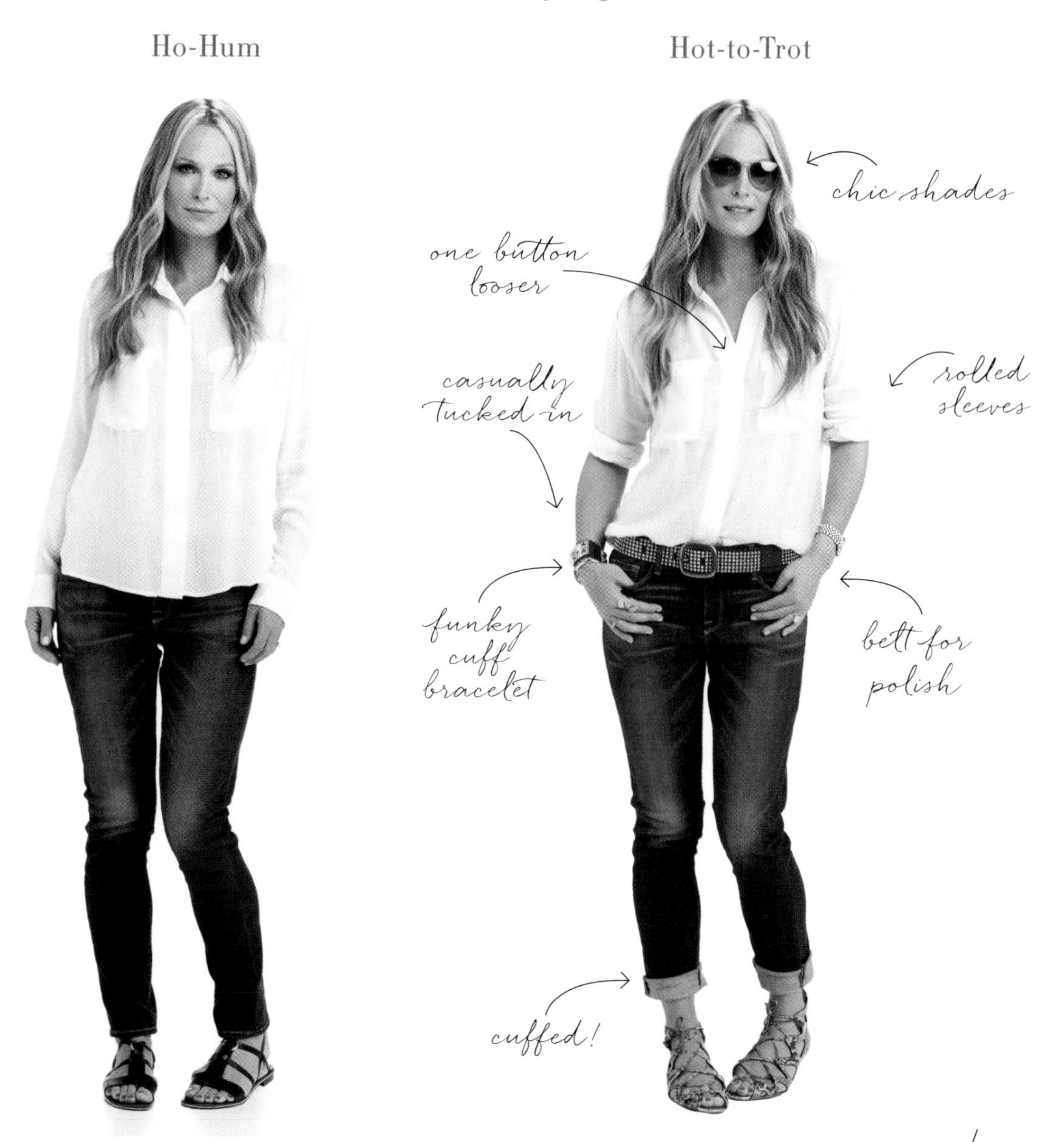

6 WAYS TO *rock* A SCARF

"How do I love thee, Let me count the ways." Pretty sure Elizabeth Barrett Browning was writing about a scarf when she wrote this. I L-O-V-E a scarf. Listen to me—it's another instant style shortcut—like a statement shoe. And no! You do not have to be tall for a scarf to look good. You just have to know how to wear a scarf—*and not let it wear you*. When you aren't feeling fab, a scarf in a fresh shade or fun pattern can perk you up. The right scarf worn well is the number one easiest way to add supermodel sensibility to ANYTHING you have on. And I mean *anything*. Learn how to wear it well. Go to mollysims.com for a tutorial on how to get these looks.

1. SLOUCHY & CHIC: This classic way to wrap is easy to accomplish and is both messy and polished all at once. You can wear it with a blazer and leggings, jeans and a white tee, a long cotton dress . . . pair this with almost anything and you can't go wrong.
2. KNOTTED & BESOTTED: Frames the face and has a bit of glamour girl style. A little more conservative, this look complements a tailored blazer or in contrast with a masculine, leather moto-jacket.
3. THE HALO: I love this look beneath a jean jacket or with a long linen tank dress. It's gorgeous with hair up and earrings dangling. Also looks nice with a chunky knit.
4. BAGGED & TAGGED: Honestly no time to dress up your look? Tag your bag with a scarf of almost any kind, something with color is great. A fun pattern or bright color will add a nuance to your look—even if you are in all black.
5. THE WATERFALL: This is runway chic, flowy, feminine and sexy. Gorgeous paired with a long dress or an evening look. Or try with bell bottoms, platform shoes, and a button-down.
6. THE PROFESSOR: Perfect to wear under outerwear of all kinds. Love it under a peacoat. Classic. Understated. Elegant. Excuse me, did you graduate from Cambridge or Oxford?

the re-stylists *say*

Scarf *length* is key. It needs to be long enough to be versatile. How to gauge? Place the scarf around the back of your neck and bring both sides forward. The scarf length on each side should fall between midthigh and your knee. If you are petite or shorter, measure a scarf the same way, but choose a more refined, finer-weight fabric that isn't too buxom or bulky so it doesn't overwhelm. A scarf is also a great way to disguise a large (or small!) chest. Wear something in a darker shade and go with one of the styles above that creates a vertical line and elongates (the Waterfall, the Professor, or Slouchy & Chic are all excellent options.

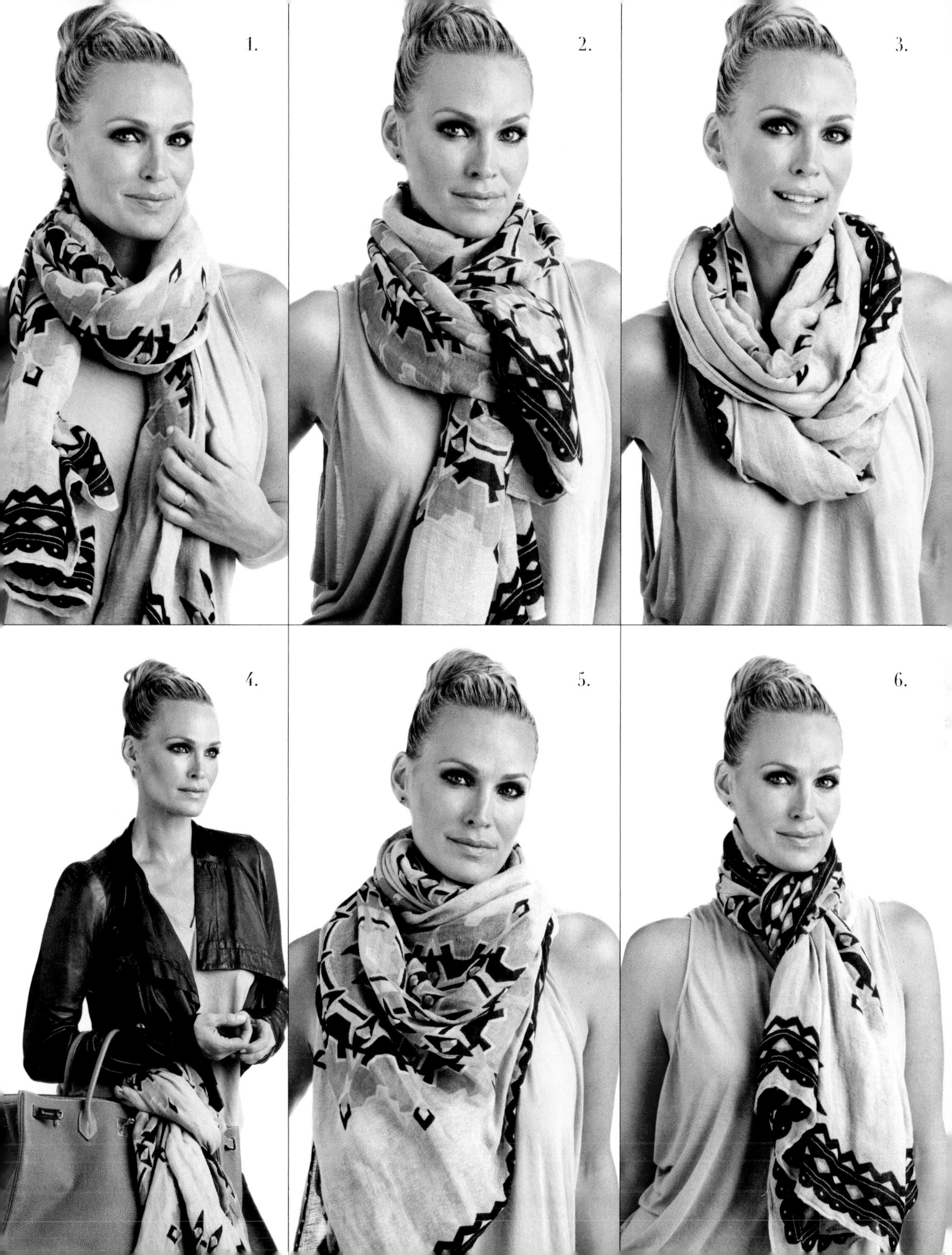
1.
2.
3.
4.
5.
6.

Fashion *mistakes* Models (Usually) Never Make

These fashion faux pas are so *not runway* and so *run the other way*!

1. **TIME WARP TRAP:** Models don't get stuck in ruts. Think Linda Evangelista. They change things up. They challenge themselves and their identity. Their closet isn't a time capsule. We dress up differently for every job we have, so we get comfortable taking risks. So should you! Evolve. It's okay to have a uniform, but don't get stuck in it. Have fun. Clothes are not tattoos. They come off.

2. **MATCHY-MATCHY:** Models will never be matchy-matchy. For example, a model won't wear pearl earrings and a pearl necklace and a pearl ring and so on. *Never.* Diamond studs, a statement necklace, and a vintage gold ring? Yes. Paisley-print capris and a nautical tee? Heck yeah! Models mix prints, styles, metals, themes, and so on, to give their look edge and interest.

3. **PERFECTION IS FOR P*$$YS:** There needs to be a flaw somewhere. (This goes along with the done/undone philosophy). Models always go for an unexpected twist. The deliberate imperfection, something that doesn't quite fit. They always add their own unique take on something. A sexy fitted sheath dress . . . and a beanie. Nothing is overworked, overthought, or contrived. It all just works.

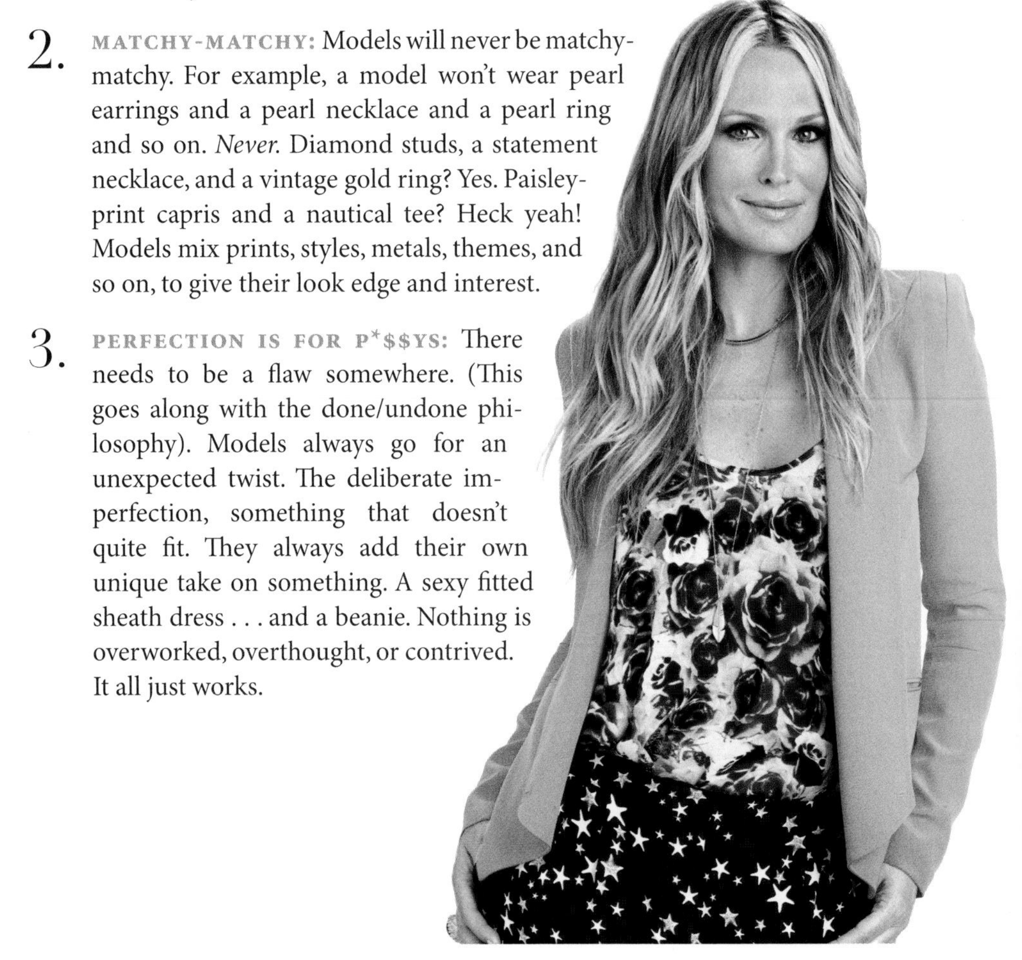

4. **DON'T GO OVERBOARD ON SEXY:** Model sexy is definitely different from what day-to-day divas think should be worn to seduce the opposite sex. Model sexy is about a peek, *not a porno*. Less here is *always more*. A bit of the bra strap, not the entire bra . . . a skirt that shows a little leg, not all the way up to the Bermuda triangle. And pick one—a little cleavage or little leg—not both. You get the idea. And finally, every shaped woman looks sexy in a Diane von Furstenberg wrap dress. Get one!

5. **THE SUPERMODEL SWAGGER:** Whatever you wear, wear it with confidence. Rachel Zoe said this above, but it bears repeating. When you step out of the house and like the way you look, it will show. And if you don't feel good in it—do not wear it. Because that will show too.

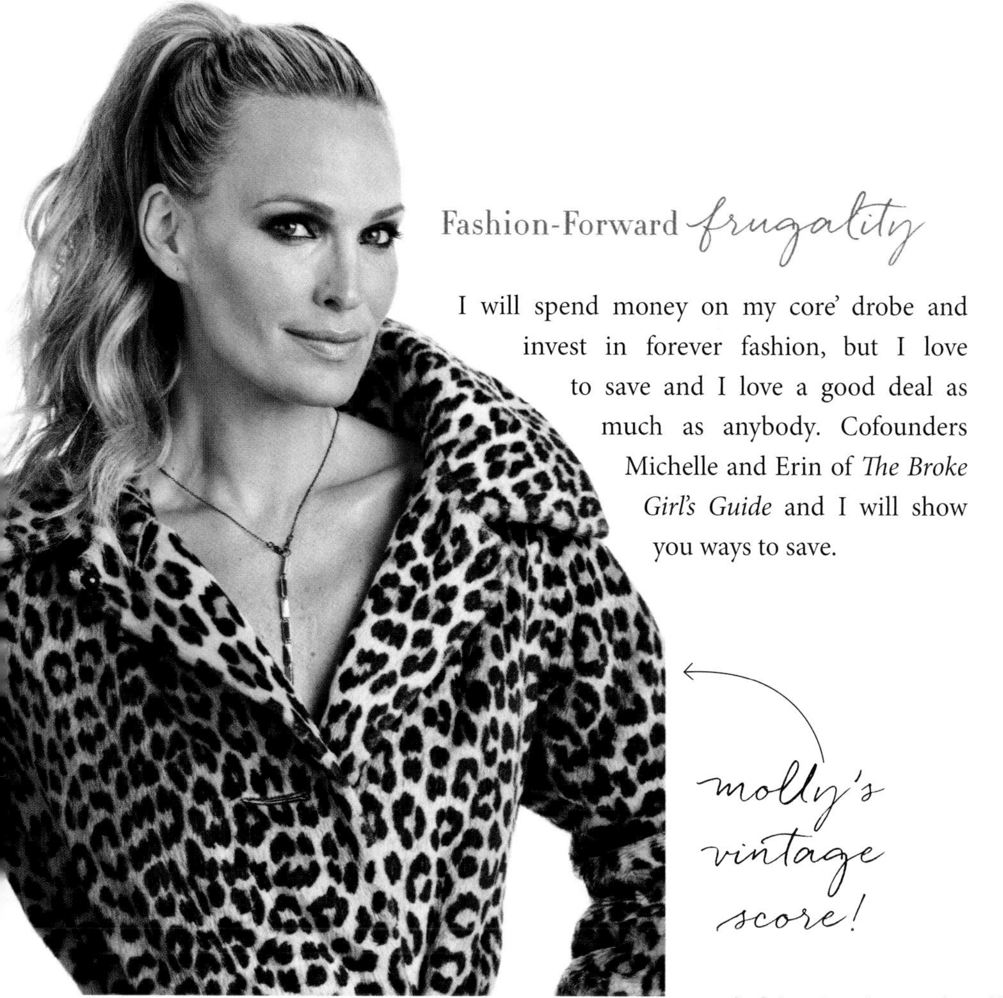

Fashion-Forward *frugality*

I will spend money on my core' drobe and invest in forever fashion, but I love to save and I love a good deal as much as anybody. Cofounders Michelle and Erin of *The Broke Girl's Guide* and I will show you ways to save.

molly's vintage score!

1. **SHOP VINTAGE, CONSIGNMENT, AND THRIFT STORES:** You have to be patient and you have to look, but you can find incredible finds and even core classics and expensive labels. This is a great way to secure signature or fun pieces that no one else will have and you will have acquired for a steal! You can often score gently worn designer handbags here at a fraction of the retail price.

2. **CLOTHES SWAP:** Get together with fashion-minded friends and have some fun. Trade items you are over for items they are over. You can refresh your wardrobe for the cost of a shared bottle of wine. Also, there are great swapping sites like SwapStyle.com and DesignSwap.com. These are fab online places to swap pieces that aren't designer.

3. **CASH OUT WHEN YOU CLOSET CLEAN:** Using sites like Ebay.com and Etsy.com is a great way to sell directly to consumers. The RealReal.com, Tradesy.com, and Shophers.com are also excellent for cashing out your clothes. They are especially good with designer pieces, not as good on your midrange clothes.

4. **FLASH SITES, SALES, DISCOUNT RETAILERS, & E-TAILERS:** This has become all the rage and you can get incredible deals. Warning: Do not buy on sale just because it's a spanking deal. Even if you are getting a huge discount, you should still LOVE it. Whether it's $10 or $1,000, don't buy anything you don't love. Think about it, all those "cheap" impulse purchases that you've never worn could have been that one designer piece you'll have forever!

5. **WAKE UP YOUR WARDROBE:** If you have a nice-fitting blouse or coat that could be beautiful if it wasn't for the cheap buttons—swap them out for nicer ones. Same goes for a skirt with a cheesy belt or poor-quality zipper—replace them with quality pieces and you'll upgrade the look.

6. **KEEP 'EM SEPARATED:** Instead of buying a dress or jumpsuit—*buy separates*. You will always get more use out of them because separates are simply more versatile.

7. **LEASING LUXURY:** Websites and stores like RentTheRunway.com and WearTodayGoneTomorrow.com allow you to "lease" fancy designer pieces for a few days at affordable prices, usually around 5–15 percent of the retail cost. You can look like a million bucks without spending it. Another word of advice: Have *social media savvy*. If you know you are going to be photographed a lot, and splashed all over Facebook, Twitter, and Instagram wearing something, don't spend a lot on it. You likely won't want to wear it again. This is when a great knockoff, or rental dress comes into play.

supermodel *secret*

Yes, I've been on "best-dressed" lists. I've also been in the Fashion Police section as "what not to wear." Everyone makes fashion mistakes. I've certainly made a few. And if I am a true fashionista, I will again. One thing I've learned the hard way, always check yourself before you leave the house—do a 360. No one wants a skirt tucked into the top of her stockings or . . . to wear something that is actually completely see-through . . . like I did here. Oops!

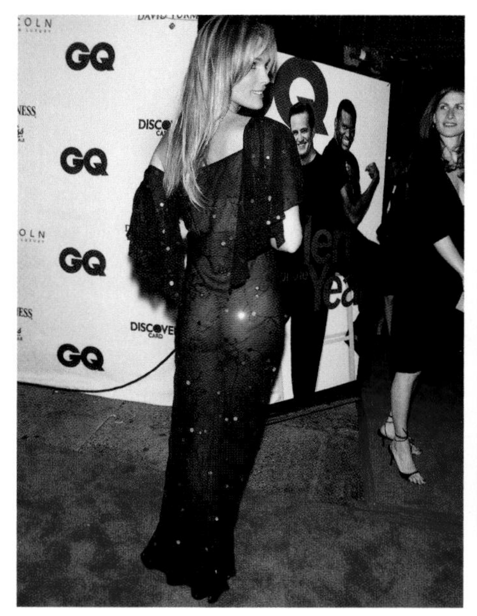

Under the lights and flashes . . . totally see-through.

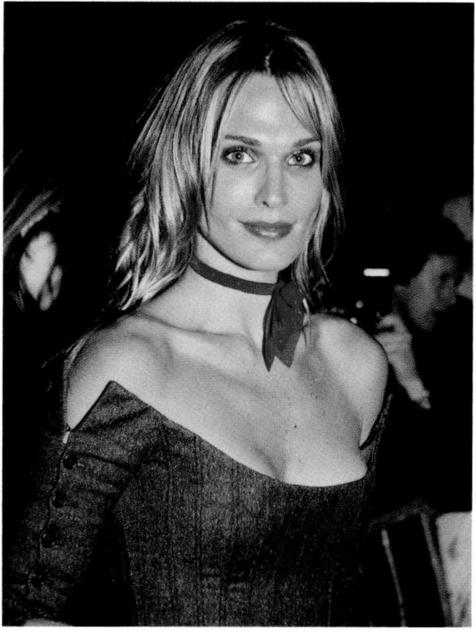

Bless my heart. Channeling Dolly Parton circa 1979.

let's talk *trends*, baby

The core 'drobe definitely incorporates trends—fashion has to be fun. But don't be a sucker! While I ALWAYS pay attention to what trends are happening, it doesn't mean I indulge in them all. Here are some *everyday supermodel* rules when it comes to fast fashion.

Trend It *like* Beckham

1. **DON'T SPEND A LOT:** Trends can be finicky. They come and go. If you really love a trend, go for it. But don't empty your wallet. Many of them are in for one season and *so over* the next.
2. **DON'T GO OVERBOARD:** Just because orange is the new black does not mean you buy heels, a purse, a headband, a bandage dress, and a motor vehicle all in this shade. One piece with punch is almost always enough.
3. **AGE IS NOT A FACTOR:** A lot of women feel they are too old to fly the trendy skies. Nonsense! Trends keep things interesting and can be classy and sophisticated. If zebra print is "in," that doesn't mean you have to wear a zebra striped bikini. Something as simple as a zebra print scarf tied around your handbag will do the trend trick.
4. **TAILOR THE TREND TO YOU:** Let's say short-shorts are all the rage, but you don't like your legs. *Make it work for you.* Pair the shorts with tights or buy a longer short and wear it with a sky-high heel.
5. **IT'S OK TO DISS A TREND:** All trends are not made equal. Be selective. Work the ones that suit you and skip out on ones that don't. Let's face it, we aren't all Steven Tyler and meant to wear feathers in our hair.

Trends That Are *timeless*

There are a few "trends" that never die—or at least never stop coming back. Which makes them Classic Trends. It's okay to pay good money for something in this category because they are here to stay.

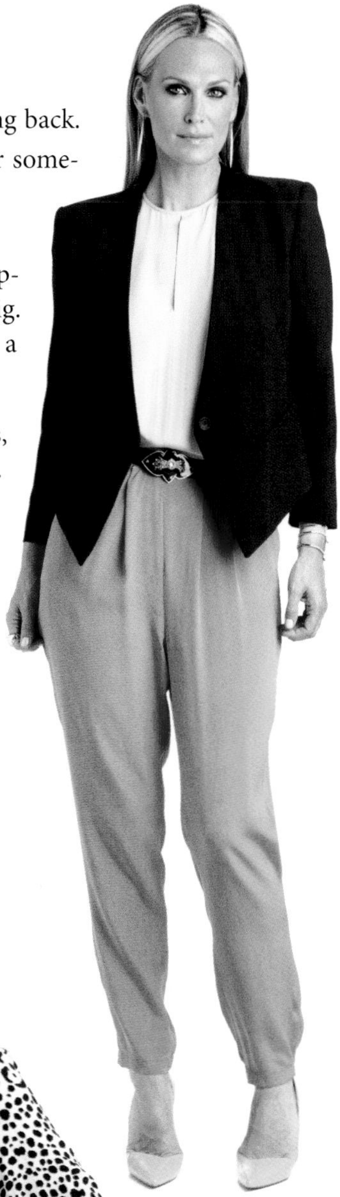

1. **LEOPARD:** There's something eternally sexy and primal about leopard print. Some years it's really big and other years it's just . . . big. Whether you invest in a leopard accessory, like a great clutch or a pair of shoes, we promise this look never goes extinct.

2. **STUDS/ROCKER:** Remember the '80s, the '90s, and now? Studs, rocker, leather—it's all still here. I love studs on a motorcycle boot. But the easiest way to work them in is via accessories, such as bracelets and the like. They are easy to store and can be worn with everything.

3. **JEAN JACKET/JEAN SHIRT:** Some years it's the jean shirt that's in, other years it's the jean jacket. It goes back and forth. But denim is pure Americana and not going anywhere! Just be sure to invest in a classic cut and shade (i.e., not acid-washed or ombré).

4. **COLOR-BLOCKING:** I hesitated to put this in . . . but then did the math. This so-called trend has been trending for almost five years now. It has gotten so much red-carpet attention and it just won't go away because it always looks fresh, fun, and just . . . good. Congratulations color-blocking—you made the list.

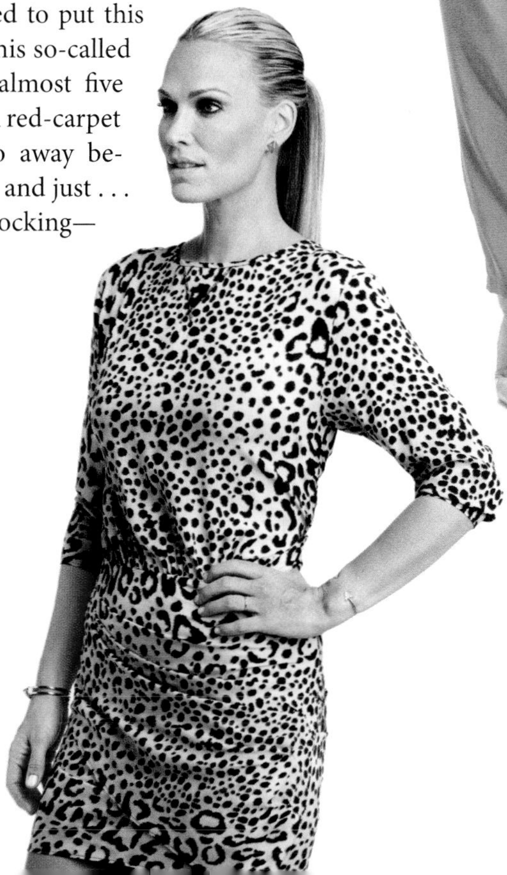

Tips for *different* Body Types

- **PLAY TO YOUR STRENGTHS:** Find ways to showcase your attributes. Do you have great calves? Beautiful shoulders? Show 'em off.
- **DON'T HIDE:** It's best not to "hide" your bigger parts under baggy clothes—chances are you'll look heavier. This is definitely true when pregnant too. Often curves need a *little* cling—but not total suction. Wear a fitted dress and top it off with an oversized blazer or an army jacket.
- **COLOR & TEXTURE TRICKS:** Distract! Wear darker colors to slim and prints or shiny fabrics where you'd like to draw attention. If you'd like to slenderize your bottom half, wear dark denim on the bottom paired with a printed blouse on top (horizontal stripes or a bold print will draw the eye to the top half). Want to minimize the top half? Try a full-coverage fitted top paired with a printed, flowy skirt or loose/cuffed boyfriend jean.

Fuller Figured? Curve Appeal *advice* from the Zoe

- I love tailored pieces that showcase the figure. Choose clothes that nip at the waist and skim smoothly (not tightly) over the body.
- Low-waisted jeans or trousers deemphasize a generous backside (just don't go so low that you risk exposure).
- For a voluptuous top: Avoid anything with prominent details on that zone of your body, including oversized lapels, chunky knits, or double-breasted anything.
- For fuller arms, choose looks with a three-quarter sheer or opaque sleeve.

fashion LOOKS

I love, love, love

Everyone should have "go-to" looks. Looks you love. Looks you can count on. No-brainers. They just make life easier. My friend has a "first date" look and she wears it on *every* first date. That way—she doesn't have to stress, doesn't have to worry. She knows she'll feel and look good in that get-up. Have yours. Here are mine.

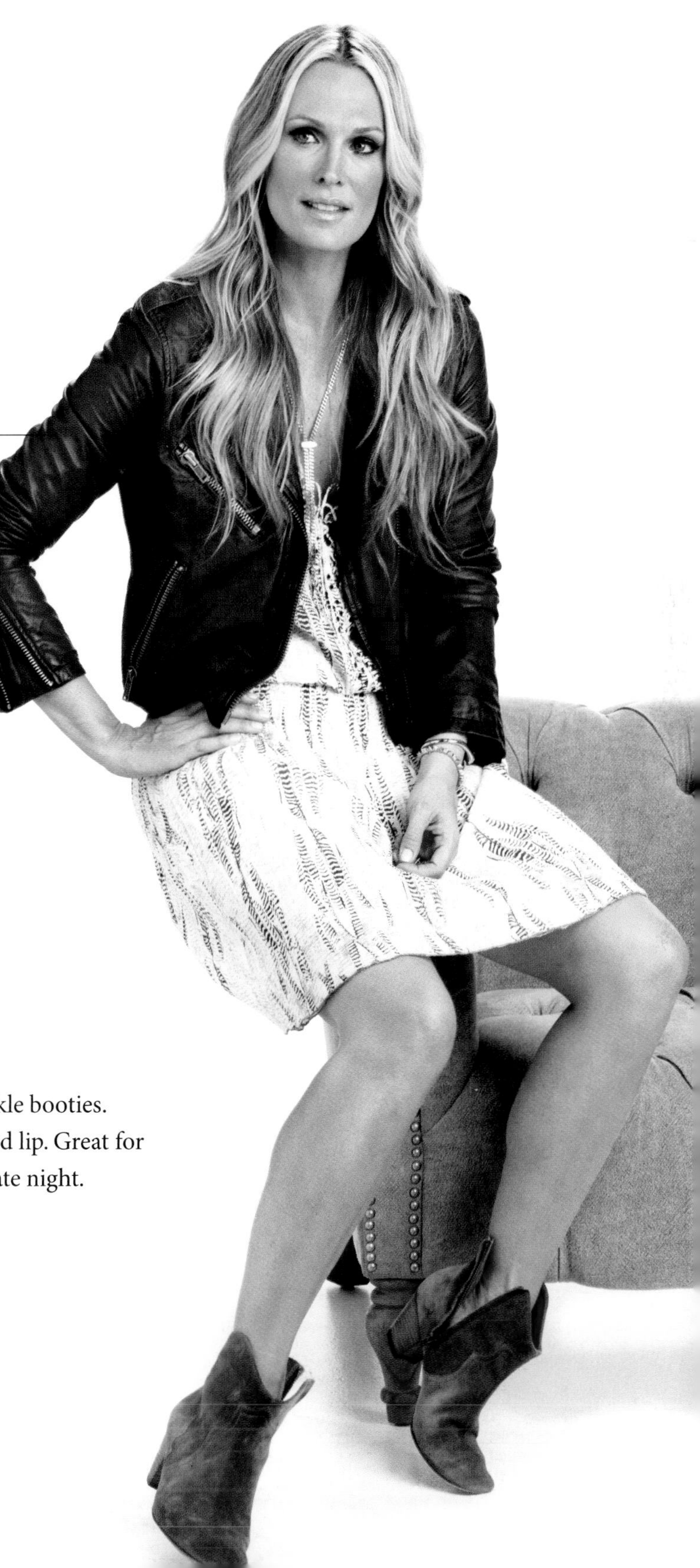

1. boyish boho

Floral dress, leather jacket, ankle booties. Give it a classic twist with a red lip. Great for lunch with friends, a casual date night.

2. city chic

Boyfriend blazer or midlength fur, fitted coat. Skinny jeans or leather leggings, and a suede bootie with some gold accessory. Love this for dinner in the city, art opening, or whenever I want to feel supermodely.

3. my "i feel hot" dress

Every woman needs that dress that makes you feel amazing. Sexy. Smart. Sophisticated. In control! And if you just aren't into dresses, then you need that suit or that something that works for you.

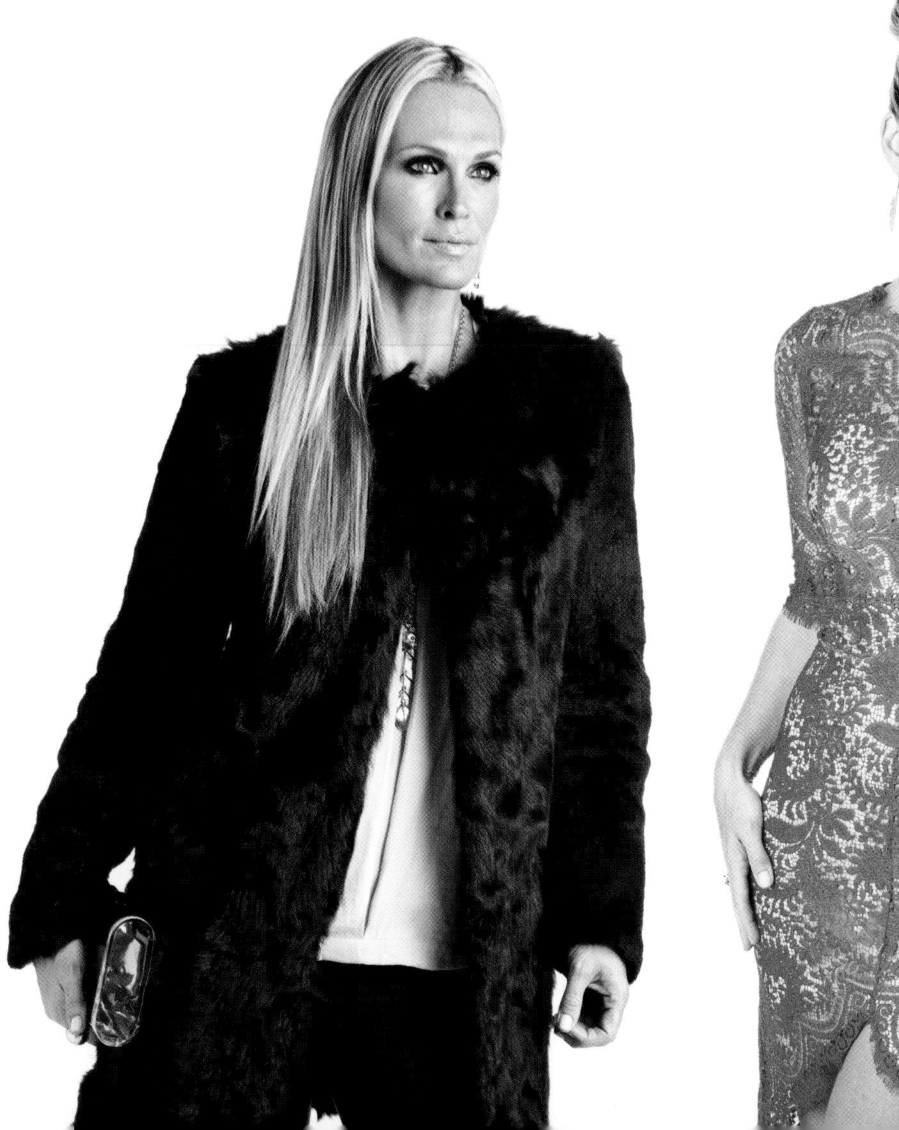

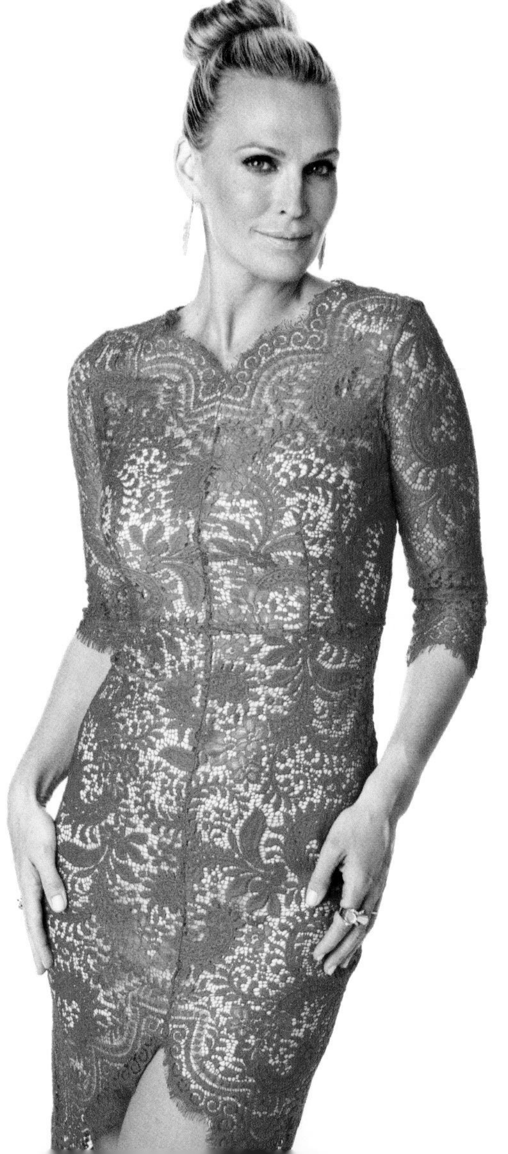

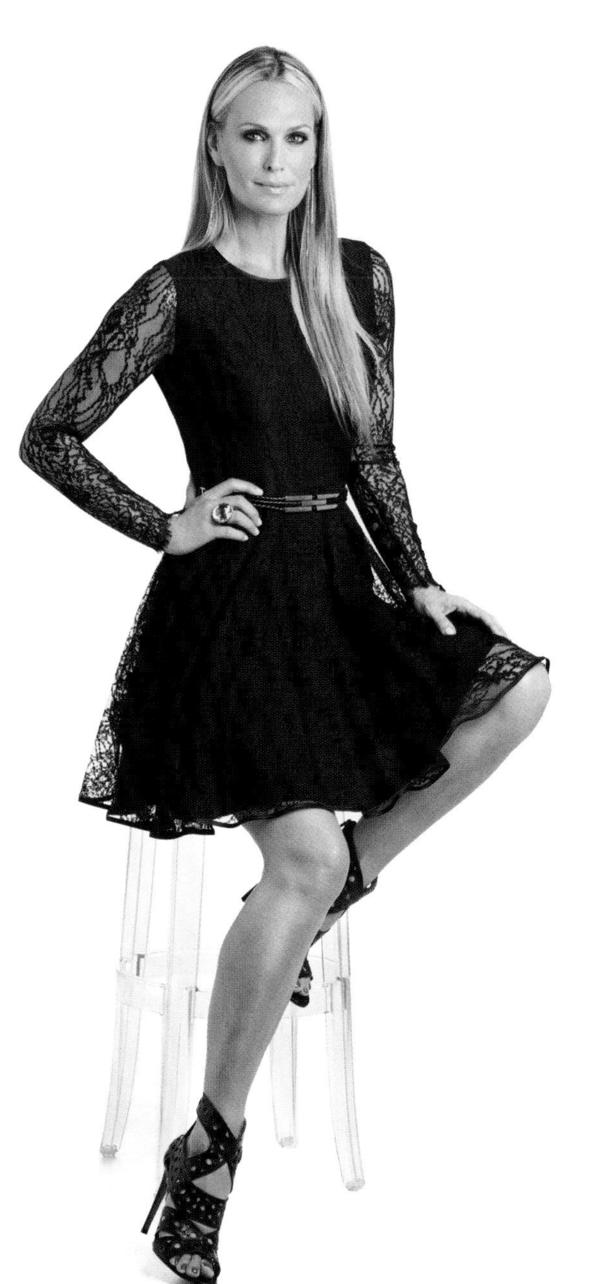

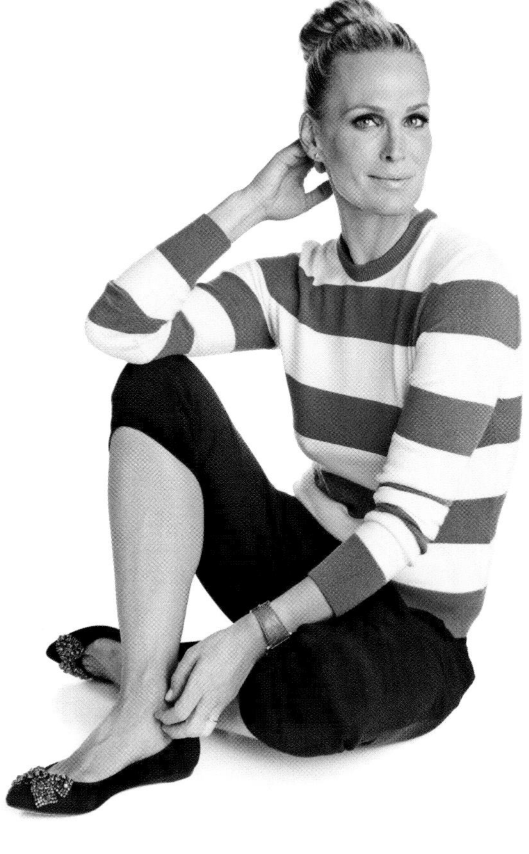

5. frenchie nautical

Striped tee, pedal pusher, ballet flats, and you are golden. This look goes anywhere. It's fresh, ageless and effortless. If you want to make it a little more rock 'n' roll—swap out the pedal pusher for a leather short. Models love the naughty nautical.

4. i love the lbd!

A definite go-to that always saves the day. It's an essential part of the *everyday supermodel* wardrobe and gets a lot of wear in mine. I've worn mine to weddings, luncheons, red carpets. It's time-tested.

pregnancy OUTFITS & THE EXPANDING WARDROBE

Some days it was a struggle to get dressed when I was pregnant. To make it easier, I mapped out my outfits in advance and had all my go-tos. When I tried to just throw something on, I'd feel (and look) terrible. Planning and preparation was key to avoid a meltdown.

what to wear When Supersized, Swollen, and Pregnant

1. **STAY OPEN TO ALL BRANDS:** In other words, you don't have to only shop maternity stores and brands. I bought a few things from the Pea & the Pod, but apart from that, I actually continued to shop regular brands. I didn't even buy those expandable preggers jeans everyone does. My legs got too big, and, frankly, jeans were the last thing on earth I wanted to wear.

2. **LONG, LAYERING TANKS:** I lived and breathed by these things. First off, I was always hot and sweaty, so I'd layer them for that—so even if I was soaked (which I likely was)—you'd never know it. Also, they were slouchy and covered my ever-expanding belly. And I love them still. Wear them all the time. Money well spent.

3. **HIPPIE SKIRTS:** My favorites were the kind that were banded at the waist, that I could pull up or down and were übercomfy on my belly. I wore this one tie-dye-patterned skirt so much I should probably burn it. They are just supercozy and soft.

4. **LONG, FITTED TANK DRESSES:** My favorites were by Rachel Pally, really soft and comfortable and perfect. Even if you are big, if you do what some women think you should do, and wear those tent dresses, you will look like a *tank*. Don't.

5. **BLAZERS OVER FITTED THINGS:** This was another go-to. I'd wear a fitted pant and tank (or a fitted tank dress) and then an oversized blazer or coat. Honestly, this somehow made me look leaner and longer and not as gigantic. A jean jacket works as long as it's not a stiff, uncomfortable one.

6. **OVERSIZED MEN'S SHIRTS:** My button-ups wouldn't fit around my little finger. So I bought oversized men's shirts and wore my husband's. I paired them with long skirts, or leggings and a cardigan.

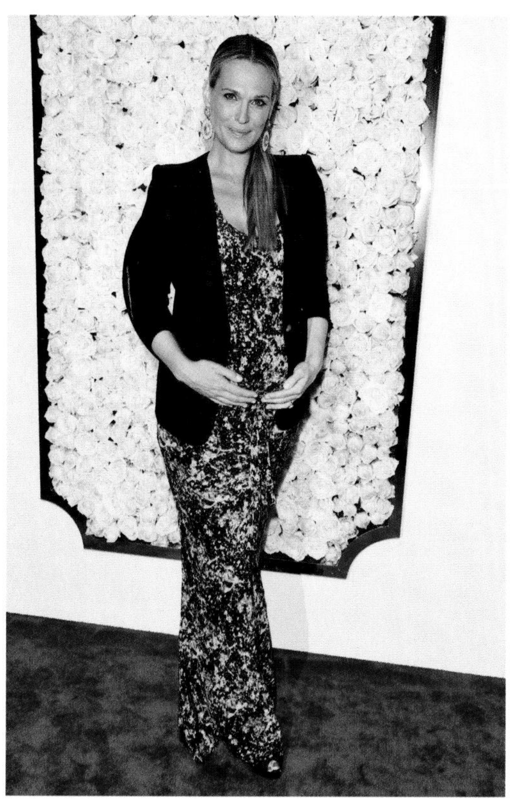

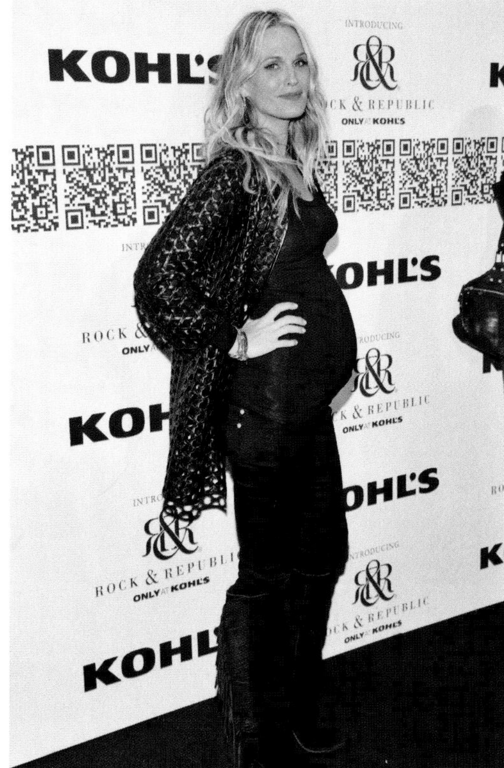

7. **MAXI DRESSES:** Basically, maxi dresses were glued to my body after month six. Dressy maxi dresses were about the only thing I'd be photographed in. They were flowy and feminine, breathable, yet still hugged my curves enough.

8. **SNUG CARDIGANS:** I must've worn my J.Crew leopard cardigan a million times. These also look great over tank dresses and with the long, hippie skirts.

9. **LEGGINGS:** Duh. No pregnant woman can live without these. I'd wear really big oversized sweaters over them—or I'd pair them with a boyfriend-style slouchy cardigan and a superlong tank underneath.

10. **BALLET FLATS & FLIP-FLOPS:** Both a must. I had a great pair of studded Havaianas and of course my Lanvin flats. I actually had to throw some of my shoes away after my pregnancy because I just wore them out. Birkenstocks are good too, adjustable to fit fat feet, and they now come in all kinds of stylish, fun looks (metalics and florals).

11. **AND LAST BUT NOT LEAST:** ALL BLACK! You can never go wrong.

the closet *edit*

If you want to get serious about being an *everyday supermodel* . . . you must closet edit. Building a core wardrobe should start with a little fashion foreplay. The Re-Stylists helped give my closet a makeover. Here's what we did and how you can do one at home.

1. CLOSET CLEAR OUT: A cluttered closet is like a cluttered mind. First, take everything out. Next, try it all on. Ditch the crap you never wear. Determine what items make it back into the closet by asking a few more questions: Is it still cool, but needs to be tailored or repaired? Is it past its freshness date (as in the white shirt or tee)?

2. WHAT TO DO WITH THE DISCARDS: Decide immediately so it doesn't sit around. Decide what to *donate* to charity, what to *gift* to friends and family, and what to *sell* or consign.

3. IDENTIFY NEEDS: This is a great time to make a list of the core 'drobe pieces, shoes, and accessories you are missing. Keep a working list in your wallet and refer to it when shopping. That way you'll be less inclined toward impulse purchases.

4. SEASONAL SWEEP: The general rule is to do it twice a year, in the spring and fall. Also, when consigning clothes, remember that shops or online sites usually buy seasonally—so summer pieces in summer, winter pieces in winter. If you have a designer coat you want to consign, save it to sell in the winter when you'll get good money for it.

hell no . . . gotta go

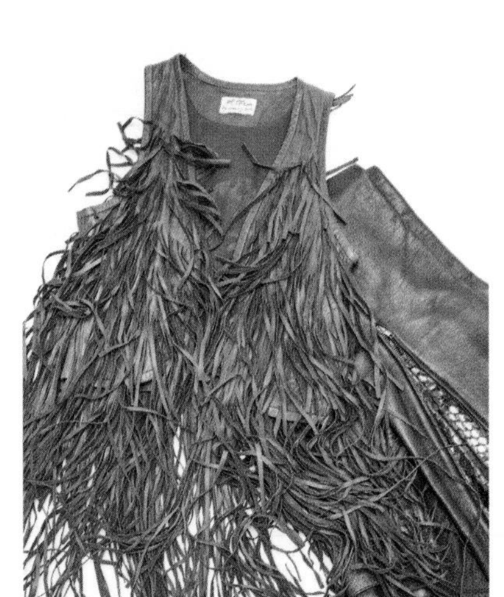

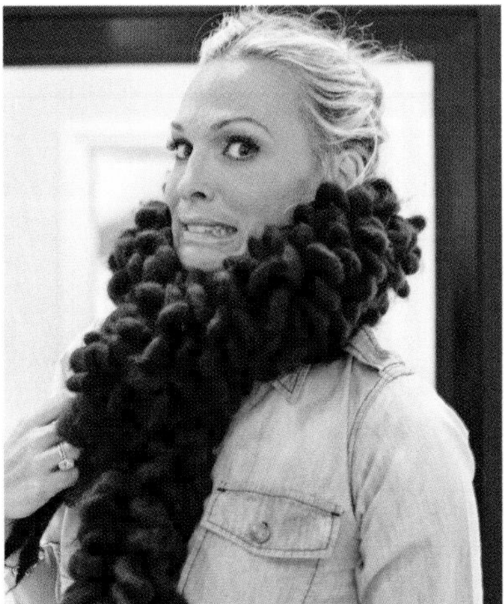

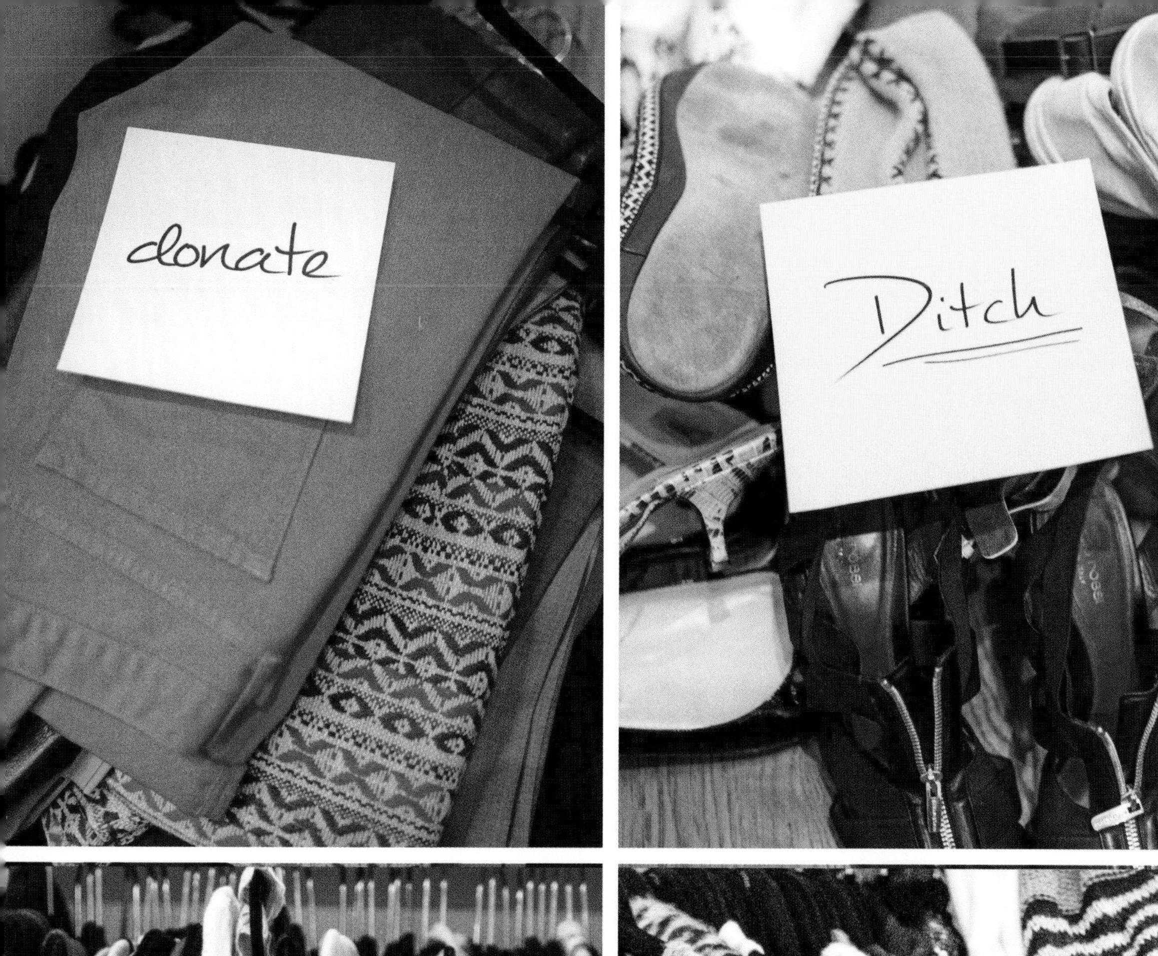
donate
Ditch

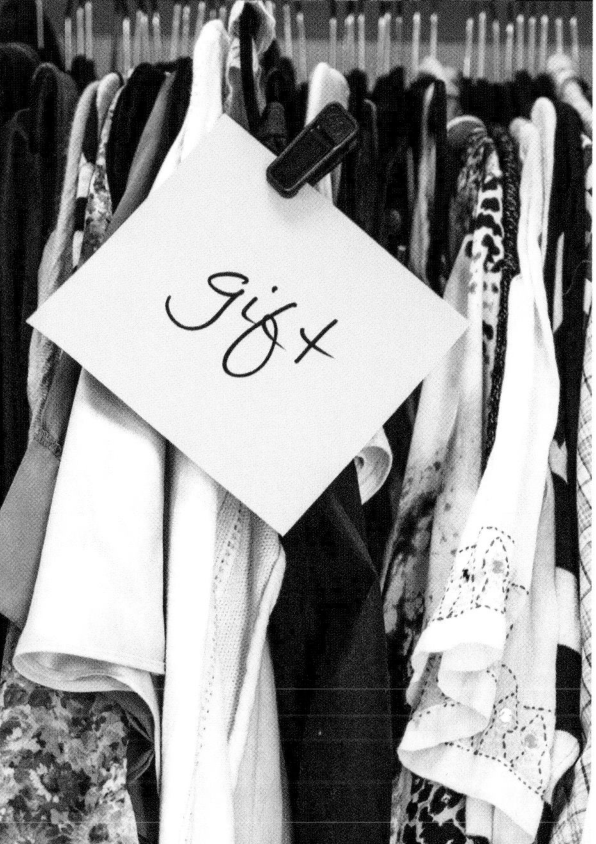
gift

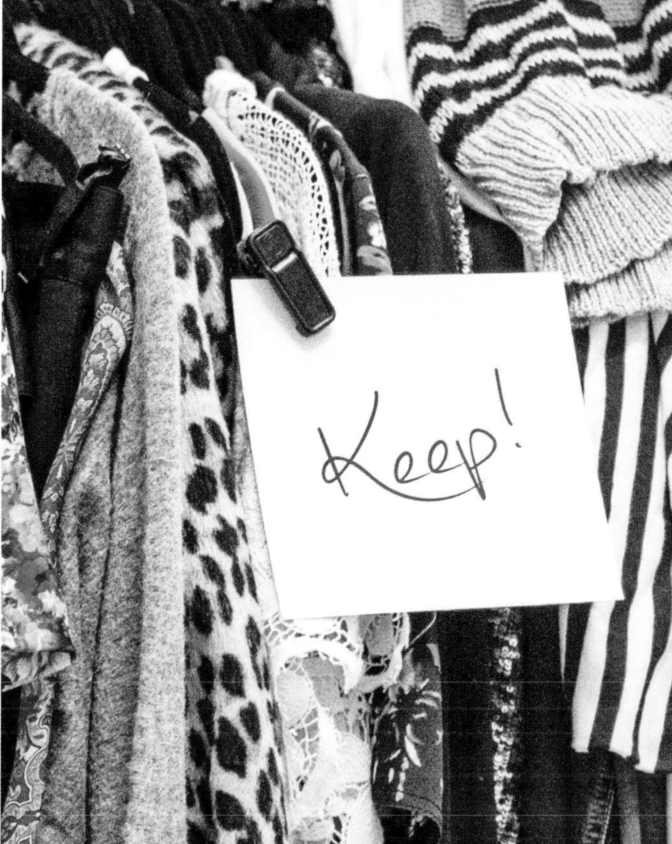
Keep!

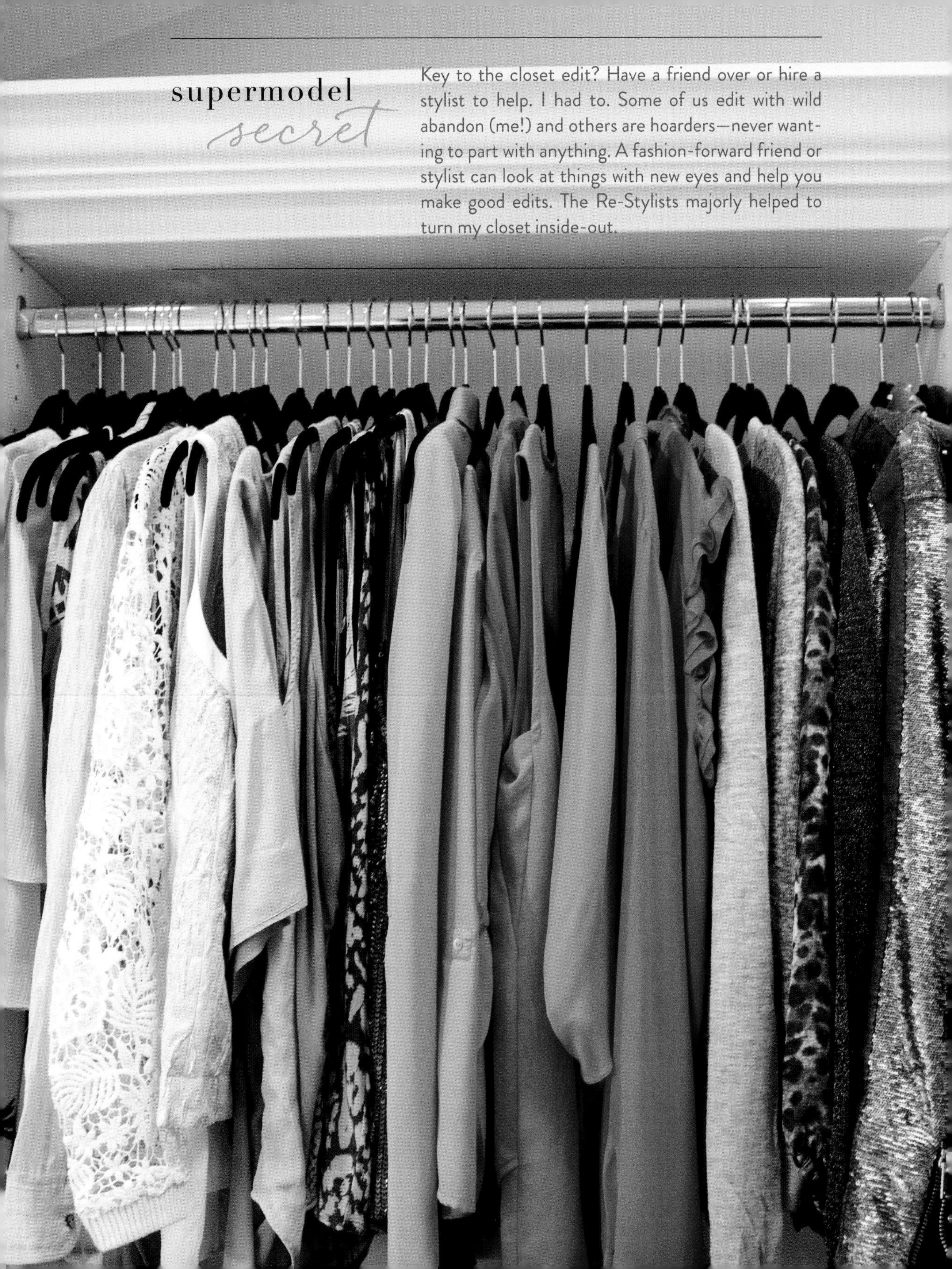

supermodel *secret*

Key to the closet edit? Have a friend over or hire a stylist to help. I had to. Some of us edit with wild abandon (me!) and others are hoarders—never wanting to part with anything. A fashion-forward friend or stylist can look at things with new eyes and help you make good edits. The Re-Stylists majorly helped to turn my closet inside-out.

Stylist Mimi Brown's *Tips* for Closet Cohesion

- CODE BY COLOR & CATEGORY: Makes your closet like a boutique or well-merchandised store. Color coding makes it easier to find things too.
- NO MORE WIRE HANGERS: The narrow velvety hangers are the bomb. Clothes stay put and won't end up in a puddle on the floor. Padded ones are good for special pieces.
- SPACE PLACE: Don't overstuff your closet. Clothes need room to breathe. Otherwise they lose shape, take on odd shapes, or wrinkle and it adds work to your morning (ironing—yuck!).
- DOS FOR DELICATES: Fold cashmere sweaters, fine wool sweaters, undies, nylons—generally anything that can snag. Place in drawers or on shelves rather than hanging. Line the drawers with embossed papers, like faux alligator, to also keep items from snagging.
- CONTAIN YOURSELF: Lucite boxes or cubbies are great for storing shoes and belts . . . you can see inside! They are also good for sunglasses, hats, gloves, and specialty pieces.
- TOUGH STUFF: Stuff bags and tall boots with tissue or loose wrapping paper so they don't lose form.
- LUXE LAUNDRY: West Elm has great lacquer bins and felt baskets for dirty laundry that look chicer than the mesh sacks you used in college.

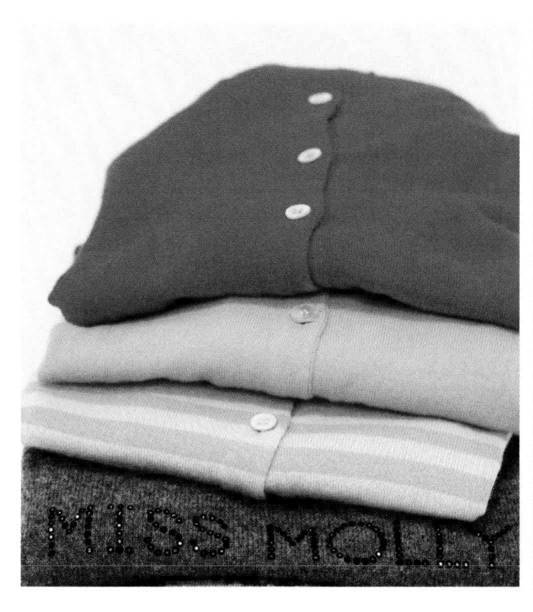

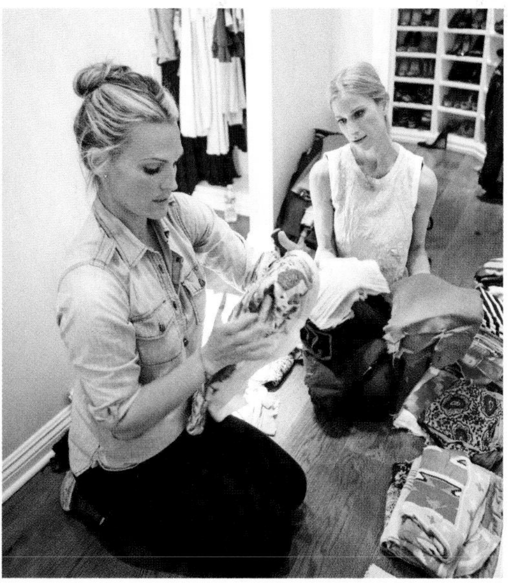

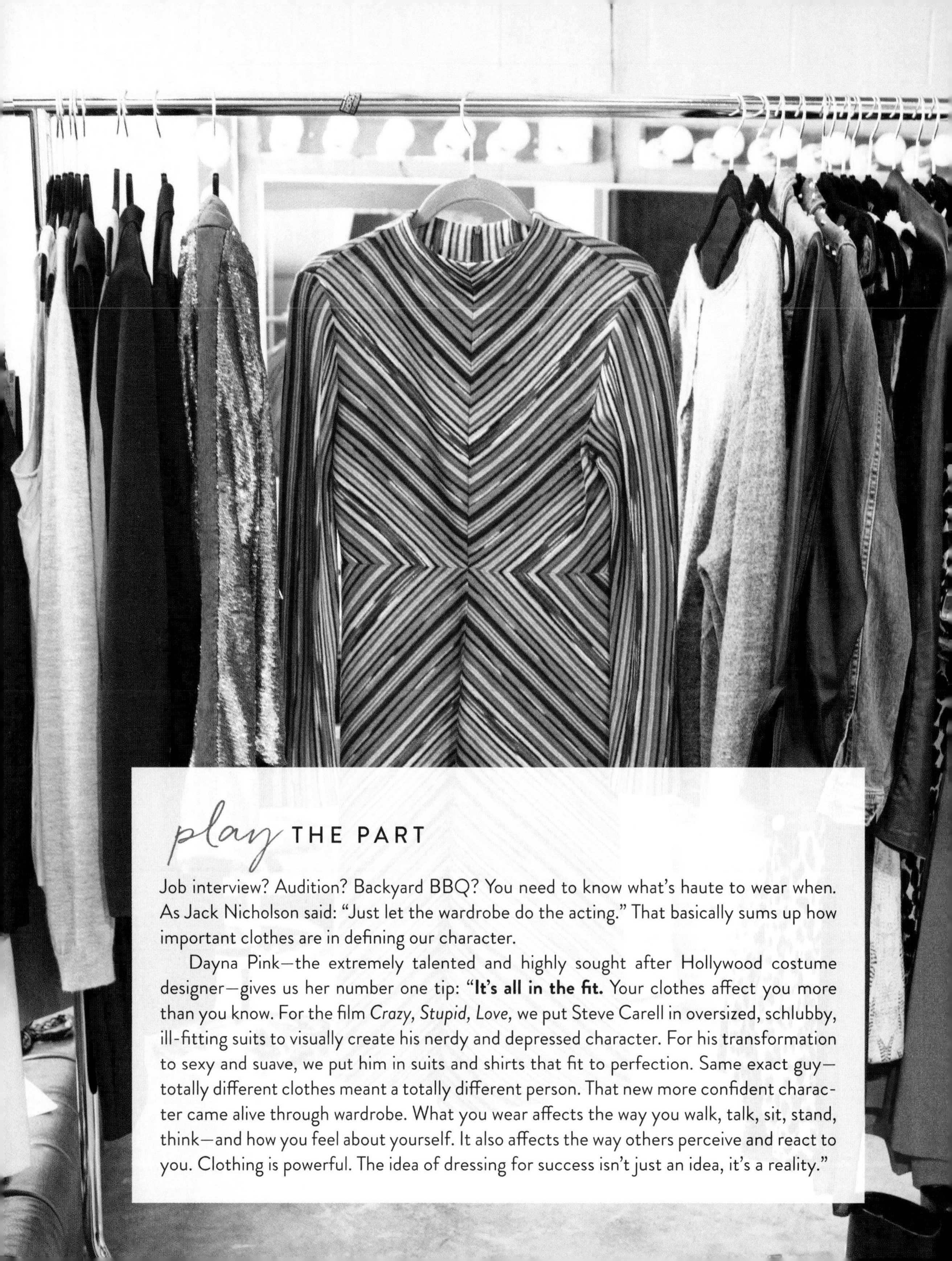

play THE PART

Job interview? Audition? Backyard BBQ? You need to know what's haute to wear when. As Jack Nicholson said: "Just let the wardrobe do the acting." That basically sums up how important clothes are in defining our character.

Dayna Pink—the extremely talented and highly sought after Hollywood costume designer—gives us her number one tip: "**It's all in the fit.** Your clothes affect you more than you know. For the film *Crazy, Stupid, Love,* we put Steve Carell in oversized, schlubby, ill-fitting suits to visually create his nerdy and depressed character. For his transformation to sexy and suave, we put him in suits and shirts that fit to perfection. Same exact guy—totally different clothes meant a totally different person. That new more confident character came alive through wardrobe. What you wear affects the way you walk, talk, sit, stand, think—and how you feel about yourself. It also affects the way others perceive and react to you. Clothing is powerful. The idea of dressing for success isn't just an idea, it's a reality."

the *everyday* supermodel
TOP 10 takeaways

1. Build your core wardrobe. Be frugal fashionistas, but don't be afraid to invest good money in those forever pieces, those pieces you wear a lot, a lot—A LOT!

2. Don't get stuck in a rut or be afraid to take chances and evolve.

3. Pay attention to the supermodel rules of the style road: almost always buy a size up, layer pieces, mix and match, and wear your clothes with attitude.

4. Rethink what sexy means. Show your stuff, but remember the rule—always hold a little bit back.

5. Cuddle up with your closet and—purge what you don't need and purchase what you do.

6. Dress to impress yourself. We are all a work in progress. Don't use your weight or your workload as an excuse.

7. Trend it like Beckham—have fun with trends, but be cautious and wise when wielding that cash.

8. Play to your strengths and always have that go-to piece, ensemble, or dress that makes you feel foxy!

9. Your tailor needs to be on speed dial. If you don't get things tailored, you need to start. It truly is the hallmark of what makes a piece of clothing look chic, sophisticated, and *expensive*.

10. It's never just about the clothes. Polish is about the total package. From hair to skin to nails to the no-scuff policy on your shoes. Always do a 360 in the mirror before you leave.

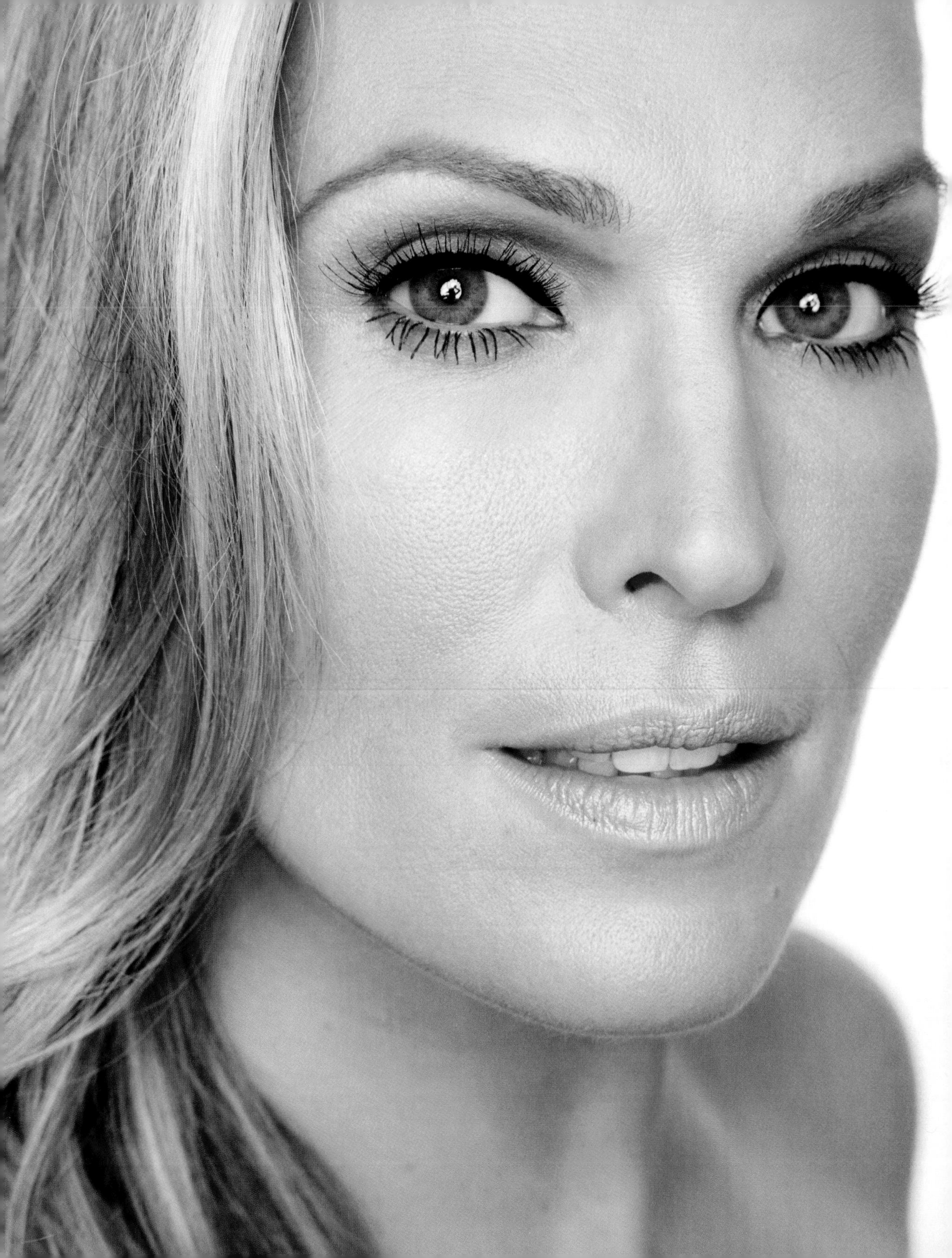

ch/4

the glow portfolio

Listen up when I tell you that I am the ultimate guinea pig—I mean it! I have tried virtually every beauty remedy out there when it comes to skin care and makeup. As a model and actress, it's part of my job to keep my hair and skin in "coming in for the close-up" shape. And for me that has not always been easy. I was not blessed with flawless skin. Quite the contrary. *My whole life I've had to fight for it*. I've been on Accutane twice for my acne. I once had a pimple so massive in the center of my cheek, it lasted three weeks. How's that for hot!?

I have struggled with acne since the age of twenty—and it does not feel good. Early on, it was a big problem when it came to my career. Back then, a blemish could get you booted off a job because there wasn't retouching or Photoshop like there is today. Retouching was expensive, so you had to show up *already* looking retouched. No pressure there. There were a few models who never had a pimple in their lives, but most of us were just normal girls with the same issues as everyone else. Not to mention, every day I worked with a different makeup artist, their brushes, their skin care, all brands of cosmetics, etc. It was a complexion nightmare. Then, and now, I do whatever it takes to get and keep my skin in shape.

As I've gotten older, I continue to face ongoing skin issues associated with life's stages and, of course, aging. During pregnancy and after, my skin was a sad sight. Pimples again. Serious melasma (it looked like someone spilled a latte all over my face!). And the lines in my forehead multiplied like Gremlins when wet (obviously I was not Botoxing). So much for the *pregnancy glow* everyone raves about. Uh-uh—not me. Who are those people anyway? The same extraterrestrials who always emerge with perfectly paired socks out of the dryer! Because of all of my issues, skin care products and treatments have become my *best friends*. And that includes cosmetics. Thank God for them!

Makeup magic has literally helped me save face throughout my career and in my everyday life more times than I can count. The day of my first-ever real TV appearance (for MTV's *House of Style*) I had a zit the size of Peru in the middle of my forehead. Seriously?! I had picked and poked at it so much, it looked like a cigarette burn. Day one on the job and I was so embarrassed. Makeup artist Monika Blunder was there to save the day and conceal it away.

And while I do love to be makeup free occasionally, most of the time I don't want to walk around with obvious blemishes and my on again/off again "pregnancy mask." Therefore, I happily rely on makeup to make me feel more like myself. Like Dolly Parton says: "Any old barn looks better with a coat of red paint." Plus, makeup is fun! It's fashion for your face. You can experiment. Get creative. And it helps bring to attention the beautiful parts of each one of us. I've been lucky to learn from the best makeup artists (and the worst of the worst). Just like there is top-shelf liquor, there are top-shelf makeup looks and techniques. Your makeup choices can make miracles *or* mayhem. They can make you look older and highlight flaws *or* . . . more youthful and flawless! There are times I don't even recognize myself in a photo because I look so good. That's magic—it's not me.

In this chapter, my beauty battalion and I give you top-shelf skin-care tips and makeup advice that will have you turning heads. You are now officially enrolled in my beauty boot camp. Consider this your Glow Portfolio.

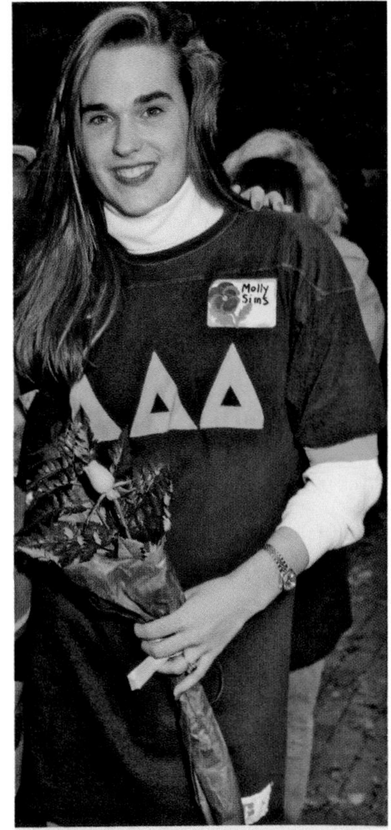

First and foremost, I'm a woman and like any other woman I have insecurities. We are all the same. I always say this, but I don't wake up looking like Cindy Crawford. There's Cindy Crawford and then there's me, Cindy. I don't always look or feel like Cindy Crawford. Cindy Crawford is two hours of hair and makeup, a stylist, the best lighting and camera angles, and so many other things that go into those images. Sometimes it's a lot of pressure being her, because I'm held up to an idealized version of myself. Fashion is a dream; it's a fantasy and I've loved being in this world. But it's not real.

—CINDY CRAWFORD, model

My Beauty *battalion*

- **DR. KARYN GROSSMAN:** Board-certified cosmetic dermatologist with more than twenty years of experience, doyenne of the dermis, my Botox banshee.
- **TRACY O'CONNOR:** Beauty biz consultant, lifestyle expert/writer, and how-to beauty video babe.
- **JOEY MAALOUF:** Rachel Zoe's and my go-to guru of glam, inspirational, sassy soul sister of style. Joey has been doing hair and makeup since he was five.
- **MONIKA BLUNDER:** Hollywood makeup artist, fellow supermomma, and makeup magician. We met on *House of Style* like a million years ago.
- **GIANPAOLO CECILIATO:** My New York–based makeup artist. He has done every runway show known to man and he is ah-makeup-azing.
- **EMESE GORMLEY:** Product whore, and my personal go-to girl for all things pretty.
- **JESSICA BERG PROSSER:** Model, makeup artist, and all-around gorgeous girl.
- **MIWA KOBAYASHI:** Celeb manicurist and genius of my toes and tips.

---

dr. karyn *counsels*

With skin-care, generally speaking, the morning is about *protection* and the evening is about *correction*. During the day, I recommend using products that protect your skin from environmental factors that cause damage, such as UV rays, pollution, and stress. You want to choose products that feature antioxidants. The evening is when you should apply products with ingredients that treat and correct specific problems, such as melasma or wrinkles. Look for formulas with corrective, wrinkle-fighting, and/or brightening agents.

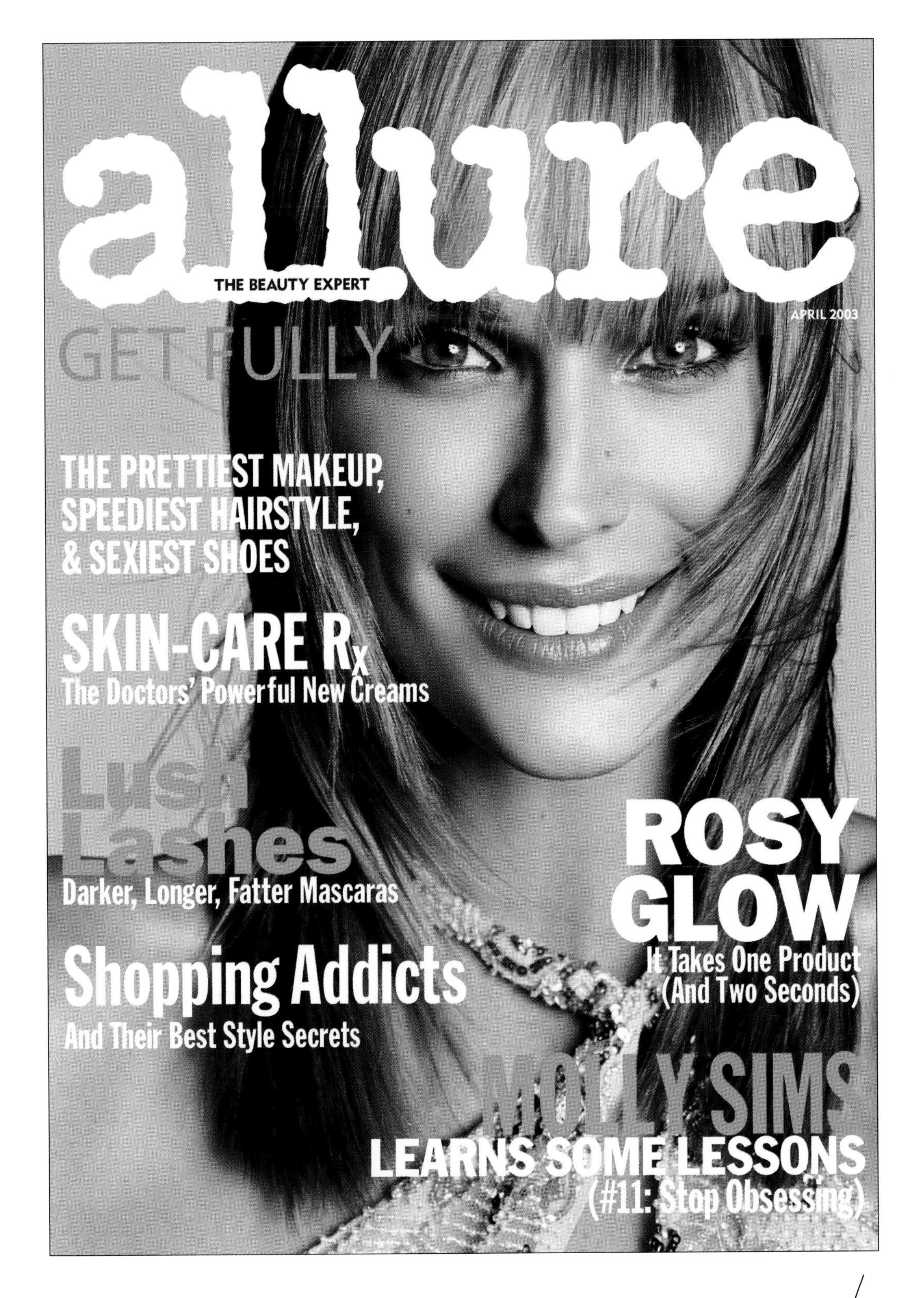
allure
THE BEAUTY EXPERT
APRIL 2003
GET FULLY
THE PRETTIEST MAKEUP, SPEEDIEST HAIRSTYLE, & SEXIEST SHOES
SKIN-CARE Rx
The Doctors' Powerful New Creams
Lush Lashes
Darker, Longer, Fatter Mascaras
Shopping Addicts
And Their Best Style Secrets
ROSY GLOW
It Takes One Product (And Two Seconds)
MOLLY SIMS
LEARNS SOME LESSONS
(#11: Stop Obsessing)

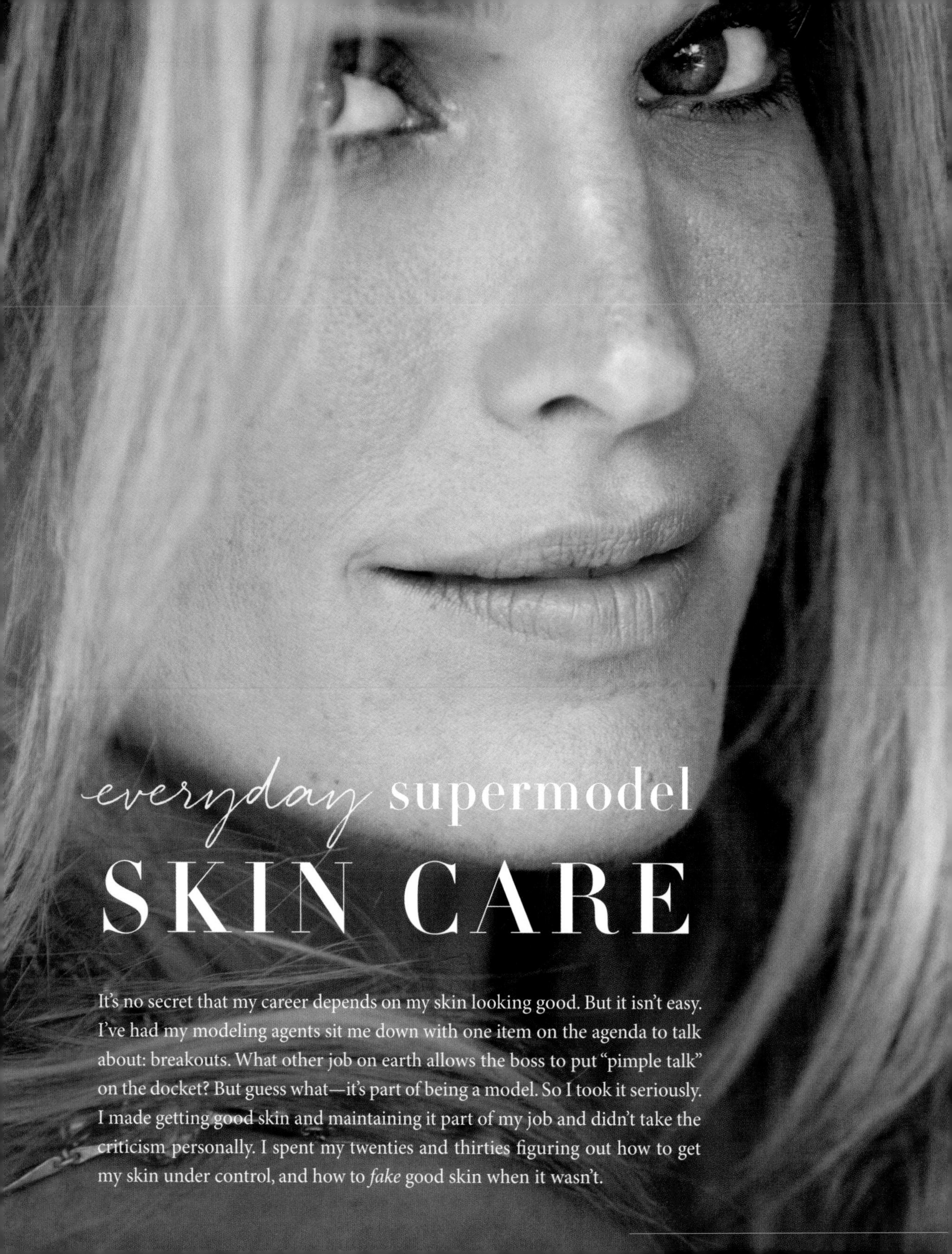

everyday supermodel SKIN CARE

It's no secret that my career depends on my skin looking good. But it isn't easy. I've had my modeling agents sit me down with one item on the agenda to talk about: breakouts. What other job on earth allows the boss to put "pimple talk" on the docket? But guess what—it's part of being a model. So I took it seriously. I made getting good skin and maintaining it part of my job and didn't take the criticism personally. I spent my twenties and thirties figuring out how to get my skin under control, and how to *fake* good skin when it wasn't.

ENROLL YOUR SKIN IN DAY (AND NIGHT) CARE: You have GOT to have a daily regimen. It makes a difference. Taking the time to spend a few minutes every morning and night will add up to younger, healthier skin. I 100 percent believe that my skin still looks young at my age because I've always taken care of it. I see dermatologists often and stay on top of new products, treatments, and technologies I will try (almost) anything as long as it's safe and the results are natural looking. Per Dr. Karyn—here is my personal regimen. Because I experience a lot of different unpleasant skin stuff, likely there is something you'll relate to.

my "Issues": Any of these sound familiar to you?

* **BREAKOUTS:** Yes. *Still.* Hormonal around jawline and occasionally small bumps on my forehead and temples. And—the occasional cyst from hell.
* **FINE LINES/WRINKLES:** Big time on my forehead and between and around my eyes.
* **MELASMA:** I started seeing it in my late twenties and have struggled with it in my thirties. It attacked with a vengeance during my pregnancy (and when you are pregnant, it's more difficult to treat).
* **DARK CIRCLES/PUFFINESS:** Who doesn't deal with this under-eye dilemma? Started in my thirties.
* **ECZEMA:** Occasional eczema on my body, small patches. My baby boy, Brooks, has it too. Sad face. It's often linked to genetics.

my Daily Routine:

MORNING

* **CLEANSE:** The Ultra Gentle Cleanser by Karyn Grossman. It doesn't strip and dry out my skin, but it does gently clean away impurities. Cetaphil is also good and you can find it at most drugstores. Never use a cleanser with harsh detergents—even if you are superoily. Believe it or not, oil-based cleansers are excellent for sensitive and dry skin types. I'm a fan of the Treatment Cleansing Oil by AmorePacific.
* **BRIGHTEN:** SkinCeuticals Phytocorrective Gel. It's the bomb for brightening. I had a pregnancy "mustache" that rivaled Magnum P.I., so

Dr. Karyn put me on this to help lighten my skin discoloration. It doesn't work overnight, but all the ingredients are natural and chemical-free so it's a brightening agent safe to use during pregnancy and breast-feeding.

- **HYDRATE:** SkinCeuticals B5 Gel. This antiaging serum is packed with hyaluronic acid and vitamins. It contains antioxidants that protect from free radicals (which age our skin). Another option, natural aloe vera gel is an affordable, low-tech way to hydrate your skin. Rodin Oil is also a favorite serum that gives skin instant glamour and glow.
- **MOISTURIZE:** Epicuren Colostrum Cream. Ah, true love. It soaks right in, doesn't feel greasy, and leaves my complexion soft, creamy and smooth as a baby's bum.
- **SUNSCREEN:** EltaMD Sunscreen SPF 50. Every day, without fail, I apply it. If you are prone to blemishes like me, this is hands-down the best sunscreen. Native Maui also formulates beautiful, organic and chemical-free sunscreens ideal for sensitive-skin. I love their Glow Potion SPF 45 and the Kid's Organic Spray SPF 45 (so easy to use!) on baby Brooks. When choosing a sunscreen, always look for broad spectrum. And—don't forget to wear dark sunglasses to protect your eyes from solar damage (and crow's-feet!). C'mon, people.

EVENING

- **CLEANSE:** DNA Health Institute MediClear Skin Lightening Wash. It has brightening agents that gently cleanse and treat the skin at the same time.
- **EXFOLIATE:** Two to three times a week. The GlamGlow Mud Mask is so good! It tingles, stimulates circulation and vacuums all the crap right out of my pores. Look for masks with kaolin clay; they are divine for detoxing and softening your skin. Other fave exfoliants and detoxers include Bliss Pore Perfecting Facial Polish, Clearasil Rapid Action Face Scrub, and Kiehl's Rare Earth Cleansing Mask.

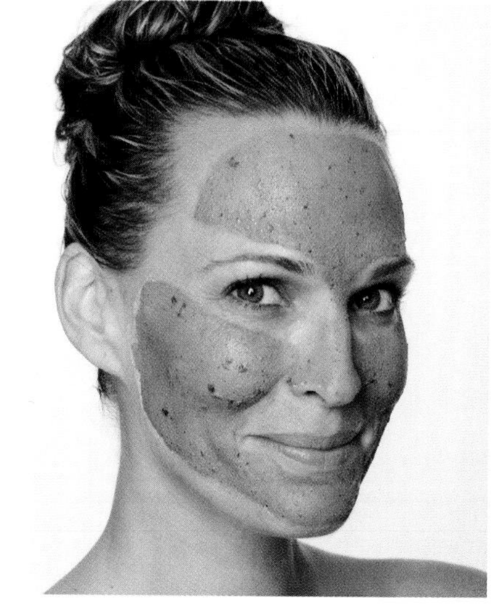

- **HYDRATE/BRIGHTEN:** SkinCeuticals Phyto Corrective Gel. It hydrates and brightens. Love it. Kiehl's Midnight Recovery Serum is another lovely evening serum. It has healing oils and calming aromatherapeutic benefits for enhanced sleep.
- **MOISTURIZE:** Pro+ Therapy MD Advanced Ultra Rich Night Repair. I slather this on my skin at night and wake up in the morning and almost don't feel like I need to apply a morning moisturizer. It contains peptides (proven collagen boosters) and other antiwrinkle agents. Some nights I also use Kiehl's Ultra Facial Cream. Just a clean, simple, supermoisturizer.
- **EYE CREAM:** Natura Bissé Diamond Eye, pricey but worth it. I use it a few times a week. My friend Emese swears by Giorgio Armani Regenessence; she says it's a lifesaver. First Aid Beauty Eye Duty Triple Remedy treats dark circles, lines and puffiness, and even slightly covers then with a tinted formula. Thank you! Note: Never apply any eye product too close to your actual eye, the tiny vessels will pull product into the mucus membrane and then, bad news . . . itchy, irritated eyeballs!
- **SPOT TREATMENT:** Epiduo prescription blemish cream is great to dab on pimples. For a good over the counter, look for something with 5% benzoyl peroxide. Don't put any spot treatment all over your face—just where you need it. A dab of prescription Retin-A microgel also works well when dotted on breakouts.

WHAT ELSE?

- **SKIN-SCRIPTIONS:** Daily prenatal supplements. I've taken them religiously since I turned thirty for all kinds of reasons. They are excellent for healthy skin, hair, and nails. They work. I take a prescription version that also has a fish oil supplement. New Chapter makes a good over-the-counter one. It takes a month or two to see results. I also believe in taking a little added zinc if my skin is breaking out.
- **SPECIALTY SKIN-CARE SAVIORS:** *Healing Cream:* I often use Traumeel on elbows, feet, or anywhere I've got dry patches. It's a homeopathic cream for very dry skin and can help soothe eczema. *Do-It-All Balm:* Egyptian Magic should be called the Do-It-All-BOMB! It's got honey, olive oil, bee pollen—and is simply delish for skin of all types. Sometimes I just smother it everywhere and call it a day. You can put

it anywhere. Well, almost anywhere—and not on your face if you are acne-prone. *Sunburn Relief*: Biafine Cream is French and a home run for calming sunburns, rashes, and irritations.

- **AT-HOME SPA FACIAL:** There's nothing an at-home facial can't fix. You get to do it on your own time and don't have to squeeze it in during business hours. Light a candle, take a bath (add a few drops of lavender or eucalyptus oil), put on Enya, and a series of face masks. It's the perfect treat to do when pregnant or on "house arrest" with your newborn baby.

---

supermodel *secret*

While we all love Thanksgiving, *nobody* likes turkey neck. So just a reminder! Moisturize your neck and chest—and while we are at it—your hands! Skin here is thinner and more sensitive, so you don't need anything too active or fancy, simple is better. A moisturizing sunscreen is a good option to carry in your purse, and have hand lotion next to your sinks at home. Always moisturize after washing your hands.

"THE MELASMA MONOLOGUES": Ugh. Melasma. Even the word itself is horrible. It's a tricky skin condition—and has been my dermatological nightmare for a decade. It results in excess melanin production and usually shows up in the form of brownish symmetrical patterns, spots or splotches on the face. Derms believe it's hereditary and triggered by heat, sun exposure, and hormonal fluctuations (the reason it's often referred to as "the pregnancy mask"). Once you have melasma, it's very difficult to entirely "kick." I've tried it all, but so far nothing works to eradicate it for good, so rather it's about keeping it as under control as possible. I do that via my daily skin-care regimen listed above, and doing a serious "antimelasma" topical program once or twice a year. I use a prescription intensive depigmentation cream for eight weeks, alternating nights, under my derm's supervision. The main ingredients are Retin-A, hydrocortisone, and hydroquinone. (Despite the controversy, most dermatologists agree that hydroquinone is safe in small doses.) It wipes out my spots by 90 percent. A dermatologist can compound a customized cream like this for you. Prescription Tri-Luma and Obagi products are also known to work. Just recently, I did the DermaCeutic program with Dr. Fusco and Dr. Wexler. A brightening mask (formulated with a combination of acids and anti-oxidants) is applied in-office, left on for eight hours during the day, and then washed off. I then use the DermaCeutic daily product regimen for 30 days. So far, my skin has never looked better. Cosmelan is a natural and effective clinical depigmentation treatment done with a dermatologist that requires no downtime (a great option for those looking for quicker results). Important—beware any type of laser treatments as certain ones can often make melasma worse (case in point: IPL). And when doing any kind of intense depigmentation program: Stay out of the sun!

BEAUTY *simplified*

Now on those days or nights when you just can't be bothered, or you are traveling and don't want to tote all the above products around, here are your *bare skin essentials.*

cleanse: Use a gentle, oil-based cleanser that cleans and hydrates at the same time, or if really in a hurry, a facial cleansing wipe. Comodynes brand are makeup artists' on-set staples. They get the makeup off (yes, even eye makeup) and are sensitive-skin friendly. Pond's towelettes work in a pinch too. (Truth be told, I keep them bedside for when I'm too tired to do anything else.)

treat: Find an effective multitasking product to address your main issues. For example, if you are acne prone and aging, SkinCeuticals Retexturing Activator treats both congestion and fine lines! If you are dry and dehydrated, use a nourishing serum like Replenishing Nutrient Complex by Tata Harper, which is like a multivitamin for the skin.

moisturize: If it's daytime, find an effective moisturizer that gives good glow and protects from UV damage. For that, Native Maui skin-care/sunscreen combos are great. If it's evening, look for something that will moisturize and repair. If you aren't acne prone, Egyptian Magic is *magic.*

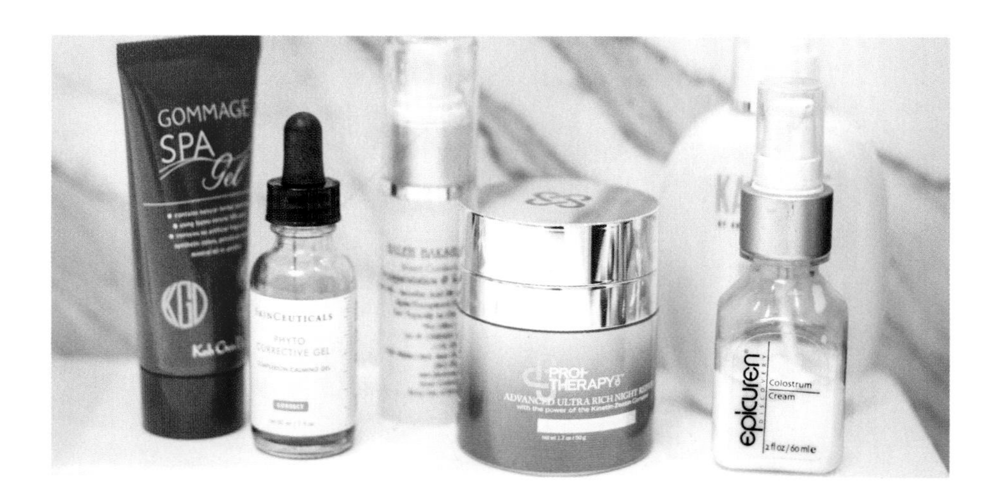

dr. karyn *counsels*

1. **Does our skin get used to skin-care products, causing them to stop working?** Well, yes and no. Products don't stop working, but our skin does plateau. If you are using a product for spots or wrinkles and you see improvement, but then over time, it appears to stop working, it's really just that your skin has improved as much as it's going to with that particular product and formulation of ingredients. It's a good idea to rotate skin-care products and have a few to switch in and out and consult your dermatologist if you are no longer seeing results.
2. **Do expensive skin-care products really perform better than those at drugstores?** Here's the truth: The FDA does not regulate cosmetics and over-the-counter creams the way it does prescription products. So even if the manufacturers claim the key ingredients in pricy products are expensive and effective, the formula is proprietary, and there isn't really any way to know how much of that ingredient is actually in there. Also, over-the-counter cosmetic products don't have to undergo rigorous clinical studies like prescription creams do, so we as consumers have to rely on the manufacturers' claims, and again, their claims aren't strictly regulated. The only way to really know if something works, expensive or inexpensive, is to read direct consumer reviews and to try the product out for yourself.
3. **When it comes to skin-care products and treatments, where should you invest your money?** The solution is really different for everyone, because it depends on what your core issues are. If you struggle with spots and melasma, they can be effectively treated with over-the-counter topical products and treatments. If your problem is deep under-eye circles and bags, you can spend all the money in the world on products, but the real solutions will be injectable treatments and fillers. Talk to a cosmetic dermatologist about your budget, and he or she can help plan the best program for your budget and maximize your investment. One thing is for sure—don't buy a bunch of products and use them all at once. You should only introduce a new product or two at a time to your skin. Otherwise both your skin, and your wallet, are likely to freak out.

skin services

WHAT I'VE *tried* AND KNOW *works*

I see several dermatologists for their unique specialties. One thing I'm always doing is asking them what is new in the skin-care world. Like most women, I want to know about things that will prevent lines and wrinkles and correct them, especially treatments that can be done in the morning (no knife needed!) and make my skin look younger by that night. Who doesn't love instant gratification? I'm up for giving most things a shot, as long as it's not too uncomfortable or the effect is unnatural.

I also get the scoop on skin services that have worked for other actresses and models. If someone looks better than she did the year *before,* I will go to the end of the earth to find out what she did. (Because I know she's done *something.*) With the help of my sources and superderm Dr. Karyn, I've done all the work for you—here is what really works.

---

supermodel *secret*

To Botox or not to Botox is not the question for me. *How, where, and when to Botox is.* When I was thirty-two, Dr. Karyn sat me down and said to me, verbatim: you NEED Botox. By the time I was thirty, my forehead had more lines on it than a football field. I am just very "expression-y"! So, ever since then, I've gotten Botox every three to six months like clockwork (with exception to when I was pregnant). Boyfriends/spouses/significant others can be funny about Botox, I know. My husband used to tell me not to do it, but he's come around. (I still kind of keep it a secret—a girl's gotta have some mystery.) The key is subtlety/not freezer face. And for those who are Botox averse, more power to you! A few lines add character. More than that? I'll leave that to Dame Judi Dench, thank you.

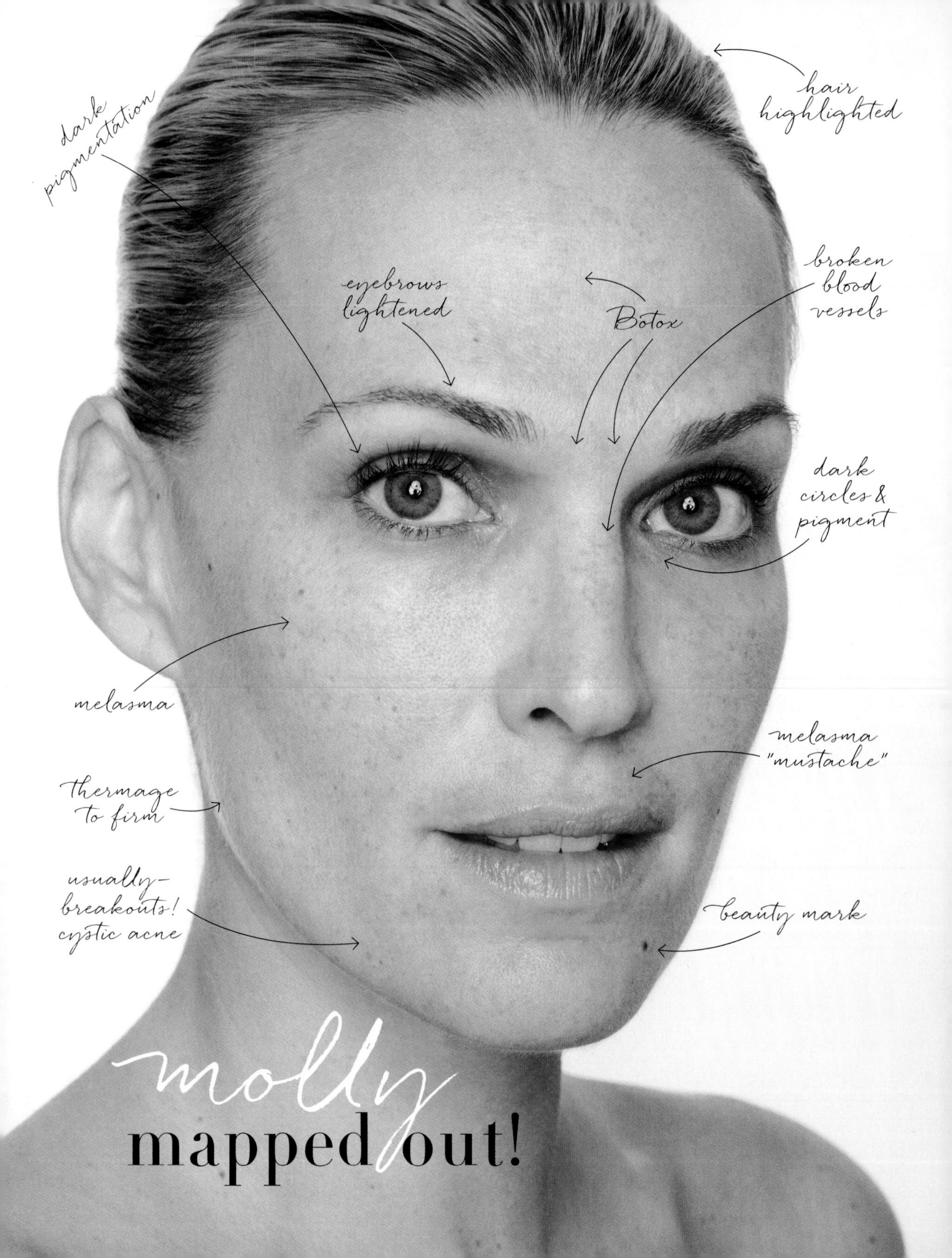
dark pigmentation
hair highlighted
eyebrows lightened
Botox
broken blood vessels
dark circles & pigment
melasma
melasma "mustache"
thermage to firm
usually- breakouts! cystic acne
beauty mark
molly
mapped out!

worth the Green and Part Time-Machine!

Magazines these days seem to recommend every cosmetic treatment out there. It can be really confusing to wade through it all. Here, Dr. Karyn and I focus on our favorites that deliver healthy skin and turn back the clock.

1. **PEELS:** There are a variety of effective peel options out there that address discoloration, wrinkles, acne scarring, and fine-to-deep lines. Dr. Karyn loves a low-concentration TCA peel (10%–20%) a few times a year. It's excellent to brighten superficial discoloration and instantly gives the skin a taut, smooth complexion. Low-concentration chemical peels are even okay to do the morning of an event to tighten and firm skin.

2. **THERMAGE:** Dermatologists use this radiofrequency device to heat the skin and encourage collagen and elastin production. Results are tighter, tauter, firmer skin and jawline. I loved my results! So far, I've done four treatments. There's no downtime (maybe minor swelling/redness); the effect is immediate and gets even better over time. They definitely take a few years off your age. Dr. Karyn recommends Thermage treatments be done in a series of two to four, spaced about six weeks apart.

3. **FRAXEL:** Fraxel involves a gently ablative laser treatment that helps to improve skin texture and tone. It's a little uncomfortable, but highly effective for reducing sun spots, sometimes melasma, and even acne scarring and pitting. It can help to shrink the appearance of pores too, which is a bonus. In general, it smoothes skin, delivers a collagen boost and reduction in fine lines. Depending on the intensity level, Fraxel can require a little downtime. Depending on your skin type, Fraxel is also most effective in a series of two or three treatments spaced about a month apart.

4. **LASERS:** There are a lot of different kinds of laser treatments out there. Depending on the wavelength of the laser, they can be effective for a variety of skin concerns. Lasers can treat acne and some scarring, shallow wrinkles, fine lines, and feathering around the eyes and lips. Talk to your dermatologist about the laser treatments he or she offers and if they are right for you. Some lasers require downtime, some you can do on your lunch break!

5. **BOTOX, OBVIOUSLY:** Botox wouldn't be one of the most popular cosmetic procedure if it wasn't doing something good. It's effective for softening forehead lines, tightening mild sagging around the jaw, and it can be used to treat a too-gummy smile. Go to a professional—not to a strip-mall or your friend's living room—and get it done right. In the hands

of an experienced dermatologist, Botox can be used off label for serious antiaging.

6. **FILLERS:** These do what products and lasers can't. Simply put—they are injected and therefore can go deeper. Juvéderm is a safe and natural looking, hyaluronic-acid-based filler. Dr. Karyn likes it for laugh lines, thin lips and lip lines, and under the eyes. It "fills in" where you've deflated. In the right hands, it's so natural looking, no one has to know. Be judicious, too much in the cheeks or under the eyes and *hellooo* Alvin, Simon, and Theodore. Botero is a new filler. Dr. Karyn has been using it successfully to fill deeper lines, including forehead wrinkles.

7. **LIGHT THERAPIES:** Intense pulsed light (IPL) or red photodynamic therapy is a treatment effective for sun damage, brown spots, broken capillaries, fine lines, and redness. It usually requires a series of treatments for best results and requires no real downtime. Unfortunately, IPL is not recommended for melasma (and could *make it worse* . . . beware if that's you!), and doesn't address skin sagging or deep wrinkles. Blue light therapy is effective for acne and helps kill specific bacteria associated with breakouts—also recommended in a series.

8. **AT-HOME TECHNOLOGIES:** Today, more and more technology is at our fingertips, even when it comes to skin-care. Silk'n makes safe, effective, and FDA approved at-home light therapy and hair removal devices. According to the American Academy of Dermatology, such devices do yield comparable results, but may take a bit more time to work. Myotone is a facial microcurrent device for home use that we love for lifting and toning the skin.

Chemical peels are a great way to improve your skin because they treat a variety of conditions, are customizable, and are generally affordable. Talk to your dermatologist about your concerns, your budget, and your work schedule, and you can create a peel plan that will improve the quality of your skin. If you can't sacrifice time off, you can plan to do a series of lighter peels more often that don't require downtime. After a peel, it's good to maintain the result by using products that continue to stimulate cellular turnover. By doing that, you will continue to see improvement.

—DR. HALEH BAKSHANDEH, dermatologist

---

supermodel *secret*

For a quick fix before a special event, I'll always do under-eye moisturizing and firming strips. Even if the effect is temporary, it works to calm, tighten, and brighten the eye area. A little tip: put them in the fridge before you use them. The cooling effect will help further reduce puffiness and swelling. (Green Tea Eyes by ToGoSpa are like a drink for your under-eyes!). Sleep-deprived mommas, take note.

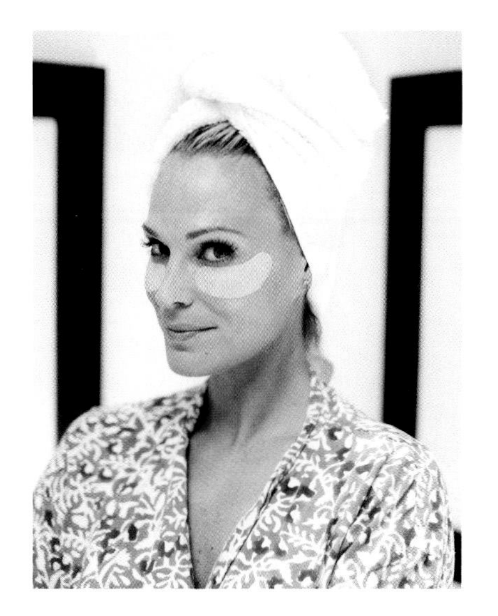

How to Find the *right* Skin-Care Doc?

Be a derm detective!

1. **CHECK CREDENTIALS:** Make ABSOLUTELY sure your doctor is board certified—and is a dermatologist, a plastic surgeon, or a facial plastic surgeon. Dentists and pediatricians are doing Botox these days! Be aware.

2. **NUMBER CRUNCH:** You want someone with a good amount of experience in cosmetic treatments. Find out how many years your doc has been working in his or her field. And if you are thinking about doing a peel or injections or any of the treatments I listed, confirm that these services are the specialties of the doctor you select.

3. **SCOUT THEIR WORK:** Ask to see the before/after pictures of patients they have *actually worked on*—not just stock images the manufacturers provide them.

4. **DON'T DISCOUNT-DOCTOR HOP:** Whatever treatment you choose, your physician will chart it and create a medical record for you. For example, if you're getting Botox, she'll chart your dosage every time you go in, making sure the *cumulative* dosage is safe. When you bounce around from practice to practice or doctor to doctor, responding to the best deals in your in-box, you won't get the benefit of long-term records. This makes for a risky result, even if you do save a few bucks.

HOW TO GET THE L.A. *polish*

British beauty journalist Newby Hands wrote an article about how and why women look so flawless in L.A. and I loved it. She specifically cited how a few British actresses arrived to L.A. from the U.K. as rather ordinary "pretty girls" and after a few years in Hollywood, transformed into certifiable movie stars. She called it the "L.A. Polish." Well, I know how they did it.

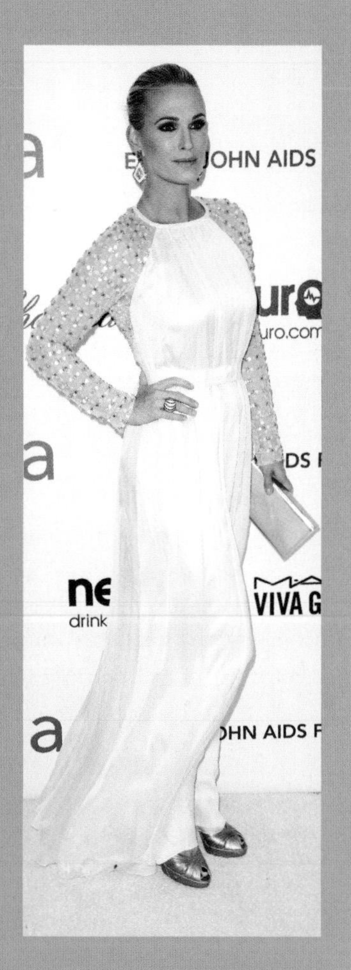

1. START EARLY: The best defense (to acne, aging, and the like) is a good offense. This is the *Hollywood way*. Back in the day, it was a face-lift at fifty. Today, everyone starts young. Now, that doesn't mean you need to obsess over wrinkles as a tween. And that doesn't mean that if you are fifty and haven't done anything, you are a lost cause. There are natural-looking solutions even if you've waited to start a beauty plan. It's just more work that way.
2. THINK IN 3-D: As Dr. Karyn says, it's never about just one thing. Using a multi-dimensional approach will present the best and most natural results. Here is your three-pronged attack:
   - Products: Having a daily regimen does improve the present state of the skin, prevent new issues from forming and help correct issues leftover from the past.
   - Treatments/Procedures: Will correct and address problems that emerge as we get older that topical products cannot treat.
   - Diet/Lifestyle: Staying healthy and active will also work to keep aging and other skin-related issues at bay.

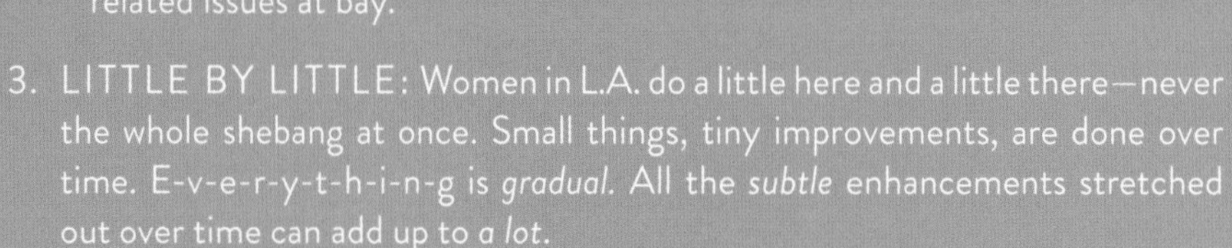

3. LITTLE BY LITTLE: Women in L.A. do a little here and a little there—never the whole shebang at once. Small things, tiny improvements, are done over time. E-v-e-r-y-t-h-i-n-g is *gradual.* All the *subtle* enhancements stretched out over time can add up to *a lot*.

THAT is the L.A. Polish.

supermodel *secret*

MY THOUGHTS ON SURGERY.

We've all watched people in the spotlight go overboard and willy-nilly with plastic surgery. To be clear, I am not a surgery advocate nor am I antisurgery; I honestly believe it's a very personal issue. We need to embrace and accept ourselves for who we are—but if who we are wants to make a change, we should also accept that person too. My momma chose to have a little nip/tuck and she looks and feels fabulous! Nip/tuck or not, my momma is a beautiful woman inside and out. Bottom line: If something about your appearance is truly standing in the way of your self-confidence, then why not correct it and move on if that's what it takes?

skin-care by decade: *dos & dont's*

teens

Runway *dos!*

* START A REGIMEN: Cleanse and moisturize in the A.M. and P.M. Wear a broad spectrum sunscreen daily, at least an SPF 30. Pack it in your school bag, especially if you play sports outside, so you can reapply. Always wash your face after gym or sports.
* ZIT ZAP: For the blemish prone, consider a salicylic-acid-based cleanser, and an organic/non-comedogenice/simple moisturizer. One with a low dose of benzoyl peroxide works too. If you do have acne, get on top of it. Ask your parents to see a dermatologist to set up a personalized acne-punishing plan.

Run-the-other-way *dont's!*

* DON'T SCRUB-A-DUB-DUB! Contrary to popular teenage belief, for those with acne, scrubbing your skin a million times a day will not help. It will disturb the natural pH balance of your skin. And do NOT use alcohol (or Listerine or toothpaste, for that matter) on pimples either—

they can burn the skin. Finally: Do. Not. Pick!! It can lead to scars later. And most of the time, say no to cortisone injections for cystic acne. Use these with extreme caution as cortisone can eventually break down proteins in the skin, leaving a crater in its place.

twenties

Runway *dos!*

- START TO EXFOLIATE: Cell turnover slows once we get into our mid to late twenties. Exfoliation speeds the process. Start to incorporate lightweight antiaging ingredients into your regimen. A hyaluronic acid serum, like SkinCeuticals Hydrating B5 Gel, is great.
- PRACTICE SAFE SUNSCREEN: I really didn't wear sunscreen in my twenties and I tanned a lot (one of the reasons I suffer with melasma), so learn from Molly's mistakes! Always. Wear. Sunscreen. Hands down, daily use of a broad spectrum SPF is the number one preventative antiaging method.
- TREATMENT TALK: Get a good referral and start to see a facialist or a dermatologist occasionally. Be proactive and ask questions. They'll let you know what products and services are right for you.

Run-the-other-way *dont's!*

- MAKEUP WILL CAKE UP: I don't care how tired you are, how drunk you are, or how hot the guy is sleeping next to you—*take off your makeup* before you go to bed. Your skin will thank you.
- THINK BEFORE YOU INK: I'm sneaking this in! Tattoos are not a rite of passage. Please don't get one impulsively. Wait. Wait. Then wait some more. And only then, if after all that waiting, you honestly believe you'll want a tattoo of a butterfly or a shooting star on your shoulder when you're fifty years old, by all means, *go for it.*
- DON'T SMOKE. PERIOD: I did. It was stupid. Smoking makes you stink. It is terrible for your health, teeth, eyes, hair and skin. Don't do it.

supermodel *secret*

ACNE ADMISSION

When it comes to treating it, I've tried every antibiotic out there, but they just didn't work for me. As a last resort, I got on Accutane for the first time at about twenty-five. Afterward, for about ten years, my skin was more or less under control. And then, at thirty-five, it came back with a vengeance. I went back on Accutane for the second time. Isn't that sexy? See . . . I told you I had to work at this supermodel stuff! I took a low dose and within a few weeks my skin cleared up and my pores appeared smaller. A word of caution: Accutane is a serious drug and it's not to be taken lightly. It can be safe and effective if closely monitored by you and your doctor—and it works. But it's no fun.

thirties

Here's where people really start to break away from the pack. If you've taken care of your skin up to this point, it will show. And it you haven't, it will show.

Runway *dos!*

- **USE THE FANTASTIC FIVE:** In your thirties, skin cell turnover continues to slow. Lines form and get deeper. Spots show up. Skin just isn't as firm or tight. Experts agree and research supports the antiaging benefits of five powerhouse ingredients—*start using them!* (See our Fantastic Five list.)
- **TREAT YOURSELF:** Consider treatments that will freshen up your skin: a series of light peels to brighten, lightly tighten, and stimulate cellular turnover. Maybe a bit of Botox to treat frown lines and help prevent future lines from forming.
- **SUPPLEMENT, SISTER!:** Get serious about taking supplements. As I've mentioned, I did. Make sure you are taking a multivitamin (or prenatals).

Run-the-other-way *don't's!*

- **STOP THE EXCUSE CABOOSE:** This can definitely be a busy-bee decade. But don't make excuses for not taking care of yourself and your skin. Do not give in to the: I'm a busy "mom/studio exec/*fill in the blank whatever you are* and therefore have no time" syndrome. Take time for you. Moisturize. Put in the effort. You are worth it.

THE *fantastic* FIVE

The *everyday supermodel* superingredients. Don't get too caught up in the hype of trendy ingredients. These five complexion commandos are scientifically proven heroes in the war against aging.

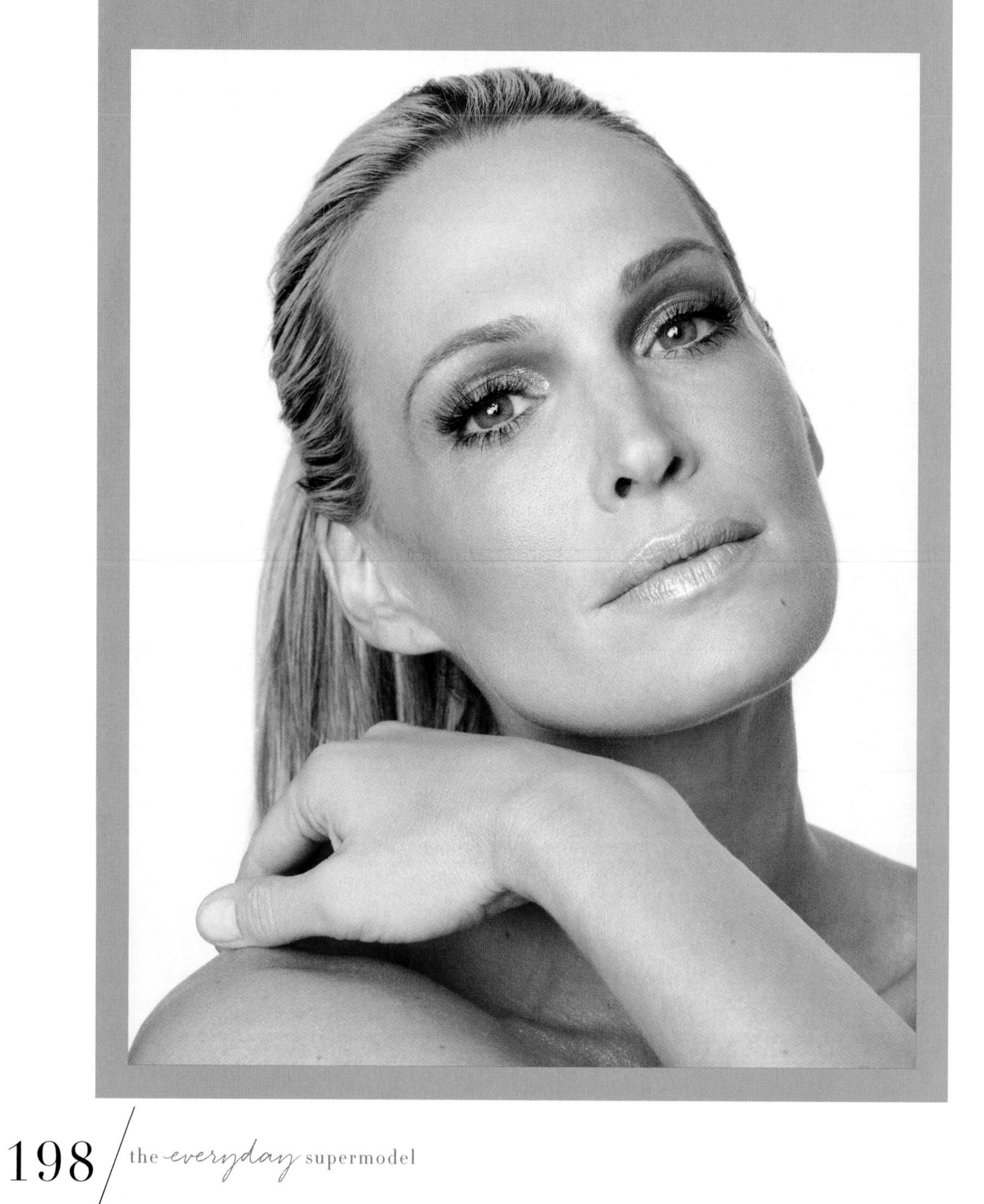

1. PEPTIDES: Scientific research has shown they help heal the skin and stimulate collagen and elastin production. Peptides perform when it comes to fewer lines and firmer/tighter skin. Some peptides have even been found to slow muscle contraction and help prevent wrinkles from forming (ingredients such as arginine). Look out for copper peptides, matrixyl, and other ingredients that usually end in "tide."
2. RETINOL: This form of vitamin A is able to penetrate several layers of skin to effectively exfoliate and reveal younger skin cells. Retinol is also a proven collagen/elastin stimulator and helps to regulate hydration levels. It is highly effective for everyday supermodels with the adult acne/maturing skin dilemma. Look for retinol on the ingredient list. If you want something stronger, the prescription version is Retin-A or Renova. (Retinyl palmitate is also a form, but it's not as strong and results are slower.)
3. ANTIOXIDANTS: These skin defenders fight free radicals, assist in healing the skin, and are effective on so many levels, depending on the unique properties of each antioxidant. Vitamin C is a proven antiager, great for lightening spots and brightening dullness. The most stable and effective form of vitamin C is usually listed as L-ascorbic acid. That's the one you want to look for. Watch out for the phoneys! Alpha-lipoic acid is believed to be one of the strongest, and studies show it boosts the strength of the other antioxidants. Alpha-lipoic acid is sometimes listed as ALA.
4. HYDROXY ACIDS: AHAs and BHAs have been around a long time but are still at the top of the skin-care game—they are major multitaskers. Hydroxy acids are stellar at speeding cellular turnover and work at the surface level and deeper to soften and smooth skin, improve fine lines, clear junk out of pores, and help your skin maintain healthy hydration levels. Look for glycolic, lactic, citric, and salicylic acid in the ingredient list. Acids can be slightly irritating, so be aware.
5. HYALURONIC ACID: This superstar floods skin cells with hydration and then holds and locks it in. As we age, we lose naturally occurring HA in our skin cells, and our skin loses the ability to hold water in the cells as effectively. Hence the dryness as we get older. Hyaluronic acid has an immediate plumping and smoothing effect on skin cells and binds water to the skin. Look for glycosaminoglycan or sodium hyaluronate in the ingredient list.

AND . . . maybe even one more? Stem cell science is no longer fiction—but it's now fact! Skin-care formulations are starting to emerge using the proteins produced by stem cells (so not stem cells themselves, which can be controversial). These stem cell proteins have been proven to help skin naturally repair itself, by undoing wrinkles, spots and the like. So be on the lookout!

forties & fifties

Back in the day, forties seemed . . . *old.* And now I'm in my forties! Today, we are more beautiful than ever. All the advice from the thirties applies . . . just turn it up a notch.

Runway *dos!*

- **MOISTURIZE:** I read Bobbi Brown moisturizes the heck out of her skin, and she's a beauty biz icon; she must know what she is talking about. In our forties, hydration levels drop drastically and we are more dry and crepey. At-home moisture masks and steam treatments are great for bringing back the pinky glow that starts to go.
- **TREATMENTS TOWN HALL:** In your forties, bones start shrinking and you begin to lose fat under the eyes. (And we gain it everywhere else?! What a joke.) Injectables such as Restylane and Juvéderm are great for those hollows and shadows. Thermage combats the sag that starts and helps tighten around the mouth and the "turkey neck." Everybody is different and needs different things.
- **THE EXERCISE EQUATION!:** Don't stop exercising because your life feels like a blur with kids and work. Studies show that those who exercise actually have thicker, firmer, more elastic skin. Plus, you now have a whole list of ways to sneak in exercise courtesy of my earlier chapter.

Run-the-other-way *don'ts!*

- **DON'T FREAK OUT . . .** and then do everything all at once. Remember the L.A. Polish—it's all about little stuff here and there.
- **OR TRY NEWFANGLED TREATMENTS:** Avoid jumping on the bandwagon of new, *untested/unproven* beauty solutions. Don't do anything unless it's been tried, evaluated by professionals, and you really trust it.

sixties, seventies, and beyond

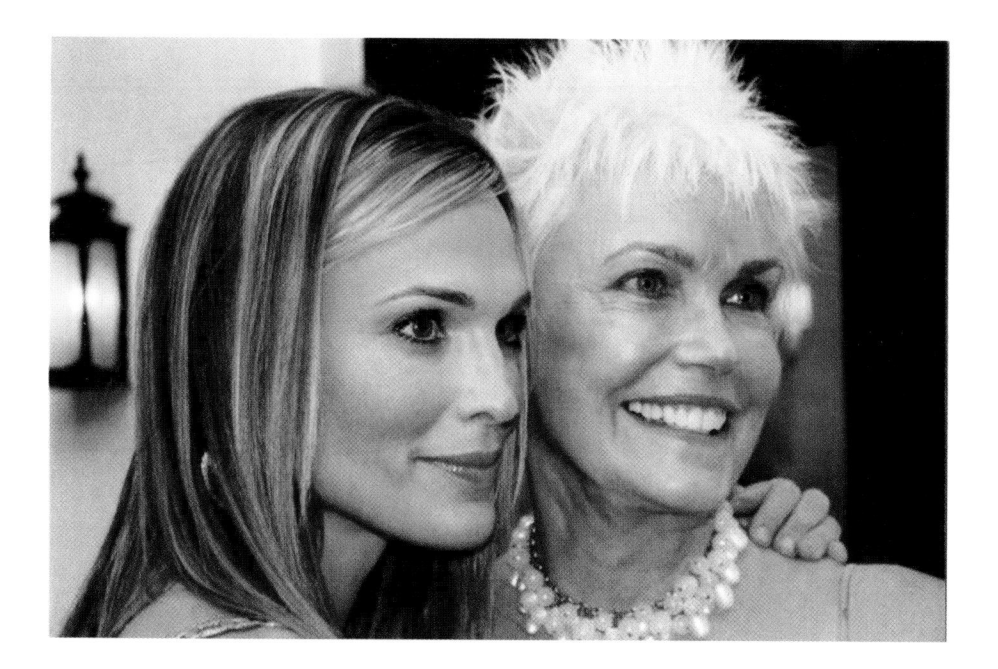

We *everyday supermodels* (and my momma is one of them!) are only as old as we let ourselves feel. Big Momma, that's what everyone calls her in Kentucky, doesn't look or feel a day over sixty. However old she really is, is her little secret!

Runway *dos!*

* **EMBRACE YOUR BEAUTY:** You've earned it. We are stunning as we age. Anxieties of youth are traded for the wisdom and experience of living. Take a step back and appreciate the woman you are.
* **REGIMEN:** The skin continues to thin and lose elasticity and moisture, so products that firm and moisturize are all key. The Fantastic Five ingredients should be front and center.
* **TREATMENTS:** Stronger peels and laser treatments are good for the deeper lines that develop around the mouth and under the eyes. Injectable fillers, such as Restylane and hyaluronic acid, take quite a few years off and leave a natural look. Very subtle nips and tucks might be warranted as the jawline loosens and eyelids tire.

Run-the-other-way *don't's!*

- **DON'T BECOME A SPLIT SCREEN:** Some women do treatments that create a disconnect in their face. Smooth forehead and cheeks and then the opposite toward the jaw and the neck. Look at solutions that will work together to address the entire face and neck as a whole.

BEAUTY TIPS FROM ONE OF *my besties*

Tracy O'Connor (also my co-author) is the beauty expert for Fox's *Good Day LA* and an industry consultant. She knows a thing or two about products, ingredients, and treatments. Before I do anything skin related, I get her approval. Here's a few of Tracy's top tips:

* FOR SENSITIVE SKIN: Whenever possible, choose skin-care products with fewer than a dozen or so ingredients. The fewer the ingredients, the fewer opportunities for one to freak your skin out.
* GREEN TEA OR BUST: I'm so beauty-obsessed with green tea, I wrote a book about it! (*Green Tea Secrets* on Amazon) When I ditched coffee and traded up for the green stuff, I noticed my skin looked dramatically better and *less stressed*. A supersipper, green tea is high in antiaging antioxidants and stress reducers and has a long list of proven beauty/body benefits (studies show it actually fights belly jelly!).
* HYPE DOWN: Learn to read ingredient lists the same way you read food labels. There is a lot of hype when it comes to skin-care products and cosmetics. Be your own cosmetic cop.
* FROM MY MOM: Don't forget your teeth, people! My mom always told me to "get your teeth professionally cleaned yearly and always smile." Easy DIY? A baking soda mask brushed onto teeth helps polish and lighten stains. GloScience makes a great at-home whitener.
* TO SHOP BEAUTY: I've been all over the world scouring fresh and innovative products. Hands down, my all-time favorite spot is the original C.O. Bigelow in New York's West Village. Praise be, you can shop it online. (www.bigelowchemists.com)

For more of Tracy's beauty tips, check out her e-books and blog online.

THE *everyday* SUPERMODEL BODY BEAUTY

I've tried a lot of products and services. When I was a model, I got occasional injections in my rear to get rid of fat. Weekly, I'd put myself through deep, painful body massages (yes, that left bruises) because I believed it worked to break up cellulite (and I do think it worked and does work). More recently, I did a series of cold laser treatments that melt fat (it worked pretty well for me). What I'm saying here—I've almost done it all. From the low-tech to the high-tech. You might just find your *everyday supermodel* body secret somewhere in here. Let's start with the basics.

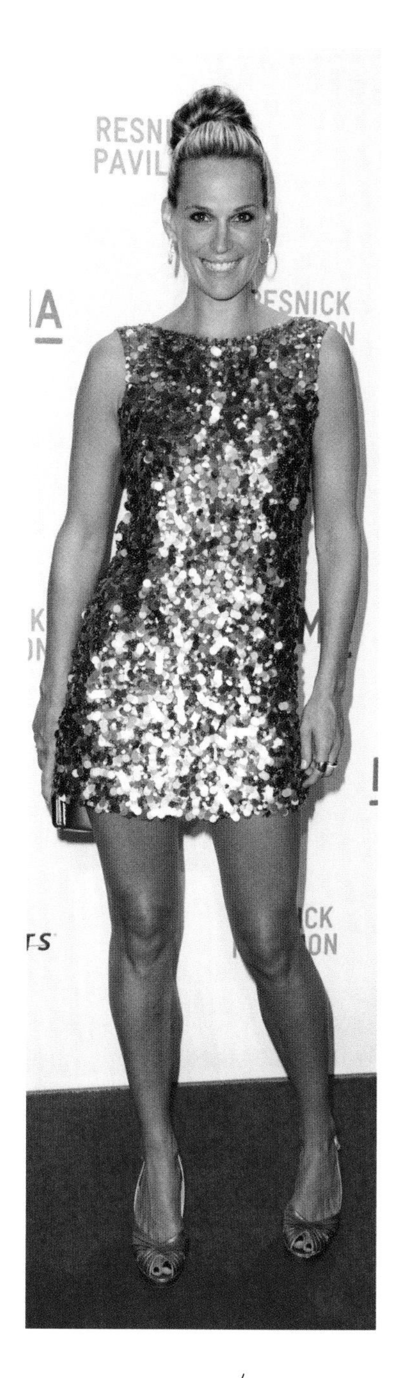

My *body beauty* Regimen

1. **CLEANSE:** First off, simmer down on the hot water. That's a no-no and dehydrates the skin. Eucerin Calming Body Wash Daily Shower Oil is my daily go-to. It cleans without stripping or drying skin out. It's also excellent for shaving any Sasquatchy areas.

2. **EXFOLIATE:** I'm obsessed with making my own scrubs. Try your own DIY version by mixing brown sugar or sea salt with olive oil—and get scrubbing once a week!

3. **MOISTURIZE:** Because of my eczema, I am religious about lubing up. I use Curel and Eucerin Body Lotion and occasionally apply natural oils, like olive or coconut, if I'm feeling daring. But then I go straight to bed as they can be a bit greasy.

4. **DRY BRUSH:** Two to three times a week I dry brush head to toe with loofa hand mitts or a "dry body brush" (you can find one at select Whole Foods Markets and beauty supply stores). I started doing this at home after I learned about it at We Care. Start at your feet, work upward and always stroke toward the heart. Devotees of dry brushing will tell you it reduces cellulite, improves your skin's hydration levels, and is fantastic for your general health (kinda like body-flossing!*)*. It leaves your skin *seriously soooooooooft*.

BODY *services*

Being a model, you are body conscious. You might have to be bikini-ready at a moment's notice. Can you imagine? Showing that much skin every day equals a lot of prep. Whether you're gearing up for your wedding, a major event, or your own day out in a one-piece or two, here's what I've done that works.

1. MASSAGE: Cellulite is a b*tch. But I believe massage can work to break up the stored fat and toxins that some believe contribute to lumps/bumps. While your body therapist shouldn't go all "Whac-A-Mole" on you, there are some who *specialize* in punishing the cellulite out of you. I used to do it, but it's just too painful. I believe regular, consistent, deep tissue massage is just as effective.

2. ENDERMOLOGIE: A vacuumlike roller machine sucks up and kneads your trouble spots like a baker does dough. It's fairly painless and is believed to break up toxins/stored fat and tighten the skin. Six to twelve treatments are recommended, and you will see results—but they are temporary.

3. WRAPS: They will help you shed excess water weight and definitely work to temporarily sculpt the body. These are go-tos for celebs and models before big events and photo shoots. But again, it's not a long-term solution.

4. THERMAGE FOR THE BODY: YES. This is good. We talked about it earlier for facial tightening, but it's effective on the rest of the bod too. Radiofrequency works to heat and contract tissue. It's uncomfortable feeling at first, but effective for tightening tummy skin postpreg (was for me!) or anywhere your skin is a bit saggy, baggy, or flabby.

5. ZELTIQ: This cold laser treatment has helped diminish my postpregnancy pooch and saddlebags—a great alternative to the traditional tummy tuck. Sometimes you need a series to see results, but you will see results, and experts say they last. I'm pretty sure all of Hollywood is doing it. It even works on back/arm jiggle.

6. LIGHT THERAPIES: For those with "Country Club Chest"—that is, freckles and spots all over the neck and décolleté—IPL uses wavelengths of light to banish these sun splotches. It works on hands, forearms, just about anywhere!

7. MESOTHERAPY: It's been around forever, and it worked for me. Shots are administered wherever there is fat, and the fat eventually dissolves and is absorbed by your body. I did it when I was younger. NO, it's not the most comfortable experience getting shots in your bum.

BABY-ON-BOARD BEAUTY *tips*

Lord have mercy, lots goes on with our skin during pregnancy. Obviously melasma was my main event. I was also so preoccupied about getting stretch marks that I greased up day and night. Not to mention, lots of products are off-limits due to the safety concerns of certain ingredients—so you've got to overhaul your life and your beauty routine, temporarily. Here are a few of my key tips:

all forms of sun protection are a must: My most important tip. The influx of hormones during pregnancy can leave your skin more sensitive to the sun and heat. Choose a physical block, with zinc, instead of a chemical block. Try and stay out of the sun as much as possible and always wear a broad-rimmed hat and glasses when outdoors.

be an ingredient sleuth: Do your research on what ingredients to avoid. Most experts agree you should steer clear of retinols, hydroxyl acids, peptides, and synthetic fragrances and colors (as they may not be healthy for the fetus). Ditch the toxic nail polishes (use the greener versions we recommend a bit later) and wear natural essential oil fragrances for a while. Try to use more natural brands when possible. (A few include: Dr. Hauschka, Tata Harper, and Dr. Mercola skin care Wen hair care. RMS beauty and Vapour cosmetics). Some of your favorite brands may also have natural, chem-free products in their collections; just ask. Visit the Environmental Working Group's website (www.ewg.org/skindeep) for recommendations, more information, and safety guidelines for skin-care and cosmetics. You can punch in current products you use and see how they rate on the safety scale—try it—it's fun and informative!

skin shift: Everyone is different, but my skin would honestly change from day-to-day during my pregnancy. If you always had dry skin? Look out—it might get oily. Be prepared for changes, and switch up your tried-and-true routine if you need to. I noticed that drinking a lot of water really helped keep my skin hydrated and more balanced. Carry a giant bottle with you wherever you roam.

Supermomma Beauty *treatments*

You can't go crazy with treatments, but there were a lot of natural therapies and tips that I chose to do to limit the havoc happening to my body. Here's my go-to list.

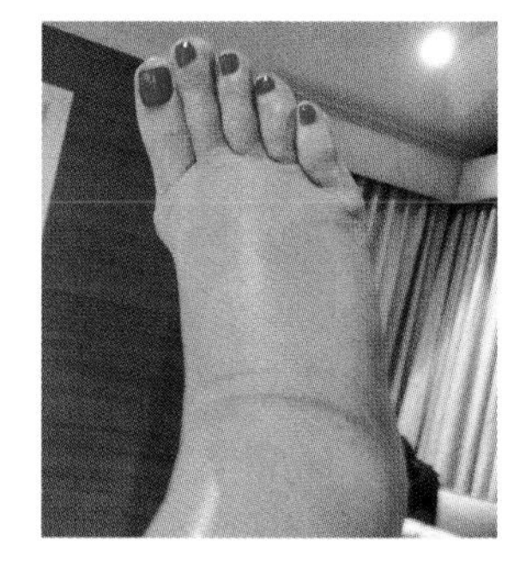

1. **MANI/PEDI MUST:** Even though I could barely see my feet (by month six, *I could not*), and they were swollen to extraterrestrial proportions, I got regular pedicures. They made me feel somewhat normal.

2. **BATHTIME BONANZA:** I bathed almost every day, especially in the third trimester. (I still bathe a few times a week, but now it's *with* my baby). Epson salt baths were my jam. High in magnesium, they helped reduce soreness and swelling. Even if not pregnant, baths are a great detoxer, and a good soak before bed will help you sleep.

3. **EVERYBODY, LEGS AGAINST THE WALL!** A few times a day, lie with your back on the ground and put your legs up the wall in a giant L shape. This alphabet move is especially effective for relieving leg pressure and can reduce your chance of getting spider veins. If you travel—always wear compression hose or socks to prevent swelling.

---

supermomma *Tummy talk*

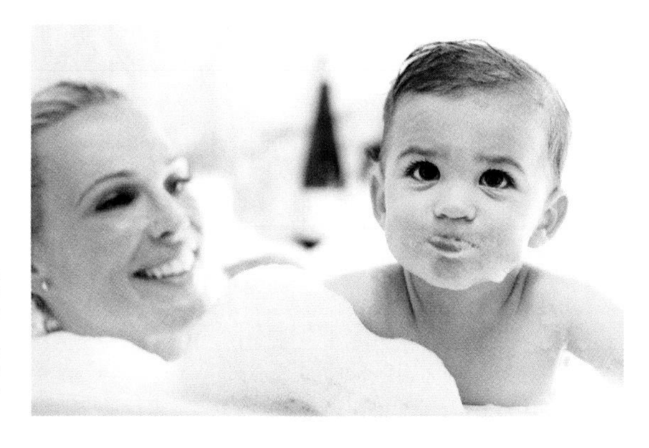

Stretch marks are a pretty big concern. The second you know you are pregnant, begin balming up your belly with whatever you've got. Castor oil will work! I lubed up every morning and every night and always right after I showered or bathed. My holistic pregnancy coach, Lori Bregman, made me a homemade belly balm (recipe here to make it yourself). I love, love, loved it—and did not get ONE stretch mark. Thanks, Lori! (Bio Oil and Mamma Mia Balm, which is all natural, are also excellent.)

Breggy's Belly Butter

INGREDIENTS:

- 1 jar of organic coconut oil
- 1 container of organic cocoa butter
- 1 container of organic shea butter
- 1 small bottle of 400 IU of vitamin E

DIRECTIONS:

Place all ingredients except for the vitamin E in a pot of boiling water in their separate containers, letting them melt (the cocoa butter will take the longest). After everything is melted, pour into a large bowl and mix together with the vitamin E. Put the mixture in a glass container and store in the refrigerator or another cool place.

Use on belly, hips, breasts, and bum. Massage in and start mothering early.

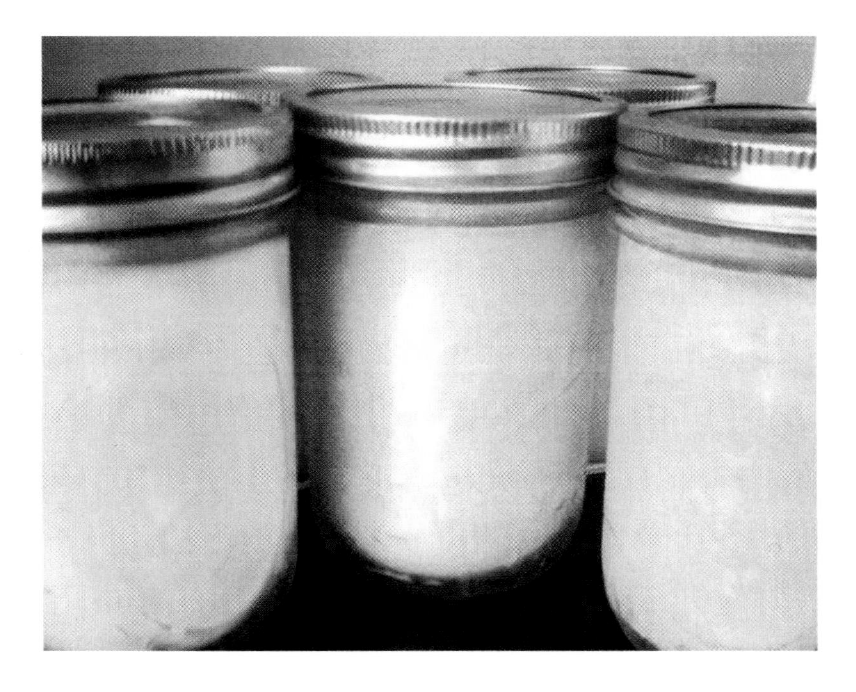

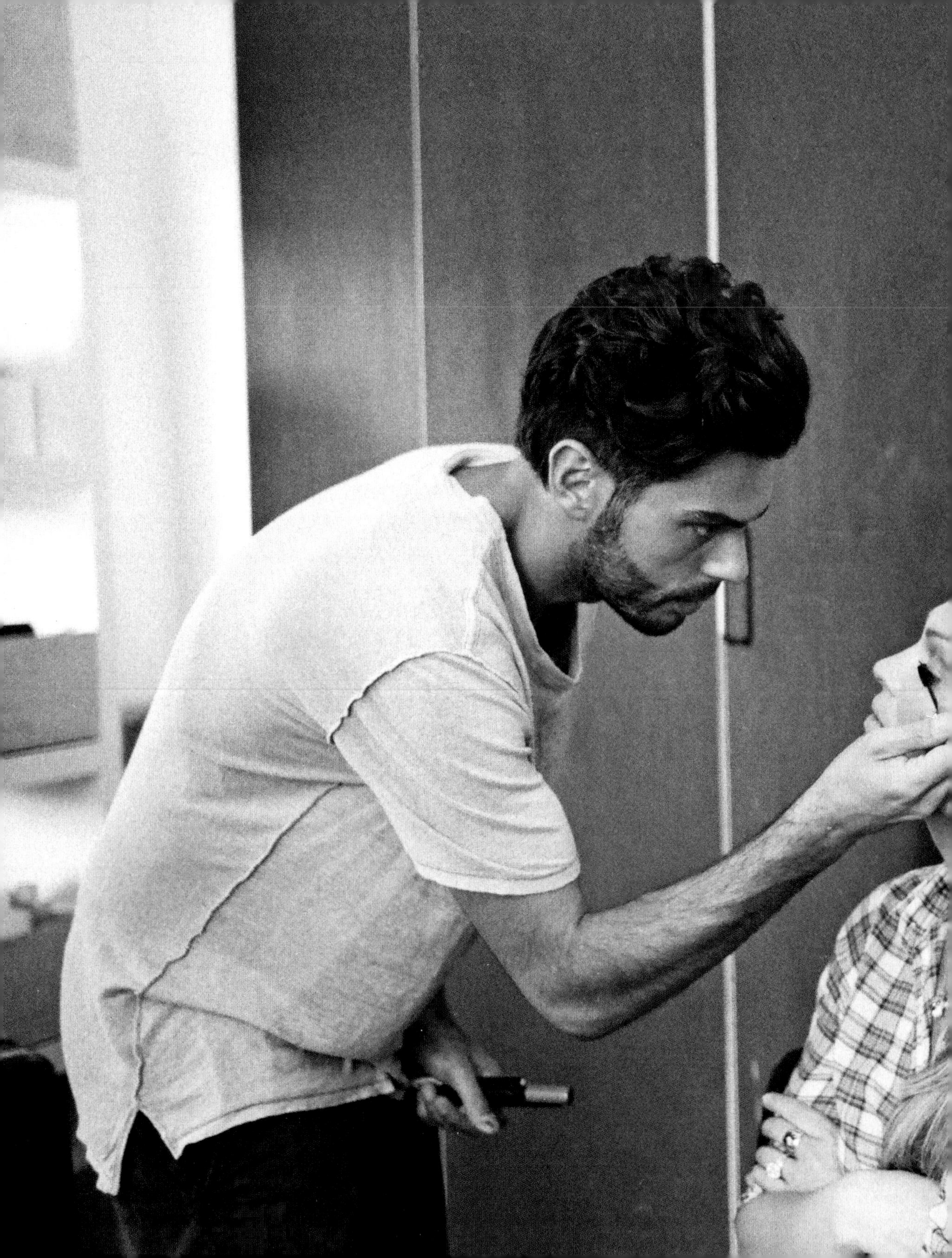

everyday supermodel MAKEUP

We've talked a lot about priming the skin. Now it's time to learn from the professionals and gab about makeup. Do you know how many hours I've spent in a makeup chair? More hours than I care to admit. But one thing is for sure—I've learned every trick. I started wearing makeup in high school and have ever since for work and play. Knowing how to wear and have fun with your makeup can be transformational, and I love me some transformation.

---

foundation

No one does foundation like my friend and makeup artist Joey Maalouf. If you want to turn back the clock on your complexion, try his application technique.

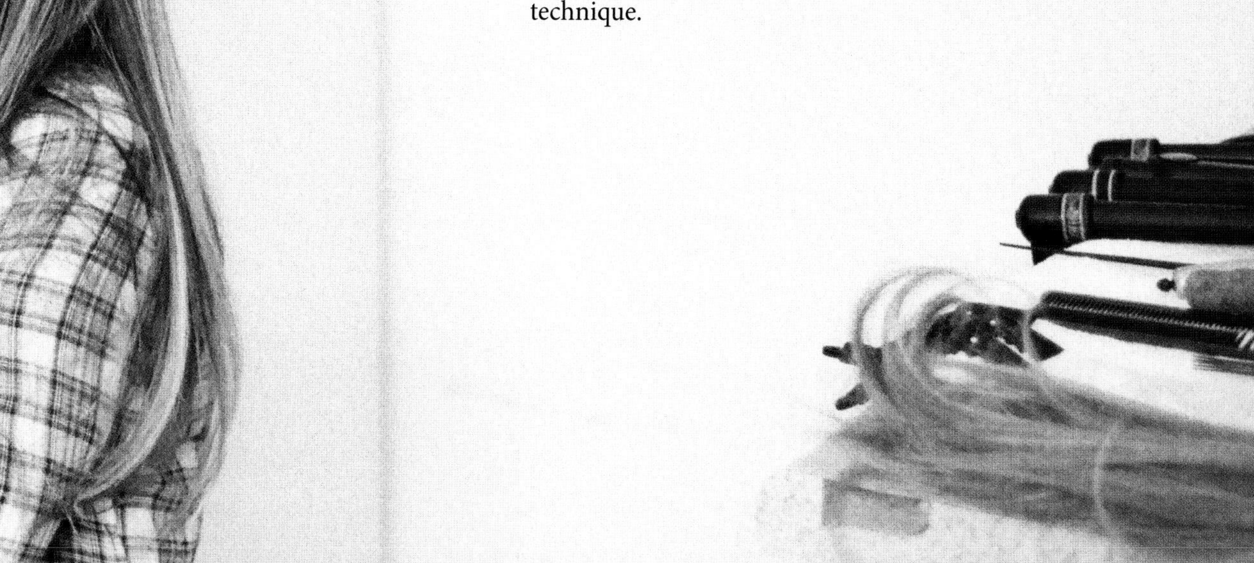

flawless foundation by JOEY MAALOUF

TOOLS

- Beautyblender or egg-shaped sponge
- Your fabulous fingers
- A water-based foundation you are obsessed with. (My fave is Hourglass tinted moisturizer. Match the foundation to the neck as there are often so many tones in the face.)
- Concealer (Clé de Peau is excellent)
- Cream blush (Peony by Stila is a soft peachy-pink and universally flattering)

step 1: Wet the sponge, squeeze, and tap it on a towel until it's only damp.

step 2: Dot your foundation evenly over the skin. Less is more.

step 3: Then, stipple the foundation onto the skin with the sponge. Do not wipe or swipe—the correct motion is a gentle tapping torture treatment all over the face!

step 4: Take leftover residue on the sponge down the neck and onto the chest if visible.

step 5: Tap a small bit of light-pink cream blush (darker or lighter depending on skin color) into the corners of the eyes and on the bluish undereye circles. (I learned this backstage at *Oprah* when I had to cover a bluish tattoo for a guest on the fly.)

step 6: Then apply your neutral concealer over the pinkish cream blush you've already applied under eyes, gently tapping and blending into the skin with your ring finger.

step 7: Allow the foundation to set into the skin for a few moments. Next, apply your creamy blush to the apples of the cheeks with your fingertips. (Smiling helps!)

step 8: Finish the look by applying a sheer powder (Makeup Forever HD Powder is great for dusting high-shine spots/T-zone) with a small brush on the sides of the nose, between the brows, in the center of the forehead, and under the bottom lip on the chin.

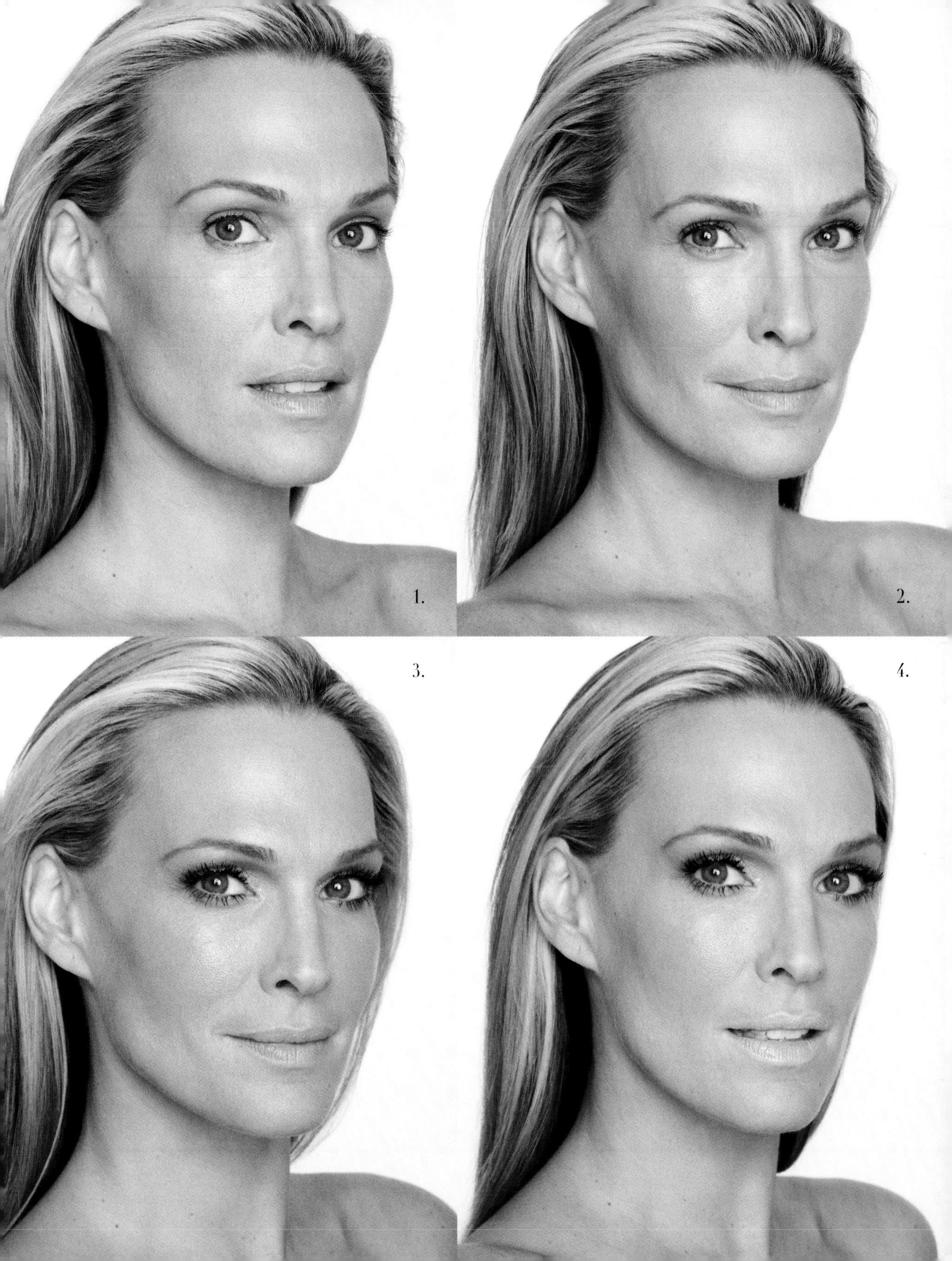
1.
2.
3.
4.

MY FIVE-MINUTE *fashionable* FACE

This is what I do day to day. This look takes about five minutes, once you have it down. And I'm experienced!

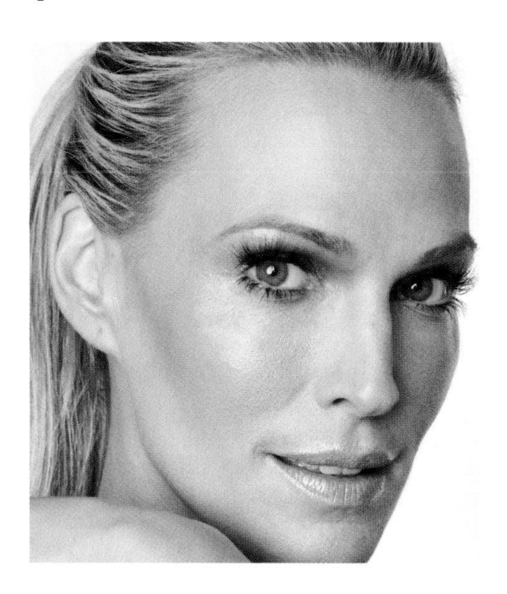

step 1: Apply a tinted moisturizer and pinky or tangerine blush to the cheeks (or Joey's Flawless Foundation Technique).
step 2: Curl lashes and add a coat of mascara.
step 3: Groom brows with a brow gel. (Try Brow Perfection Gel by Perfect—in clear or a shade lighter than your brows.)
step 4: Finish with a subtle lip tint. I love a pinky-nude.

---

supermodel *secret*

I only use powder for red carpet stuff or when I'm photographed. Why? I'm obsessed with looking dewy and glowy. Powder can dehydrate the skin, settle into lines, and give skin a dull appearance. The older we get, the worse powder-based products can look on us. I love creamy-based products so much, I'm developing a cosmetic collection around them. They might not have as much staying power as powder, but for everyday use, they feel better/look better on the skin. Dewy over dry any day = my makeup motto! And when it comes to controlling the T-zone, I carry blotting papers or dab powder just on high-shine areas.

---

day TO *night*

Occasionally after my workday, I'll have to elevate my look for a special event, and like most of you, I don't have time for a total makeup overhaul. Usually, I have just a few spare minutes to freshen my face and . . . "turn it up a notch!" Below are a few simple steps to go from office to office party in no time.

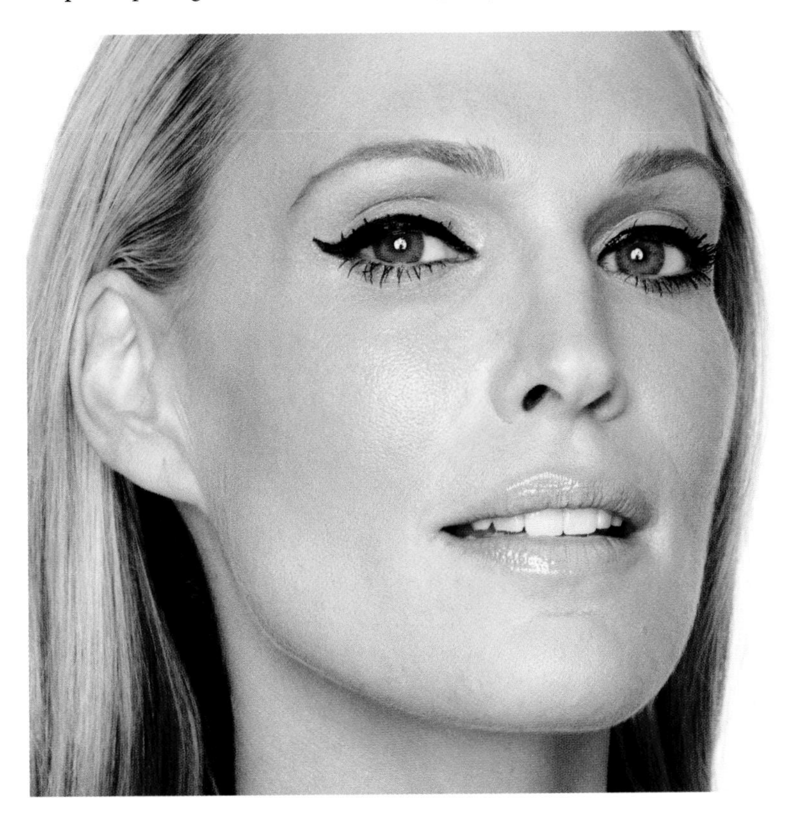

step 1: I freshen my foundation with a spritz of water and dab with the makeup sponge.

step 2: I nude out the lip with a bit of foundation and top off with a shimmery, nude gloss that reflects light. A nude lip is always sexy and sensual.

step 3: Work some eyelash magic by adding an extra two coats of deep black mascara to lashes, top and bottom, to reemphasize the eyes.

step 4: I finish the look with a bold sweep of black liner on the top lid. Try extending it out for a cat eye. It takes a little practice to master, but once you do, it's a breeze. (Smashbox Love Me Paint Pen Eyeliner features a felt-tip, and is user-friendly for beginners!)

supermodel *secret*

Want a fast, fresh look? Try applying almost any sheer balm directly onto your lids, with your fingertips. You can use a touch of Vaseline or a rose salve, as long as it's mostly colorless. It gives the all-over-illusion of fresher skin and brighter eyes (even if your skin is tired and your eyes are too). For a makeup-free look (with a bit of extra polish), simply add a stroke or two of mascara to the tips of your lashes—eyes will pop!

MAKE MAKEUP *magic*: I asked my experts, and we all agree, it's a wonderful and confusing world out there when it comes to cosmetics. Here are a few tips from my Beauty Battalion to help guide you.

- TRY BEFORE YOU BUY: Say there is a lip color you've always wanted to try, but weren't sure about. Buy a cheap version at the drugstore and wear it around vacuuming. Don't waste money buying something on impulse that you'll never wear.
- TAKE A LESSON: Go to a cosmetics counter and ask for help. Which brand's magazine ads do you like the best? Go to that counter. Blogs and YouTube are excellent resources for tutorials. Even my makeup artist Monika said she watches tutorials for inspiration. They have videos of their own too! (Search for Joey Malouff online or visit Monika Blunder's YouTube channel.)
- SUSS OUT YOUR STYLE: Your makeup choices are no different than your fashion choices. You need to know your style. You can figure it out by experimenting and copying looks you like on others. Know what makes you feel good, and always have a few go-to looks that fit your face and your personality.

Editors always ask, but I'm never going to give them tips for "doing makeup in 3 seconds while driving in the car." Take a few minutes in the morning to do your beauty routine. Even if it's just mascara and moisturizer, it matters. Those few minutes spent will make a positive difference in how you feel all day long.

—JOEY MAALOUF, makeup artist

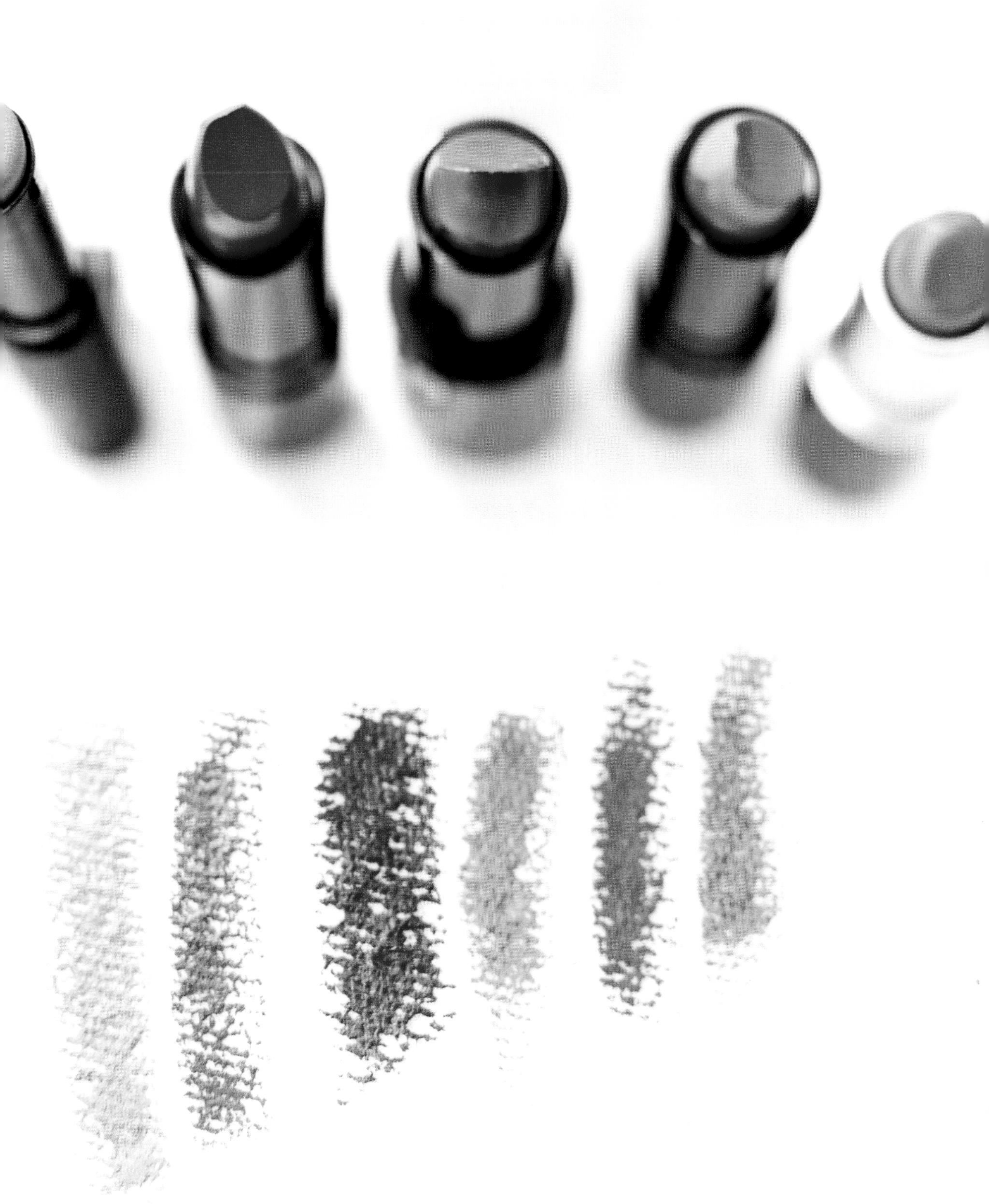

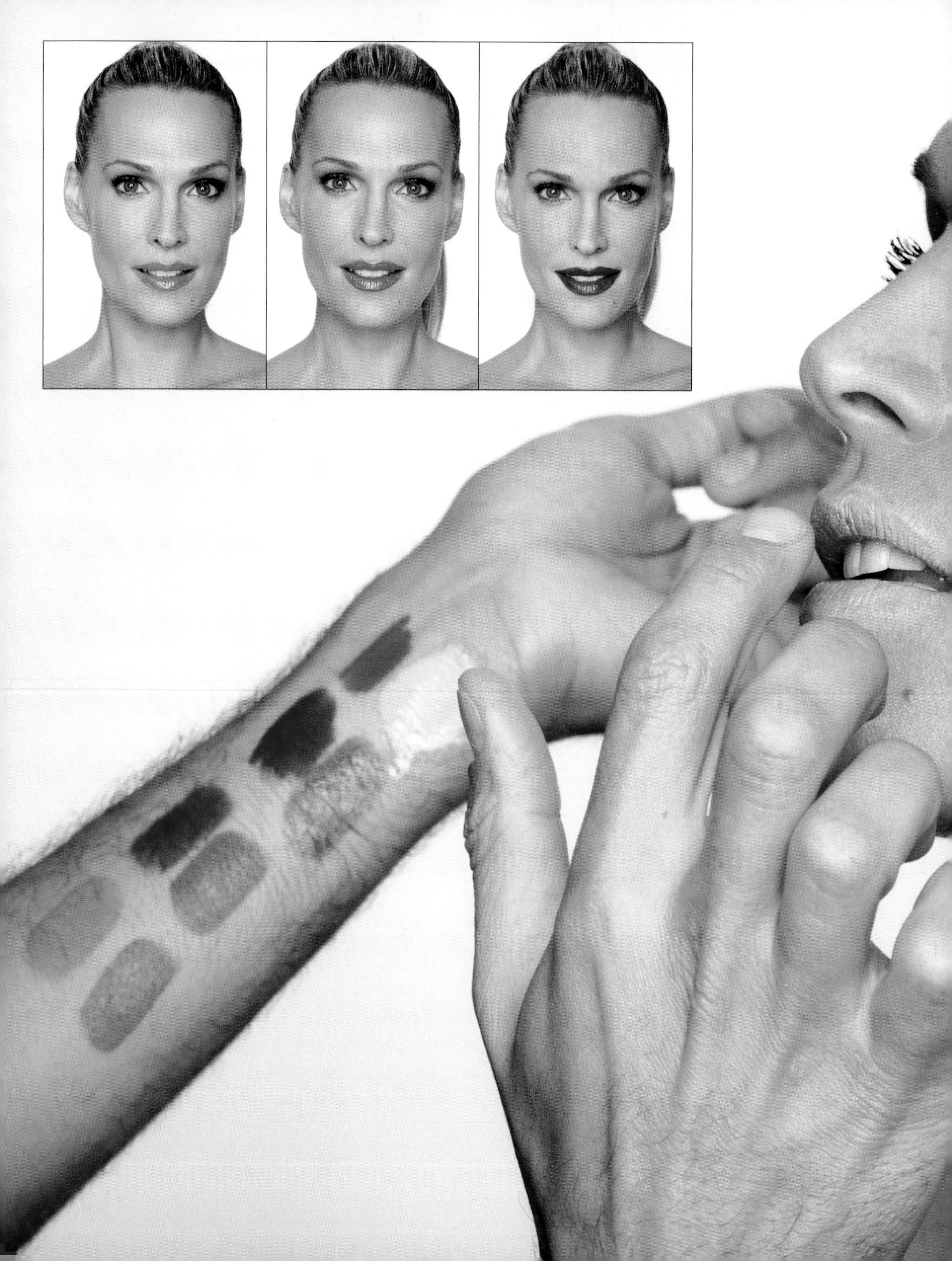

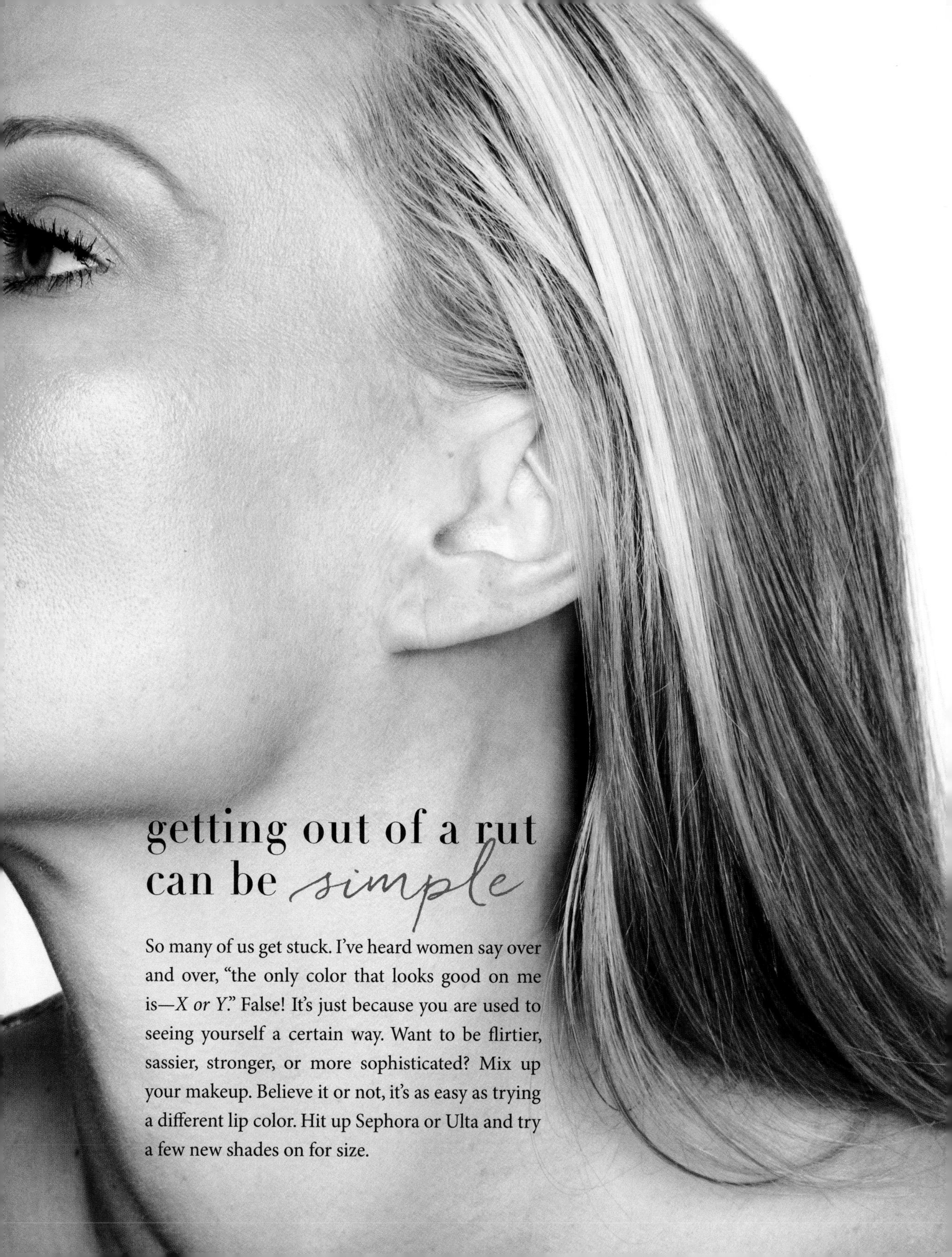

getting out of a rut can be *simple*

So many of us get stuck. I've heard women say over and over, "the only color that looks good on me is—*X or Y*." False! It's just because you are used to seeing yourself a certain way. Want to be flirtier, sassier, stronger, or more sophisticated? Mix up your makeup. Believe it or not, it's as easy as trying a different lip color. Hit up Sephora or Ulta and try a few new shades on for size.

DON'T JUST *want*, BUT *need!*

My experts and I put together a list of a few of our favorite beauty steals and splurges. Here are the products we LOVE and can't live without—your *everyday supermodel* makeup artist arsenal. Okay, so you don't need all this stuff, but a girl can dream . . .

1. **PRIMER:** First of all, if you don't know what primer is, let's chat. It helps minimize pores, gives skin a natural radiance, and helps makeup stay put! I always use primer for special events. Monika loves Clarins Beauty Flash Primer, which instantly brightens and tightens the face and is universal for every skin color. For a fresh and natural option, try makeup-artist-created Heir Atelier.

2. **FOUNDATION:** Giorgio Armani Luminous Silk and Clé de Peau are makeup artist staples. My friend Emese loves the Japanese brand Koh Gen Do Aqua Foundation for a state-of-the-art finish.

3. **CONCEALER:** I love LORAC Double Feature Concealer. Sometimes just an extra layer of your foundation will do.

4. **CREAM BLUSHES:** Stila cream blushes are ALL good. My favorites from Bobbi Brown are Pale Pink and Summer Tan. Jouer and RMS have natural shades. Keep in mind, anything in tangerine is universally pretty.

5. **POWDER BLUSHES:** Nars Orgasm and Nars New Order are classics. My friend and model Veronika Vařeková loves Lipstick Queen Blush for a perfect flush.

6. **BROW PENCIL:** MAC wax pencils are great and don't smudge, Givenchy brow pencils are soft and easy to use, as are Lancôme's. PerfeKt Brow Perfection Gels are nice for a natural, feathered brow look à la model Cara Delevingne. (You can even experiment with color and temporarily lighten or darken your brow color with them.)

7. **BRONZER:** Everyone agrees Chantecaille Gel Bronzer is a perfect shimmery bronze gel (no televangelist's wife here!). The cream-to-powder bronzer/blush duo by Hourglass in Illume is also very pretty. Monika loves Soleil Tan de Chanel Bronze Universal and Tom Ford's bronzer. ("It looks very dark." she says, "but it isn't really. Don't be intimidated.")

8. **HIGHLIGHTER:** Chantecaille, Tom Ford, and LORAC all make great versions of these. (Read on for our tutorial on how to use highlighter.)

9. **EYE SHADOWS:** Tom Ford Golden Mink shimmery neutrals palette is my all-time favorite. You can't beat Nars Alhambra in a pinky/pearly shade for a soft, eye-opening look. I also love Jouer cream eye shadow in Cashmere, which coats the eye in barely there neutral, with a satiny finish.

10. **EYELINERS:** Laos by Sue Devitt is a buttery brownish/bronze eye pencil I use a lot. Via Appia by Nars is my favorite creamy eye pencil for a rich, shimmery bronze. Generally, I love the Larger Than Life collection of long-wear eye pencils by Nars. MAC Black eyeliner is nice and blendable, and MAC Night Sky black shimmer pencil is fun! Laura Mercier Metallic Cream Eye Color in Burnished Coppers, another universal shade.

11. **TIGHTLINING EYELINERS:** These liners are for lining the water-line or the inside of the eyelid. For a nude, Rue Bonaparte by Nars is a winner. For a whiter look, I like the Benefit eye brightener. Both effectively help to open the eyes and achieve a fresher look.

12. **LIPSTICKS:** We all love Tom Ford's. They are like fashion for your face. Monika's fave is Tainted Love. Red lipstick Chanel #65 Fire is a classic. I wore Rue Coco Chanel #35 on my wedding day, a soft pinky rose. As a matter of fact, at the end of these two beauty chapters, we break down how to get my complete wedding look.

13. **LIP GLOSSES/BALMS:** Clinique Moisturizing Gloss in Black Honey is an all-time favorite. Flower glosses by Drew Barrymore are pretty and all very wearable. Bare Minerals and City Lips make gorgeous, high-shine glosses that plump too. Finally, By Terry's balm. My lips never leave home without it.

14. **MASCARA:** Dior Show gives big-time volume. Lancôme Définicils is great for lengthening. LashFood makes a great conditioner and mascara that help lengthen and thicken.

THE EIGHT *great* MAKEUP TOOLS

There are a few tools that are simply necessities. Certain brushes offer precision and keep makeup free from finger grime. And just try applying false lashes without a tweezer . . . not fun! Here are a few musts for your beauty tool kit.

1. **FOUNDATION BRUSH:** It's flat, dense, and generally has synthetic bristles so it doesn't pick up too much product. It allows for even distribution of your foundation and creates a smooth, even finish. It also is very useful for getting into the corners of the under-eye where dark circles lurk!

2. **BRONZING/CONTOURING BRUSH:** This is a medium-to-smaller-sized brush with a slight angle. It's perfect for using in the hollows of the cheek to add lift and pop to your look.

3. **POWDER BRUSH:** Find a fluffy, round brush for blending, softening, and finishing a look. It should feel light as a feather on your face! Look for soft bristles, not too stiff, so it blends and blurs, rather than sweeping it off and away.

4. **EASY EYE SHADOW BRUSH:** Choose something that fits in the crease of your eye and is firm enough strategically deposit eye shadow, but soft enough to help blend. Most of the sponges that come with drugstore shadows don't allow for blendability, unfortunately, but you can save them to soften and smudge eye pencil lines. They work well for that!

5. **EYELASH CURLER:** The Shu Uemura eye lash curler is, read-my-lips, hands down the be-all and end-all for makeup artists. Every artist owns one. Just sayin'.

6. **EGG-SHAPED SPONGE:** We love this silly-looking gadget. The sponge is user friendly and creates a poreless finish. As you learned in Joey's tutorial, it's ideal for applying foundation and cream blushes.

7. **TWEEZERS:** I can't live without my Tweezermans.These are an obvious must for shaping brows, but also come in handy when applying false lashes, snagging stray facial hairs, splinters, and (in a pinch) food out of your teeth!

8. **YOUR FINGERS:** I love my brushes. But let's be honest, sometimes, it's just faster and more travel friendly, to use your fingers! Fingers are generally great for applying most cream-based cosmetics. Not to mention, concealers, foundations and cream blushes, when warmed by the hands, often blend more seamlessly into the skin.

Tool time!

MAC, Japonesque, Sonia Kashuk (available at Target), and Eco Tools (available at Walgreens) are a few brands that make great brushes.

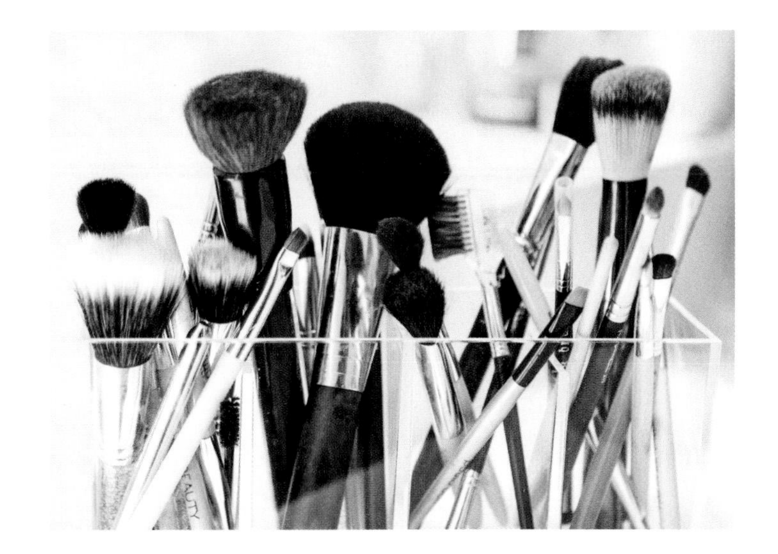

MEET MY FRIEND, THE PRODUCT WHORE: EMESE GORMLEY. I mean that in the best way possible. I love products, but ain't nobody loves products more than her. *Nobody*. Here are a few of her secrets.

EMESE'S *edicts*

- **CHECK YOUR WORK:** After you've applied makeup, always hold a mirror up to your face in natural light before you leave the house. This way you can confirm everything is blended and you don't have stray brush hairs on your face (it happens!).
- **DOUBLE THE FOUNDATION FUN:** If I love a foundation, I'll buy it in two different shades. I buy one in the shade closest to my natural skin color, and then the other one a shade or two darker. That way I can customize my own color and perfectly match my skin as it changes from season to season.
- **DOUBLE-CURL, GURL!:** Watch out—I'm a double curler. I first curl my lashes before I put on mascara, then I put on a coat or two—and then curl again. I'll even recurl my lashes in the middle of the day or after work. It's the fastest way to look instantly brighter. My favorite brand of mascara is Chantecaille Longest Lash. It has a deep black formula and lash growth serum. I had no lashes left after my lash extensions and this made them grow back in two weeks. Heaven sent!

Finally, while some people read the *Financial Times*, Emese surfs sites that talk and/or sell beauty. Her top: Intothegloss.com, Whowhatwear.com, Netaporter.com.

3 makeup looks
I love, love, love!

Meet the *Classic Red Lip*, the *Smoky & Seductive Eye*, and the *Bronzed Goddess*. They look good on everyone. The trick is to tailor the look to your skin tone, age, and style. Whether you have dark skin, light, or are somewhere in between, these looks can be adapted for everyone. They are tried, tested and makeup artist (Joey Maalouf) and model (me) approved.

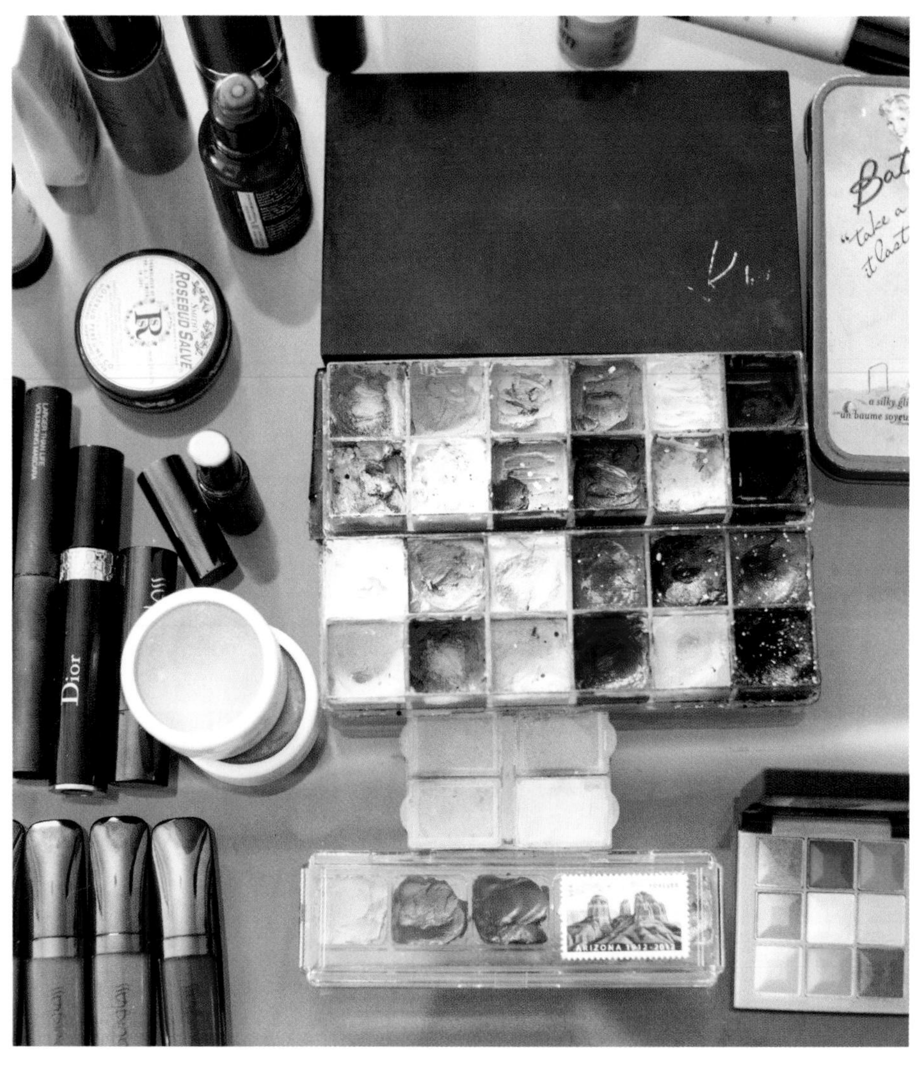

look one
THE CLASSIC RED LIP

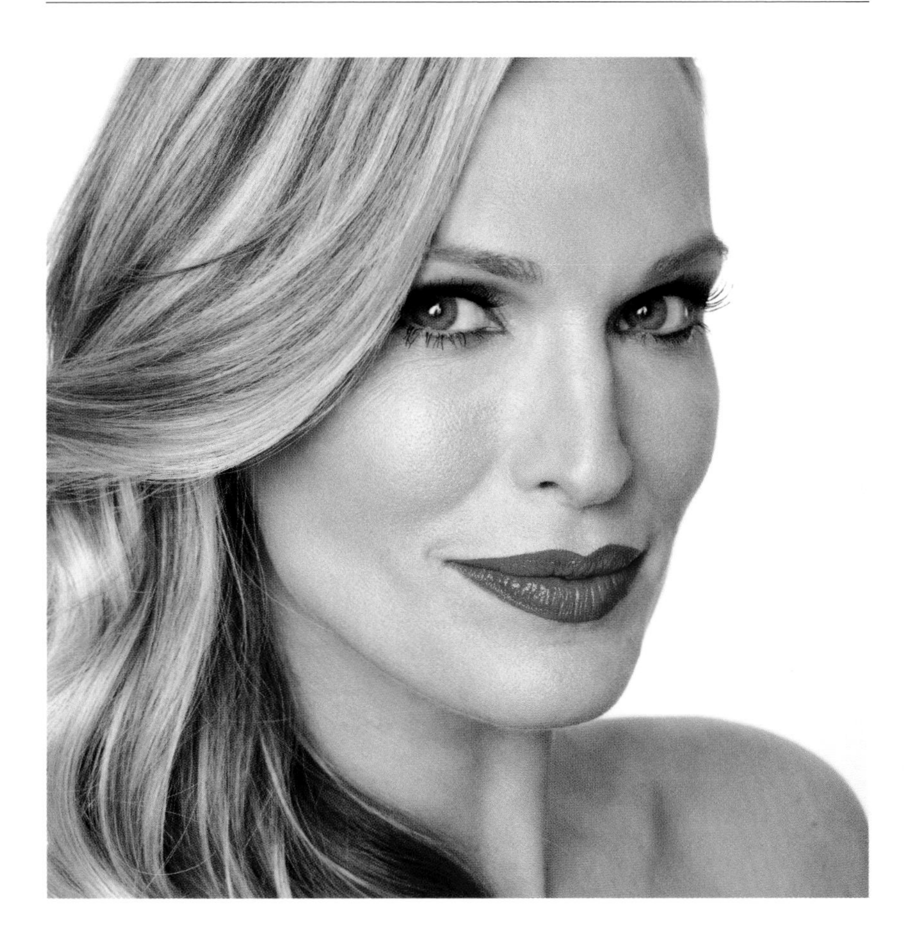

step 1: Keep skin fresh as a daisy. Simple, creamy foundation or tinted moisturizer with very subtle blush or bronzer.

step 2: Mascara and lots of it! Your eyes need nothing more. If you want a bit more pop, use a cream-colored eye pencil to tightline the inside of the bottom lashes.

step 3: When wearing a statement lip color, make sure your lips aren't chapped. Prep by exfoliating first (before applying your overall foundation). Then choose a lip color with a creamy, satiny finish for the most classic, sophisticated look (rather than a gloss-tastic-red or a matte finish). We used Raven by Hourglass. Trace with a lip liner in the matching shade if your lips lack definition.

BOLD LIP *tip*: There is a failproof way to give your lip color staying power and have it not get on your teeth. When doing any bold lip color, first dab a layer of color on straight from the tube. After, place a tissue over the lips and then, with a brush, pat a bit of translucent powder onto the lip over the top of the tissue. Then go again! Dab a bit more lip color, tissue, and powder. Finish with one last layer of color and if needed, line the lip.

---

supermodel *secret*

A red that has cooler undertones will make your teeth appear whiter, while reds with warmer undertones can make teeth seem a little yellow. Try out shades and find the one that looks best with your skin tone and your teeth. One thing's for sure. A red lip is another style shortcut!

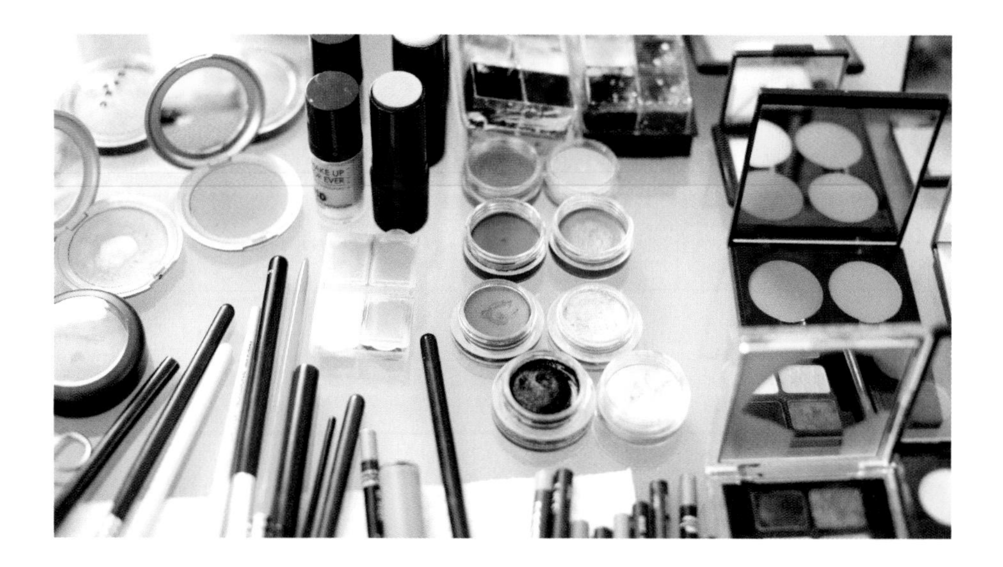

Bold lips are brave and beautiful. They have the ability to pull an entire look together and make a statement with very little effort.

—JOEY MAALOUF, makeup artist

---

look two
SEDUCTIVE AND SMOKY EYE

For a modern look, we love to smoke out the eyes with a color like navy or charcoal. We went dramatic, but you can use just one shade for a more subtle, smoky statement.

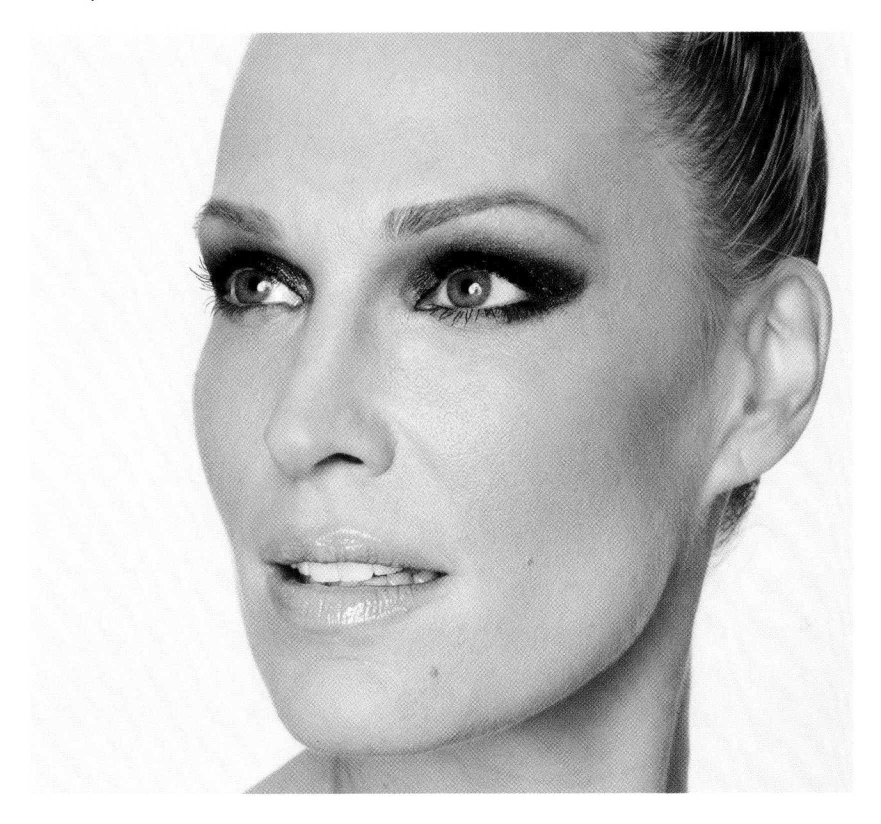

step 1: Use a simple, dewy foundation with a soft, pink blush.
step 2: Use a beige (base) shade, apply it all over the upper eyelid, sweeping it up into the brow line.
step 3: Use a wet to dry cream shadow in a charcoal with a bit of shimmer. The Chanel Mirifique Illusion d'Ombre is a one-stop shop. Apply it starting on the ball of the eyelid, then extend in a V-shape along the outer edge of the eye and into the crease. Use your fingers to blend into the crease and then lightly blend upward with a dry brush.
step 4: Use the residue from the brush to sweep just a little underneath the bottom lashes.

step 5: For extra drama, use a dark eggplant or even black shadow on the outside corner of the crease in a windshield wiper motion into the center of the crease. Using the same color, smoke out the bottom corner of the eye in a very thin line.

step 6: Lashes! Curl your lashes and apply several coats of mascara to the top and bottom. To go big, try adding a few false, flare eyelashes to the top.

step 7: Pair the bold eye with a sheer nude, pinky, or a pale lip gloss.

A modern smoky eye does not mean you need to use a million different shadow colors or black. And a smoky eye doesn't have to be overly bold. Using a khaki green or a navy can be simple, chic, and professionally glamorous.

—JOEY MAALOUF, makeup artist

---

alternate simple smoky
ONE SHADE & THREE STEPS

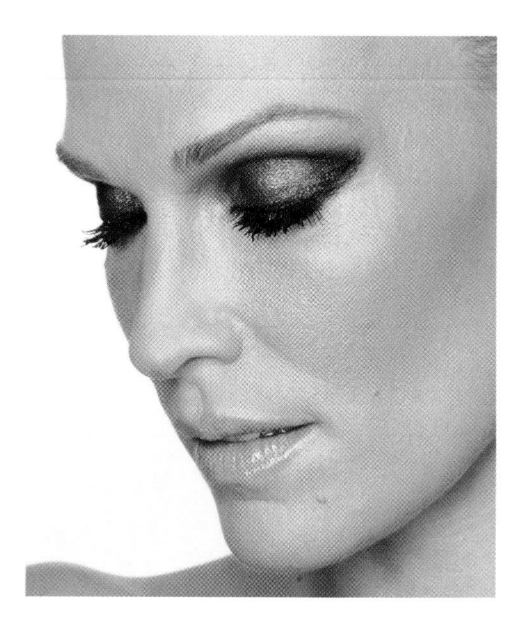

step 1: Using a cream (or wet to dry) eye shadow, smudge your top eyelid. (A cream shadow is seductive.) Then, using a puff shadow brush, smudge it from the inside corner to the outside corner.

step 2: With the same cream shadow, line the bottom lash line, start from the outside corner and finish the line to the inside corner.

step 3: Brush three coats of black volume mascara on the top and bottom lashes. *Keep everything else simple.* This look is a no-brainer for any age or eye shape.

look three
BRONZED GODDESS WITH GIANPAOLO'S SUNSET EYE

Every celeb does a bronzed goddess look from time to time. JLo, Charlize, Beyoncé, and Gisele have it mastered. Like any look, it can be turned up or down a notch. It can be natural and sunkissed or . . . dramatic like a bronze sphyinx come to life! That look is straight off the runway and out of fashion magazines.

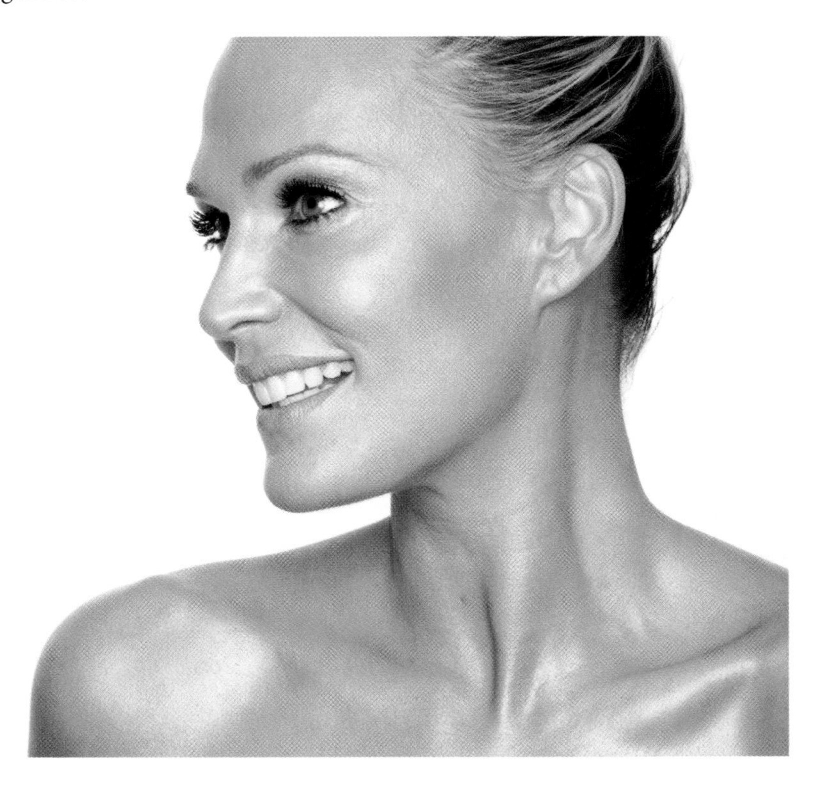

step 1: For a baby smooth canvas, start out using a foundation the color of your chest (For most, that means a shade darker than your face)—this will create a seamless look. Apply it all over your face and under the eyes as well.

step 2: Bronzer is key to this look. Use a warm shade with no shimmer; apply it to the sides of your forehead down to the temples. Also apply just under your cheekbones and along the jawline. This will intensify bone structure.

step 3: Add a touch of creamy, coral blush to the apples of the cheek; this will bring out the warmth in your bronzer.

step 4: Pair with Gianpaolo's Sunset Eye.

the sunset eye by GIANPAOLO CECILIATO

---

step 1: Line the top lid of the eye with a bronze pencil and also the inside on the bottom. We love Dolce & Gabbana Bronzo.

step 2: Take a medium brown eye shadow (we use Rachel Roy's Dark Magic), and sweep it just under the bottom lash line and along the outer corner and crease—keeping the color diffused and the line very soft. Make a soft V-shape.

step 3: Then make a V-shape in the outer crease of the eye and a little along the bottom corner with a bronze shadow (something not too sparkly, but with a nice shimmer). Blend the bronze shadow in with the brown shadow.

step 4: With a softer brush, sweep a gold shimmer shadow in the inner crease of the eye and use a windshield wiper motion to blend it in with the bronze shadow in the outside corner. The goal is to have an ombré effect, lightest color toward the inside blending to the darkest along the outside of the eyes.

step 5: Place a little bit of gold eyeliner (we love *gold by D&G*) to the inner lash line, top and bottom, to brighten and add sparkle to the eyes.

step 6: Add subtle mascara to define lashes—not too much, we don't want spider lashes to take center stage.

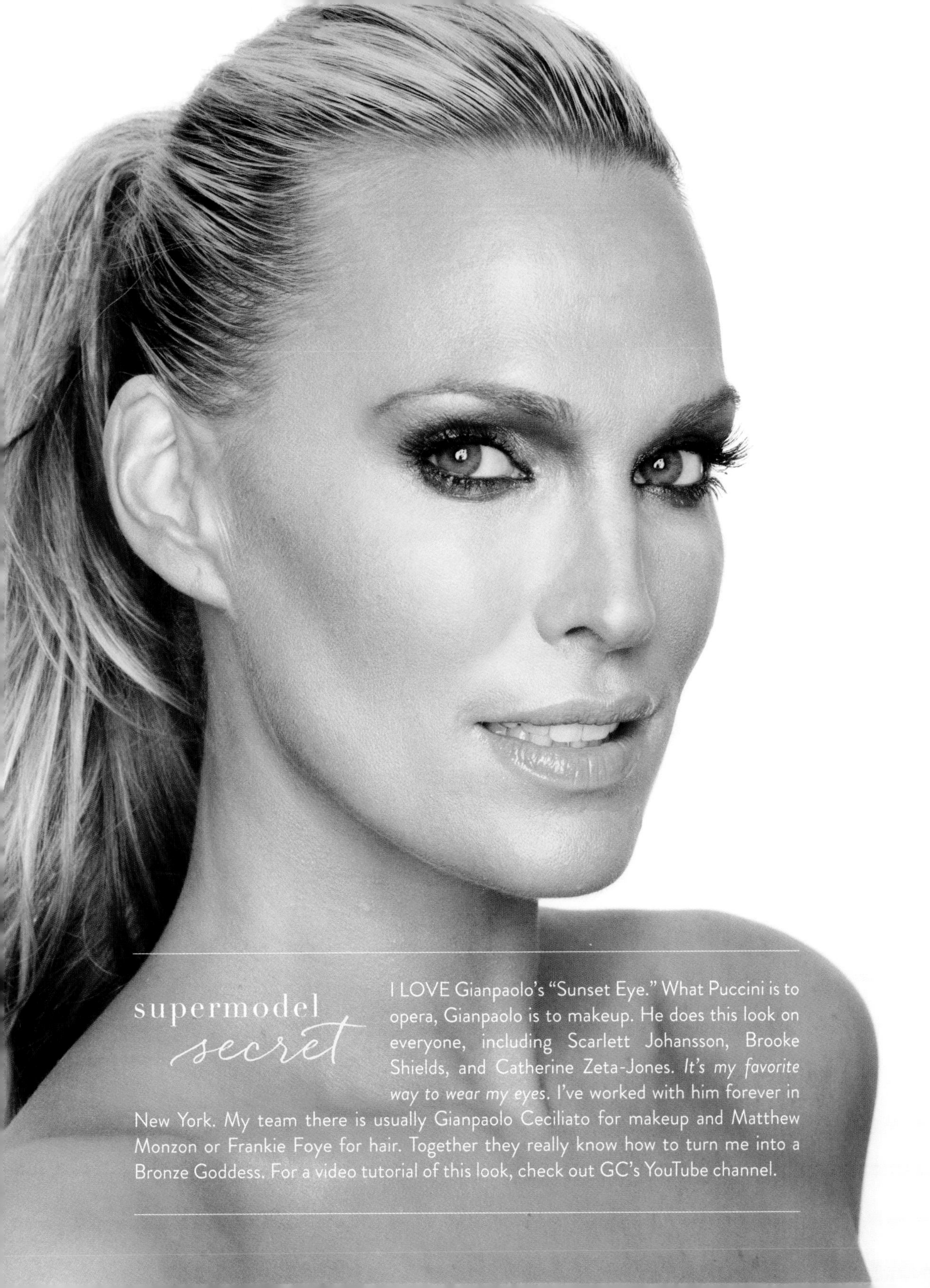

supermodel *secret*

I LOVE Gianpaolo's "Sunset Eye." What Puccini is to opera, Gianpaolo is to makeup. He does this look on everyone, including Scarlett Johansson, Brooke Shields, and Catherine Zeta-Jones. *It's my favorite way to wear my eyes*. I've worked with him forever in New York. My team there is usually Gianpaolo Ceciliato for makeup and Matthew Monzon or Frankie Foye for hair. Together they really know how to turn me into a Bronze Goddess. For a video tutorial of this look, check out GC's YouTube channel.

HOW TO *highlight*, NOT *strobelight*

A bronzed look with added highlight gives dimension and brings out the beauty of a face. Without highlighter, the look can just seem a bit dirty. Highlight can be added to a variety of makeup looks—and also looks fresh on bare, makeup-free skin. Every skin tone and color can benefit from it. There is a difference between highlighting and strobelighting. Pay attention to these rules.

> *My favorite product at the moment for highlighting and contouring is Tom Ford's Shade and Illuminate.*
>
> —**MONIKA BLUNDER**, makeup artist

- Focus on the high points of the face.
- Sweep a little under the eyebrow and a bit on the Cupid's bow of your lip.
- With a small brush, run a line of highlighter down the bridge of the nose.
- Place a dab at the top of the cheekbone, making sure not to apply any to the apple.
- Blend in with a sponge or tap in with your fingers.
- Take a clean, dry fluffy brush and sweep across the face lightly to blend any lines.
- Finish with translucent powder just on the T-zone and on the sides of the nose.
- Highlighter is also beautiful placed on the tops of shoulders and along the collarbone.

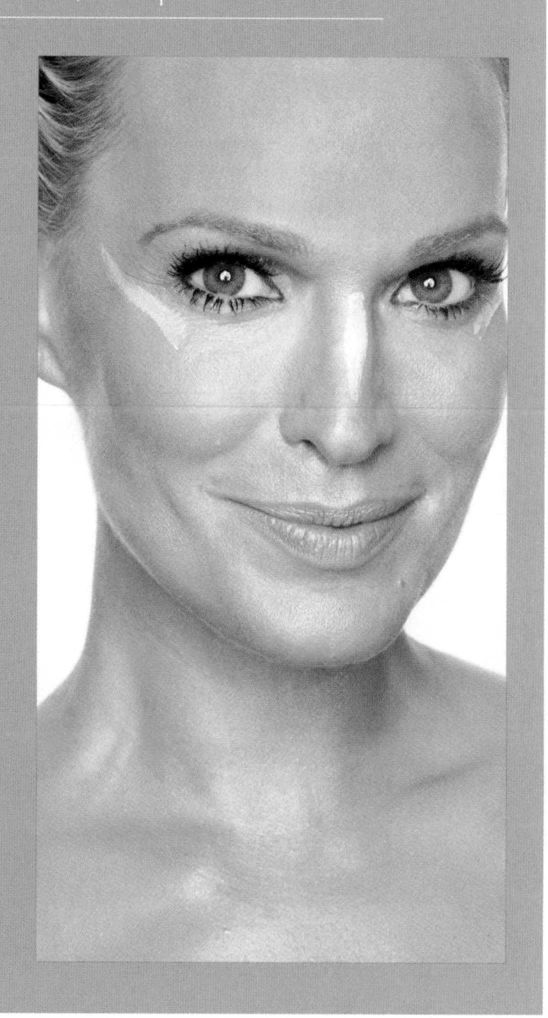

GLAMOROUS *vs* GLAMAZON

Sometimes when you try too hard to look your best, you end up going overboard. Too much of a good thing is usually—too much. I have absolutely, positively looked like a drag queen because the makeup artist was too heavy-handed. Here's how to avoid looking like a glamazon.

break up with the Following Makeup

1. **TOO MUCH FOUNDATION:** We all know this, but I still see it happening: when you can see the line around your face, you are committing cosmetic sin number one. Newsflash! You don't have to apply foundation everywhere. You can apply it just where you need it, ladies, and blend. Always make sure it's blended and that includes the jawline/neck.

2. **EXTREME EYEBROWING:** Ladies, ladies, ladies. Puh-lease don't do this. Do not line your eyebrows within an inch of their life. The goal is to enhance the brow not hunt it down, kill it, and hang it on the wall of your forehead.

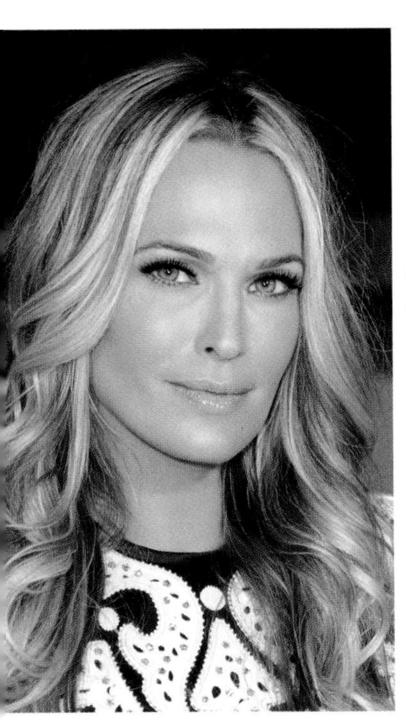

Focus on one feature: bold eyes = soft lips

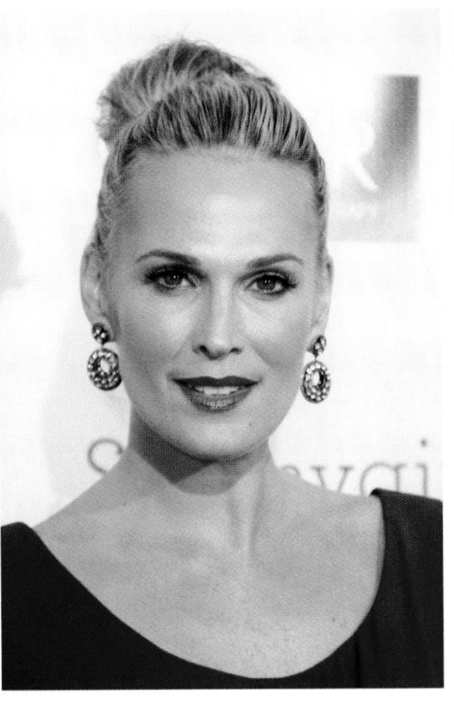

Heavy makeup can age you: case in point.

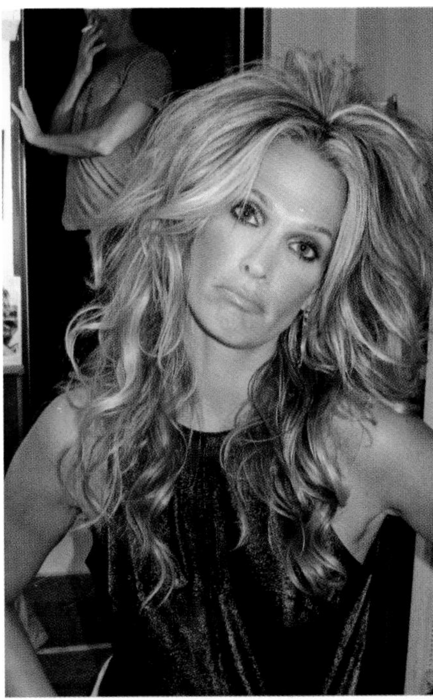

Call the color police! Yikes!

3. **EXTREME LIP-LINING:** Same goes for your lips. I only use lip liner when I'm wearing a dark or red lip color. It's more fresh and modern to go without. And never overline the lips for a bigger effect. It's just obvious and makes you look like a porn star.

4. **TROUT POUT AND GLOSS GOO:** Do not over-gloss your lips. Less is more.

5. **PUNKY BREWSTER FACE:** Stick to a color story here. It should never look like a Crayola box exploded on your face. Try to stay within a family, grays/taupes, browns/bronzes, not ROYGBIV. In general, focus on one feature of your face, not them all.

6. **DISC-OH-NO:** Practice safe sparkling. Your face should never resemble a disco ball. A little goes a loooooong way. The key with sparkle: strategically place it. If eyes are all-a-glitter, lips should not be.

7. **GO-GO-GADGET LASHES:** Yes, eyelashes are pretty. But that does not mean you should be able to jump rope with them. Spider lashes look ridiculous and clumpy and I don't know a man alive who likes this look. Stop the insanity. If you want to know how to do faux lashes right, take Monika's advice here.

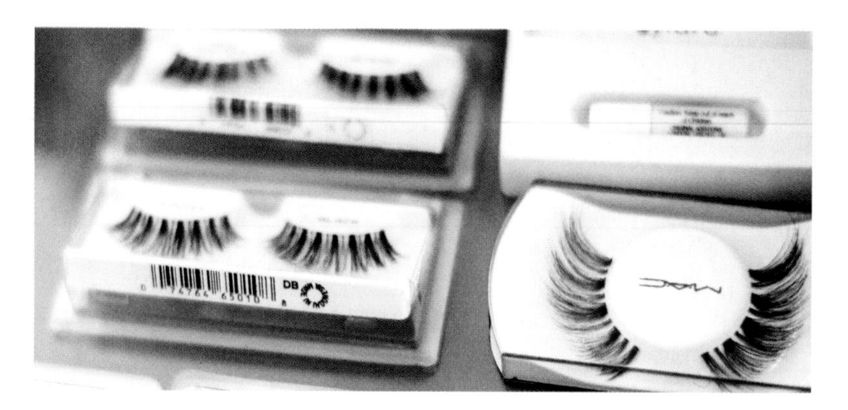

All women have insecurities and celebrities are no different. But as makeup artists, we can help each woman to feel more beautiful and confident. I know makeup does that—and that's still amazing to me.

—MONIKA BLUNDER, makeup artist

---

lash lessons WITH MONIKA BLUNDER

False lashes aren't just for photo shoots and prom. They can be easy to use and look extranatural or superglam. Not to mention, as we get older, our eyelashes get thinner, so they are great for volume in an instant. Flare lashes are fun to use once you get the hang of it. Use a variety of lengths for the most natural look. When done well, they can look like your natural lashes, only better! A strip lash is good for retro looks (think the '50s, '60s, and Katy Perry videos) and lots of glamour. Just be aware, you may have to cut it to fit the length of your eye. A few tips, use the black lash glue over the clear; it also enhances the lash line. For a nontoxic glue try LashLab. Tweezers are the best tool for maneuvering lashes onto the eyelids. Before applying the false lashes, curl your own and apply a coat of mascara. Also, fit the false lashes in between your real ones on the lash line (and not the skin) for the most natural effect. Line the top lid with black liner to conceal any glue. Lash practice eventually makes perfect! Once you master the art of lashes, you'll never get enough.

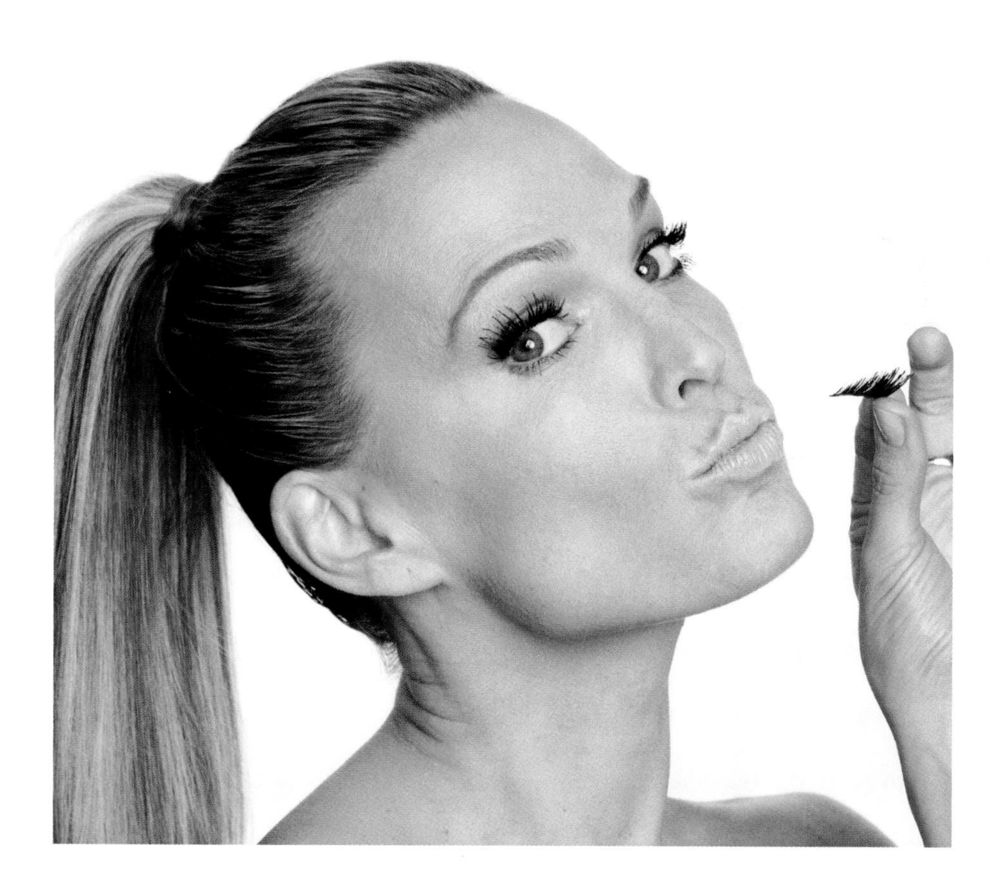

BODY BEAUTY *tips*

Believe me, my skin and legs do not wake up looking like they do in the pages of *Sport Illustrated.* Nobody's do. For looks like that, I've been spray tanned, oiled, body makeup-ed, Vaselined, and more. In reality, my skin is dry as a desert and I struggle with eczema. Never fear, you can fake great skin, like I do/they do. Here are some wearable ways you can get magazine-worthy skin.

1. **FOR SHEER COVERAGE:** MAC has a lightweight line of foundation designed for use on the body and it comes in lots of shades. It softens the look of leg veins and broken capillaries—and won't wipe off on clothes. Sold! Prtty Peaushun Skin Tight Body Lotion gives legs that silky/smooth "I'm wearing stockings" look—but you're not. It's got a pearly, soft focus finish and is beautiful for highlighting the collarbone too.

2. **GLOSSING PRODUCTS:** Nars Body Shimmer Oil and Caudalie Divine Legs give a delicate bronze glow and shimmer to the skin—and smell delicious! However, you have to apply them well in advance of getting dressed; otherwise, it can grease and stain clothes. Avon Skin So Soft and Vaseline Spray and Go are easy to use and give limbs luster.

3. **CAMOUFLAGE COSMETICS:** Dermablend is the industry standard. This highly pigmented oil-based concealer covers scars, stretch marks, birthmarks, leg veins, mosquito bites, tattoos, and even bruising from facial fillers. It's water and smudge resistant.

4. **TANNING PRODUCTS:** Tanning towels by L'Oréal and by the originator, Tan Towel, are my favorites. Avène and Bain de Soleil brands also give good bronze and don't smell awful. Rodial makes a spray for instant bronze—and it doesn't rub off. Important: Baby wipe your palms after applying any tanning products so they don't look all George Hamiltony.

SUPERMODEL *stems*

My close friend, leggy supermodelmomma, and makeup artist Jessica Berg Prosser made her living by doing heaps of sexy hosiery ads and stylish shoe campaigns. She's got legs and knows how to use 'em! Here are her tried and tested tips to getting *everyday supermodel* stems.

1. **DUNGEON OF LUNGES:** Walking lunges are the single best exercise for legs/butt, so I would do them by the truck-load and still do. I also did ballet style calf raises every day for toned calves: first with toes straight, then with toes out, and finally with toes in.

2. **GET FOOTLOOSE:** Your feet are an extension of your legs, so they should not be neglected. I'd load them up with a mixture of peppermint oil and Vaseline, then pop socks on to sleep.

3. **SPECIAL POTION:** I use this all the time on my model clients. Exfoliate the skin first; I love Pure Figi Coconut Sugar Scrub. Then, mix Nivea Silky Shimmer Lotion with a few squirts of MAC Face and Body Foundation in a shade darker than your skin color and apply. This combo gives legs a smooth, soft-focus finish and it's not sticky.

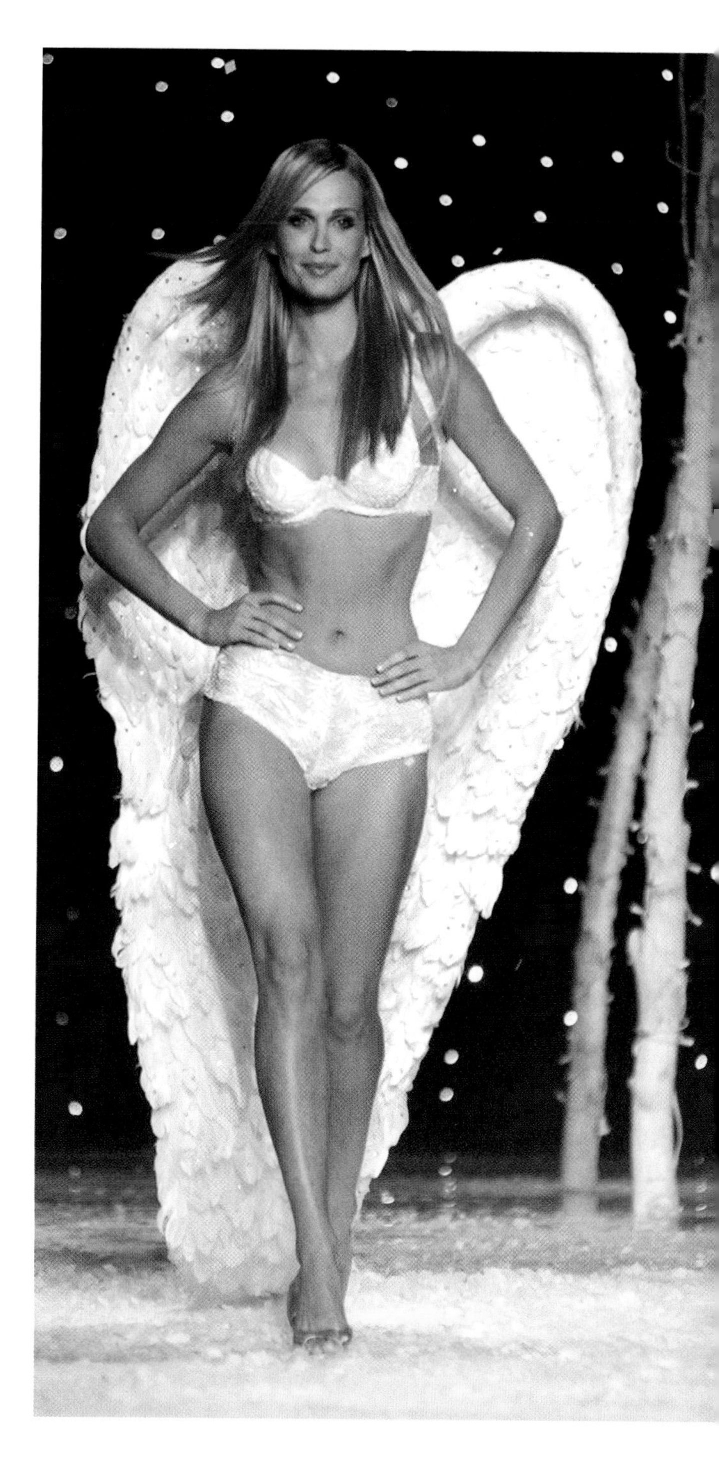

the ultimate finishing touch

MANICURE *management*

Maybe it's the southern girl in me, but you'll almost never see my nails "neked." Polished nails add, well—polish—to any look. For me, choosing my nail color is emotional. It's usually a direct reflection of how I feel, or how I *want* to feel. Your nail color can send a message! It can be sexy or sweet or somewhere in between.

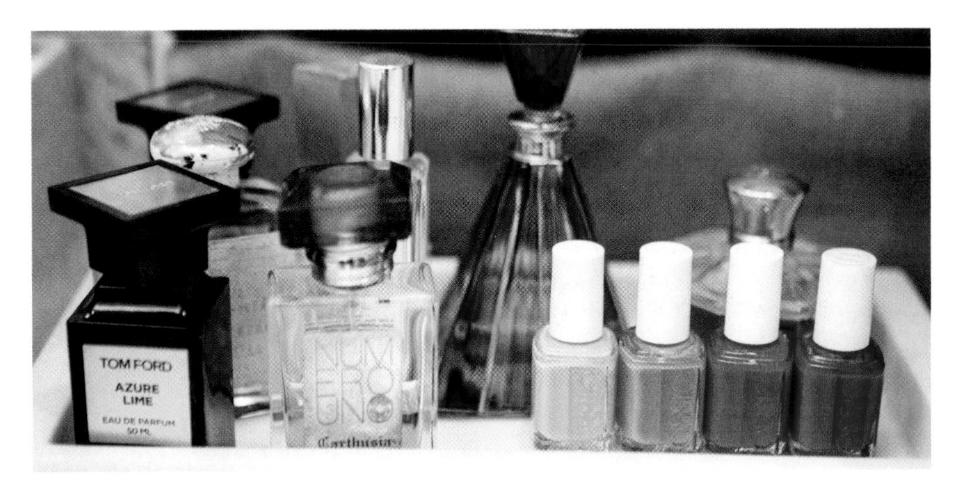

Colors that stand the *everyday supermodel* test of time:

1. ***MRS· O'LEARY'S BBQ* BY OPI:** A brownish/raisin color, à la . . . BBQ sauce! It's dark and moody but seriously sexy in a kind of mod way. A smokin' fall/winter shade.

2. ***JELLY APPLE* BY ESSIE:** It's a great orange red! Fresh, summery, and happy . . . you'll find it on my toes all summer. It's stunning paired with white and turquoise.

3. ***BIG APPLE RED* BY OPI:** The perfect red. Not too blue, not too orange—just right. It looks good on every skin tone and is a never-fail classic that glamorizes your little black dress.

4. ***WALK DOWN THE AISLE* BY ESSIE:** It is a soft, sheer pinkish-white that looks like it sounds. Feminine and soft, prim and proper, polite and fresh. Perfect for spring!

5. ***TANGERINE* BY ESSIE:** Think coral-tastic! It looks phenomenal on dark skin, pale skin, tan skin—you name it skin. It's flirty, sassy, and fun, but still chic and sophisticated.

HOW TO *nail it*

Celeb manicurist Miwa Kobayashi has been doing my nails for years. Here are a few of her tips for polish perfection:

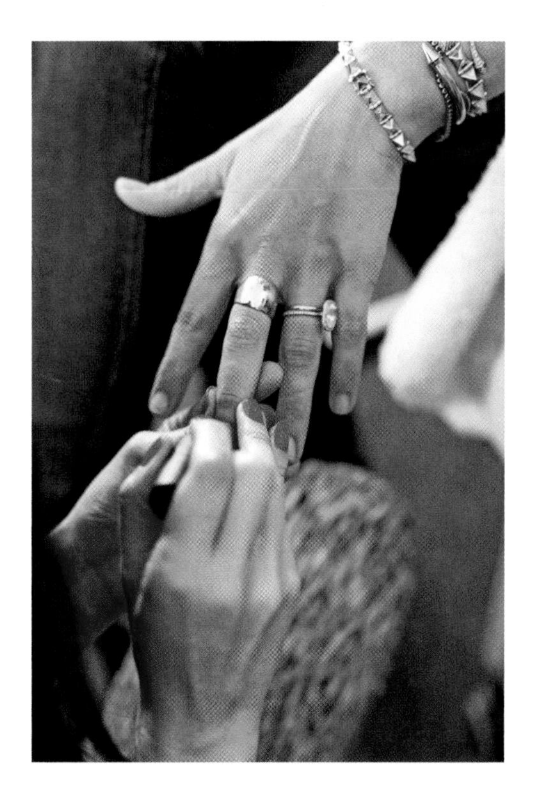

- To make hands appear younger—choose soft colors, such as pale pinks and nudes, or bright, fresh colors, like corals and candy apple reds.
- Want your mani/pedi to last longer? Apply a thin, clear topcoat to your nails each day the week after.
- To soften hands and help prevent nails from splitting and chipping, try a DIY moisturizing mask for hands once a week. It's as easy as massaging on plain yogurt and then wrapping them in plastic wrap (or thermal mitts).
- If you are looking to go green, Zoya, Chrome Girl, Sheswai, and OPI are all nontoxic and fragrance free. A safe-for-tots-and-tweens nail polish option is Piggy Paint.
- On a budget or short on time? Just ask for a "polish change" and go from glum to glam in under $10 and 10 minutes.

---

supermodel *secret*

A deep, rich, glossy, vampy nail color punctuating "people paws" is an instant *everyday supermodel* short-cut. My go-to of go-tos for this is OPI's *Lincoln Park After Dark*. Gorgeous nails are an affordable luxury that dresses you up without wearing your wallet down.

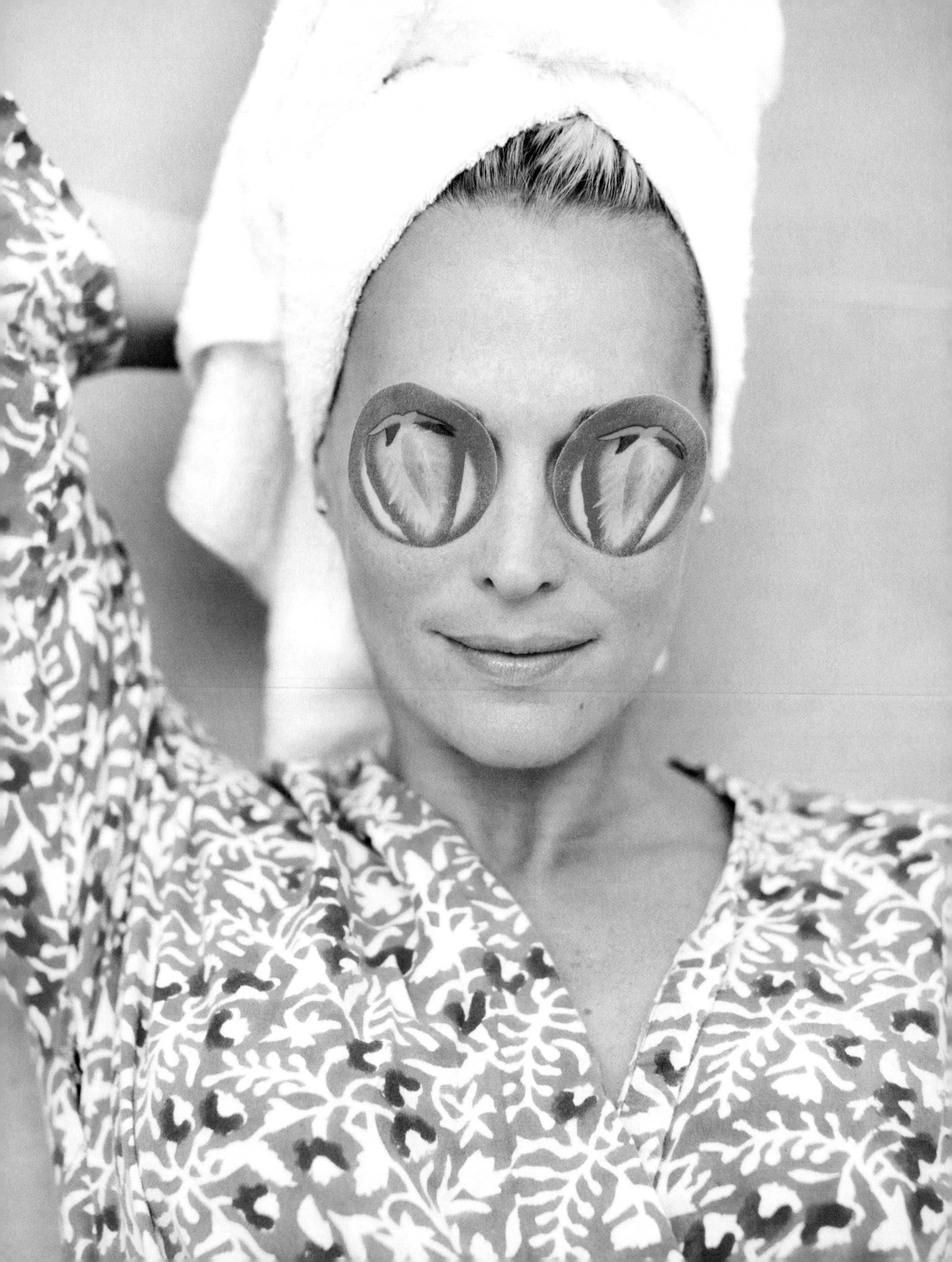

the *everyday* supermodel TOP 10 takeaways

1. Use the Fantastic Five: They are ingredients proven to work and will transform your skin, whatever your age. I promise you . . . you can't go wrong here. No gimmicks—just the goods!

2. Start taking care of your skin *yesterday*. The earlier the better, but if you haven't, then START NOW. Sunscreen, treatments, at-home beauty routines—do it. Be on top of your skin health. If you spend time on your skin, it will show. If you don't, it will show.

3. Do the research and get referrals whether seeing a facialist, a dermatologist, or anyone treating your skin. Go to the best of the best and look for the specialist who specializes in exactly what you are looking for.

4. Remember the L.A. Polish. Be subtle, and just a little at a time.

5. When it comes to makeup, play a little! Have fun. Experiment and don't get stuck in a rut. Watch videos online or have an artist at a counter teach you how. There's so much information out there to help and inspire.

6. You can't go wrong with a classic look. The Perfect Red Lip, a Smoky Eye, and the Bronze Goddess look good on everyone and at every age. Tailor looks you love to your skin color and style.

7. Dewy is always better than dry. Whatever your look, make sure it has an element of glow. Be the powder police especially as you get older. Incorporate more cream-based makeup, especially for foundation and cheek color. Dewier skin looks more youthful.

8. When in doubt, a bold lip will save the day if you are in a sprint. Throw on a scarf and some sunnies and you will be tres chic.

9. Less is always more when it comes to makeup, treatments, and products. Always choose glamorous over glamazon.

10. Thou shalt believe in yourself, recognize your natural beauty, and *work what you got*! Know you are gorgeous and work to maximize your potential. Be in charge of your life and your looks.

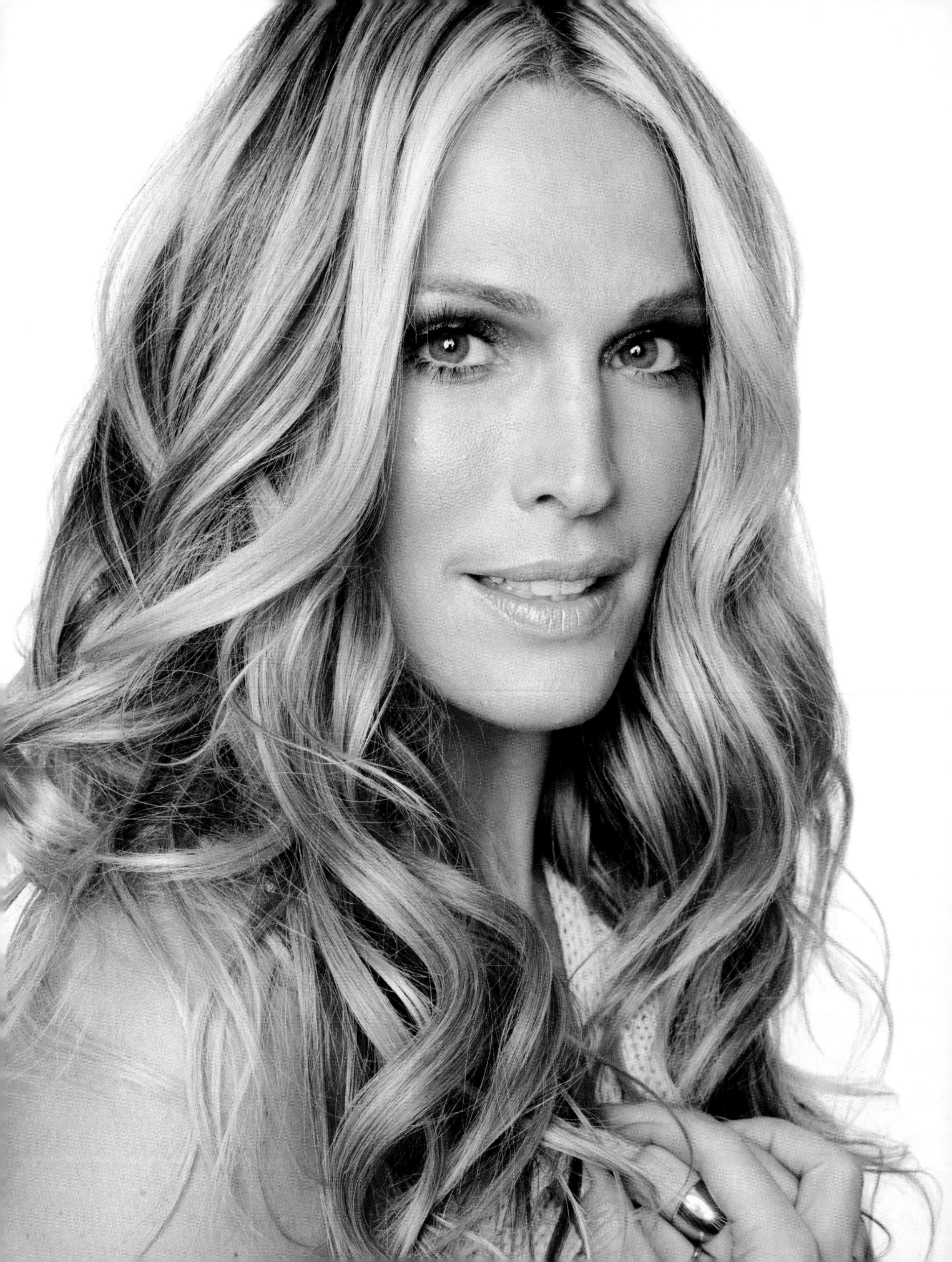

ch/5

hair, hair everywhere

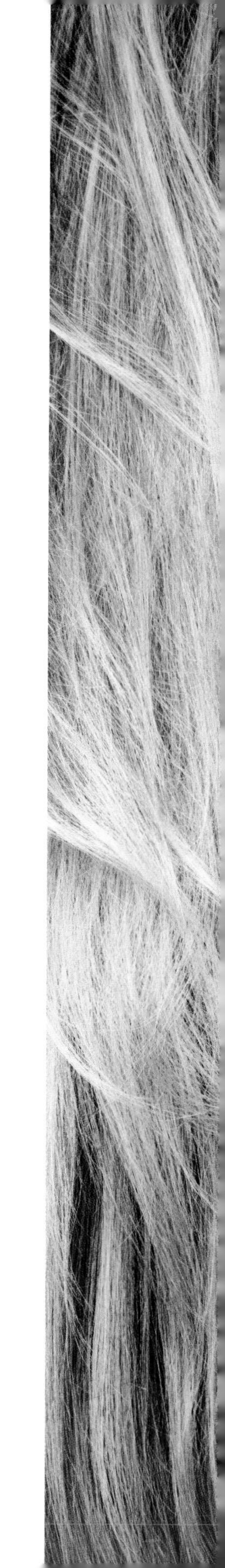

I've been obsessed with hair ever since I was a little girl with an overbite and Dorothy Hamill bowl cut. I had a doll whose hair "grew" when you pulled it so you could cut and style it. I used to cut her hair *obsessively* . . . until I ran out of hair. Without a plastic friend to style, I turned the scissors on my own locks and chopped away. Let me tell you, a homemade haircut is not exactly the best way to start to grade school.

My obsession with hair only grew from there. Being from a small town in the South, I will never forget the day my momma came back from a big city business trip up North and said to me, "Molly, *you won't believe it.* All the college girls are wearing their hair . . . *straight.*" Gasp. Double gasp. I could hardly breathe. I was terrified. It went against everything I had ever known. Flat, straight hair was unheard of in the Bible Belt. Hair was supposed to be BIG and CURLY. Our mantra was the bigger *the better.* I rocked curls piled on top of curls, teased, reteased, and finally set with ½ a can of Aqua Net. It was called the "mall pouf."

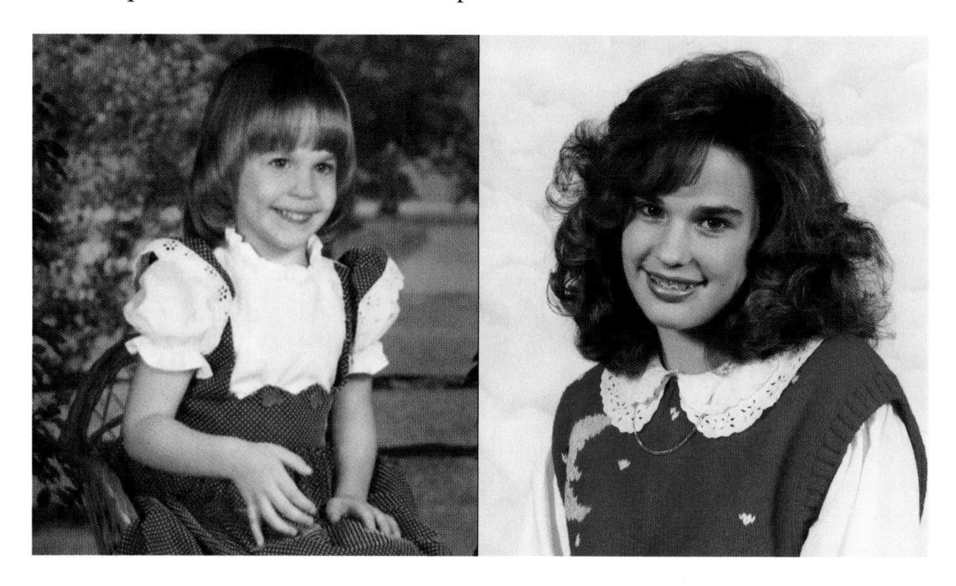

By the time I was seventeen years old I had had *at least* as many perms. Bangs rose off my head like the Second Coming. But my momma was right. The fashionable girls in the big cities had pulled a fast one on us. And God as my witness, I would not be left behind! I eventually transitioned to wearing my hair straight and have been rocking a straight hair look ever since (later, we give you a step-by-step how-to of my fave supermodel straight version).

Luckily, I've come a long way since the mall pouf, but because of the demands my career puts on my hair, I've been to hell and back with it!

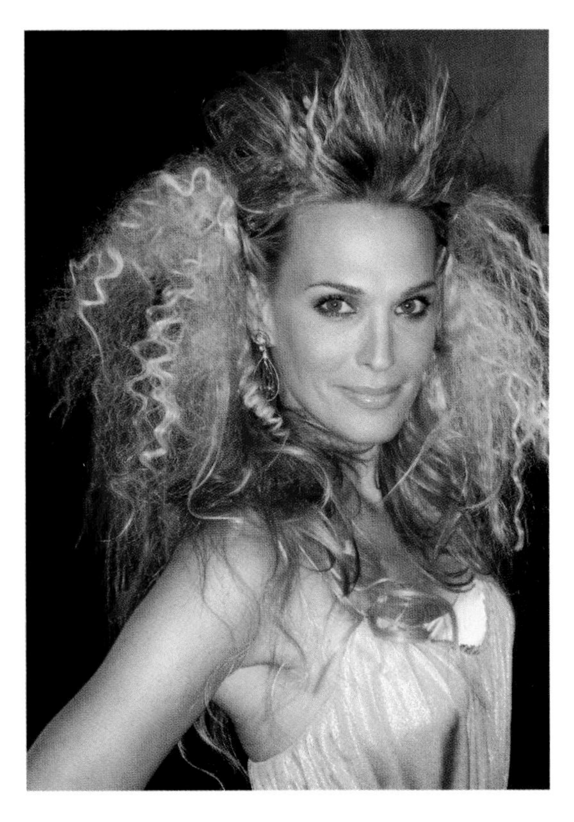

For decades my hair has been manipulated with color, styling, groping and poking. I have witnessed clumps of hair break off right in front of my eyes. Scary. In general, I've been blessed with good hair genes, but that doesn't mean I haven't had my fair share of BAD hair days. Who doesn't have a love/hate relationship with her hair? We stress out, our hair falls out. We get pregnant and suddenly we're clearing out the shower drain for *days*. And God forbid it's humid out, right? All hell breaks loose!

Whether your hair is straight, curly, long, short, thick, thin, or somewhere in between—you can absolutely make the best of what you've got. In here, my experts and I walk you through how to fake volume, get the right cut and color, grow your hair back after getting a bad haircut (or frying it off), get out of a style rut, fight frizz, secure shine, and more. We give you all the tools you need to Hollywood your hair! I don't think there is a woman out there who won't admit that when her hair is cooperating . . . she is *calm, cool and collected*!.

And my obsession with hair does not stop at the scalp. Hair-care these days is a full-time job. We've got our pits, our privates, our brows, and every other place hair crops up where it simply shouldn't (ah, the joys of aging.) We go over what to wax and how to wax, as well as when to laser and when not to. Let's go, ladies . . . *everyday supermodel* hair happiness awaits.

My Hair *harem*!

- **TRACEY CUNNINGHAM:** The best colorist on this here planet. Tracey co-owns Meche Salon in Los Angeles. There isn't a celebrity this woman has not colored. I mean it . . . she's hair-raising-amazing.
- **DAVY NEWKIRK:** We met on the set of MTV's *House of Style* and he's been styling my hair hot ever since. Davy is my hair kingpin.
- **ADRIANA TESLER:** Hairstylist, but really hair artist. Adriana always saves the day and gets me red carpet ready in a flash. Her work is stunning and you'll see it inside this chapter.
- **RIKI B:** Wizard of waxing, below-the-belt beautician, esthetician. Pruning Hollywood's down-there-hair for over a decade.
- **KRISTIE STREICHER:** Leonard(a) da Vinci of brow styling, bicoastal babe rehabbing overworked brows in New York and L.A.
- **CAILE NOBLE:** Known for his skill with shears and for creating supermodel cuts, he creates looks for magazines and red carpet events and calls Andy LeCompte Salon in West Hollywood his home.

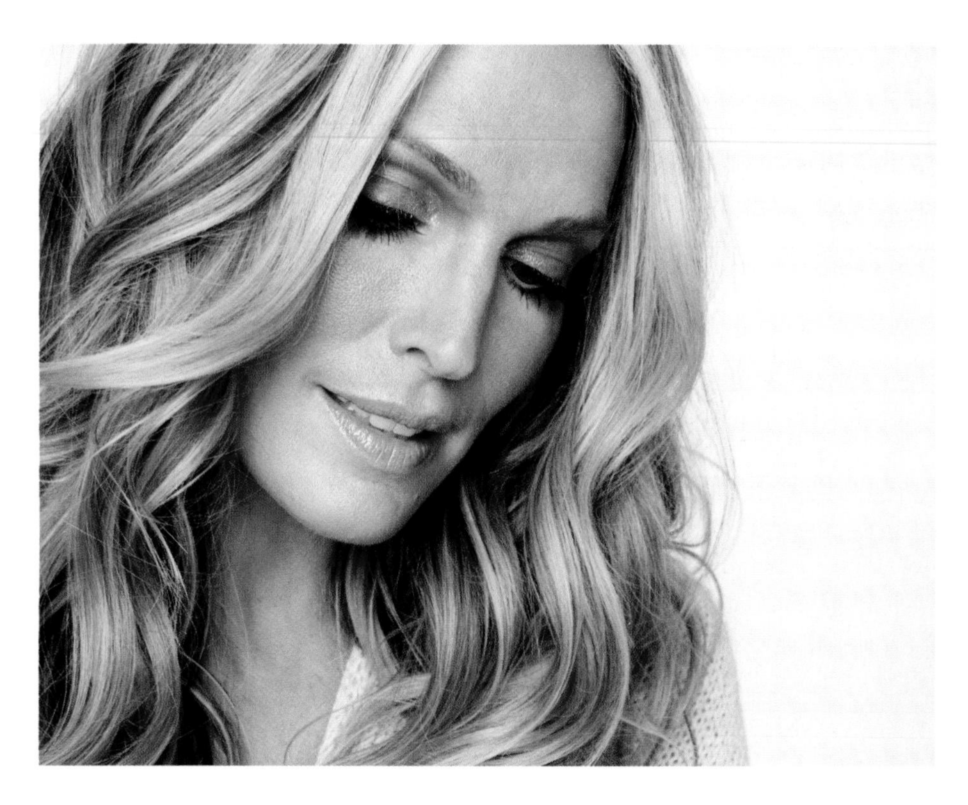

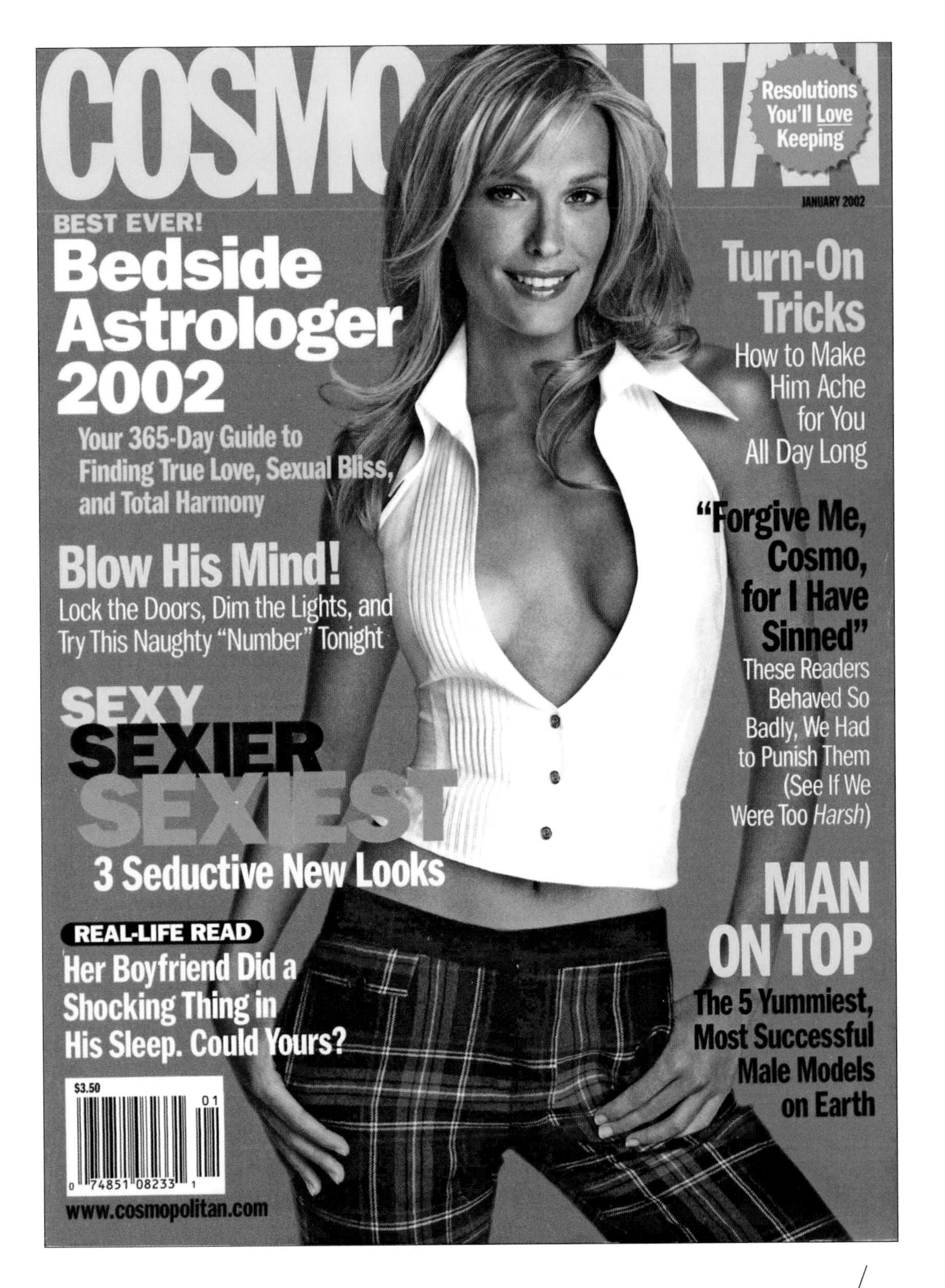
COSMOPOLITAN
Resolutions You'll Love Keeping
JANUARY 2002
BEST EVER!
Bedside Astrologer 2002
Your 365-Day Guide to Finding True Love, Sexual Bliss, and Total Harmony
Blow His Mind!
Lock the Doors, Dim the Lights, and Try This Naughty "Number" Tonight
SEXY
SEXIER
SEXIEST
3 Seductive New Looks
REAL-LIFE READ
Her Boyfriend Did a Shocking Thing in His Sleep. Could Yours?
$3.50
01
0 74851 08233 1
www.cosmopolitan.com
Turn-On Tricks
How to Make Him Ache for You All Day Long
"Forgive Me, Cosmo, for I Have Sinned"
These Readers Behaved So Badly, We Had to Punish Them (See If We Were Too Harsh)
MAN ON TOP
The 5 Yummiest, Most Successful Male Models on Earth

THE ROOT OF THE ISSUE . . . *your hair health*

Not to toot my own tresses, but I have a solid head of hair. (Thanks Momma and Daddy!) That said, I have been through really bad times when it comes to the health of my hair—mostly due to my career—but also because I like to change my style and try new things. My personal hair horror stories might scare you into keeping that outdated style (don't!), but they've also taught me a thing or two about what it takes to build strong, healthy locks from the inside out.

* **SUPPLEMENTS:** Yes, we've discussed, but for those of you who need hair help, it bears repeating! I'm a believer in taking supplements for your skin, same goes for hair. Prenatals work well here. Also, when I was a model, I took something called Viviscal. It's an over-the-counter fish oil supplement that can be easily found online and in health stores. Models still take it because it works. Studies have proven that protein and essential fatty acids (EFAs), like those found in fish oil, effectively help to regulate hormones and stimulate hair growth. Biotin and silica supplements have also been proven to promote healthier hair and growth.
* **HAIR WASHING:** Stop overwashing your hair. Drop it down to at least every other day. Always use a gentle shampoo designed for color-treated hair even if you don't color yours (this is especially important if you are a redhead or have darker hair). Tracey Cunningham always reminds me: "You wouldn't wash a delicate cashmere sweater with a harsh detergent. Same goes for your hair."
* **HAIR CONDITIONING:** I use two different conditioners. It seems complicated, but it's not. I use a lightweight conditioner meant for processed hair on my entire head. And then, just on the ends, I use Terax, a very heavy conditioner. I don't mind spending more money on a conditioner (Davy agrees) because it stays on your hair the longest and it is meant to penetrate. A mayonnaise mask is a wallet-friendly way to nourish your hair.
* **HEAT HIATUS:** You've got to do it. Avoid using too many heat tools on your hair and occasionally take a break from blow-dryers and the like. Whenever using heat tools, first work a heat protectant into the hair. Topknots and ponytails are a simple way to look stylish without excess styling or using heat (see my *everyday supermodel* styling tips on pretty ponies and buns. Just skip any steps that require heat tools).

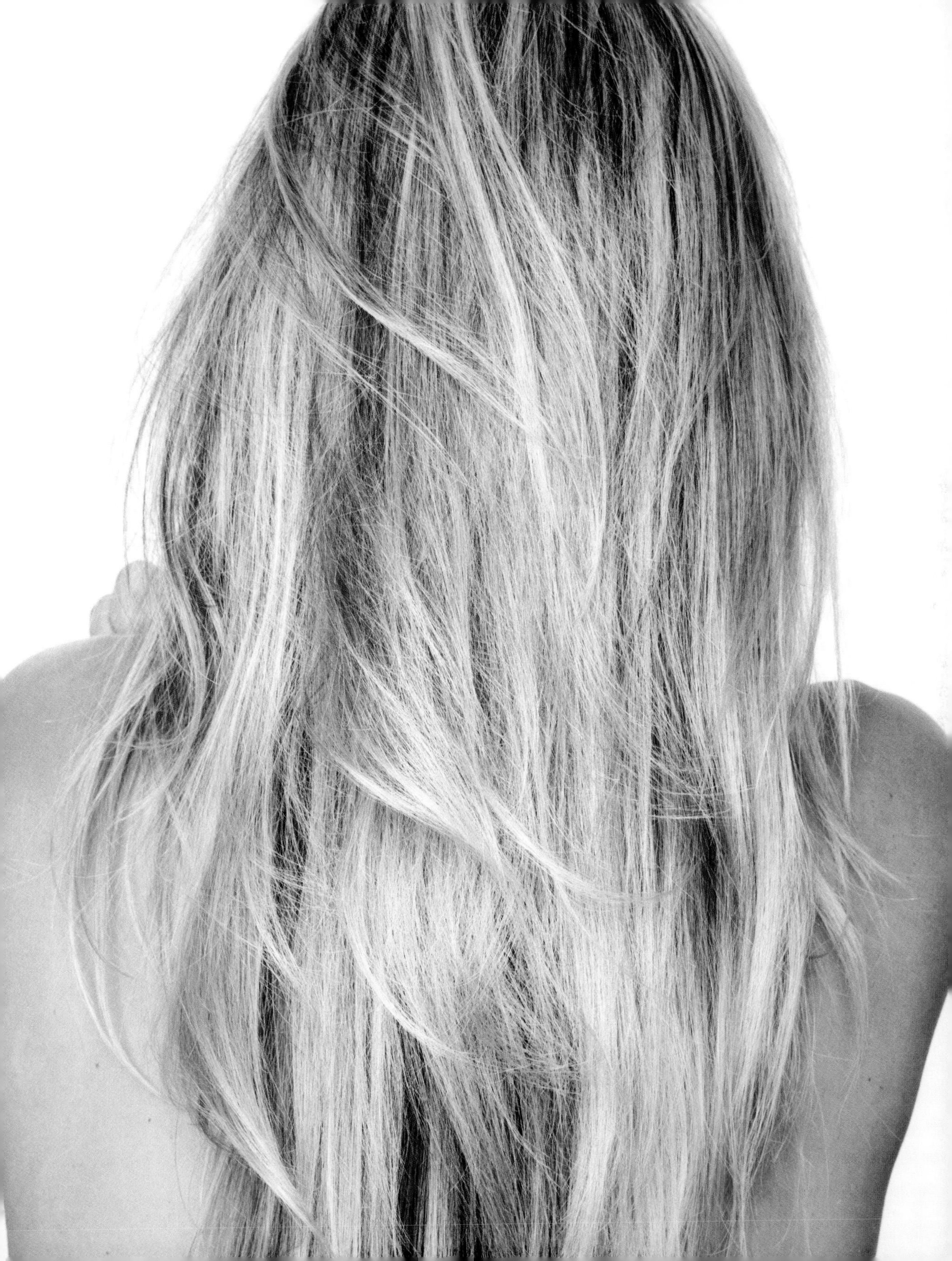

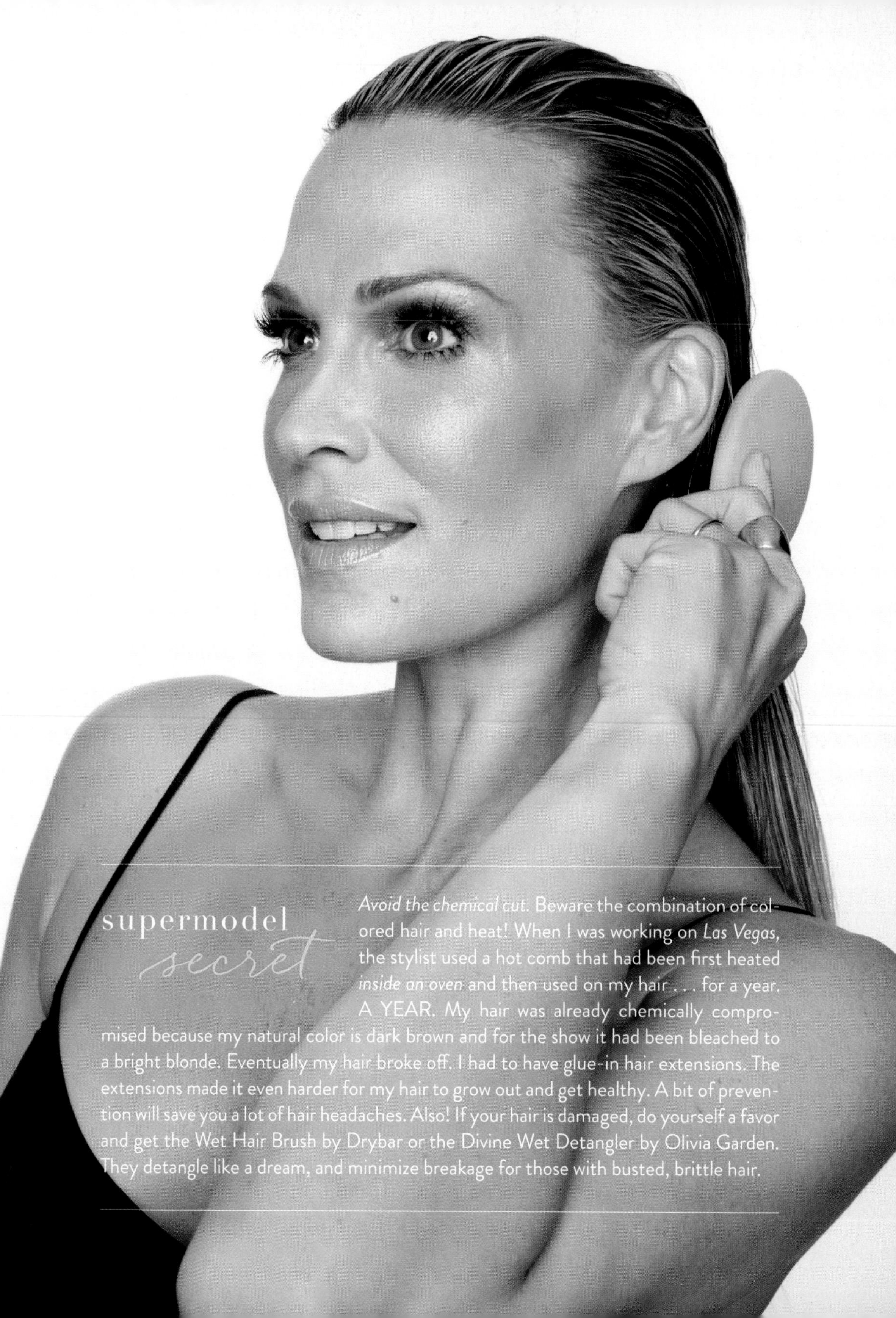

supermodel *secret*

Avoid the chemical cut. Beware the combination of colored hair and heat! When I was working on *Las Vegas*, the stylist used a hot comb that had been first heated *inside an oven* and then used on my hair . . . for a year. A YEAR. My hair was already chemically compromised because my natural color is dark brown and for the show it had been bleached to a bright blonde. Eventually my hair broke off. I had to have glue-in hair extensions. The extensions made it even harder for my hair to grow out and get healthy. A bit of prevention will save you a lot of hair headaches. Also! If your hair is damaged, do yourself a favor and get the Wet Hair Brush by Drybar or the Divine Wet Detangler by Olivia Garden. They detangle like a dream, and minimize breakage for those with busted, brittle hair.

DON'T JUST *want* BUT *need*

Hair products and tools my hair harem and I can't live without.

1. **SHAMPOO:** Nexus Color Care Shampoo. Kérastase shampoos for color-treated hair. Pureology products.

2. **CONDITIONER:** Nexus Color Care Shampoo. Kérastase Conditioners and Terax.

3. **LEAVE-IN TREATMENT:** "It's a 10" conditioning spray. So good! Dr. Hauschka Neem Oil.

4. **MOUSSE:** Drybar Southern Belle Volumizing Mousse and TRESemmé—both add volume without weighing the hair down.

5. **VOLUMIZING SPRAY:** Phytovolume Active Volumizing Spray and Bumble & Bumble Thickening Spray

6. **SEA SALT/TEXTURIZING PRODUCTS:** The Dry Texturizing Spray by Oribe or Frederic Fekkai's Summer Hair Beach Waves—Davy loves this stuff and buys boxes of it.

7. **HAIR OILS/SHINE PRODUCTS:** Moroccan Oil, Amla Oil, and Redken All Soft Argan Oil

8. **FINISHING WAX:** Magic Move—perfect for polished, clean hairline.

9. **DRY SHAMPOO:** Serge Normant Dry Shampoo, Klorane Dry Shampoo, Bamboo Uplifting Root Blast, John Frieda is excellent too! Bumble & Bumble's comes in different hair color shades for an even more custom finish. Dove's will work in a pinch too.

10. **HAIR SPRAY:** I cannot live without Elnet. I never deviate. A supermodel staple.

You don't need a hundred products to get the job done. A lot of times, you just need to find those two products that really work for you and your hair type. It does take some trial and error to find what those products are, but they are out there. Just a touch of the right product can absolutely transform your hair and your whole look.

—MATTHEW MONZON, hairstylist

DRY SHAMPOO FOR *president*

Okay, maybe I'm going overboard here, but my belief in dry shampoo is bordering on spiritual. It is the mane multitasker of the century. It usually comes in a pump or an aerosol and has a light, powdery texture. First of all, it gives your hair a holiday from washing. Dry shampoo is designed to absorb the oils at the root and instantly restores freshness, lightness, and touchability. If you are late to the game getting your roots touched up, some dry shampoos come in different colors/shades and help soften the appearance of root growth. When it comes to styling, dry shampoo works wonders when sprayed throughout to pump up the volume or add texture to even the finest of hair, even after an air dry. So yeah, that's why I nominate dry shampoo for Hair Club president. Forget that other guy.

hair helpers: These are my favorite go-tos for styling.

1. **BLOW-DRYER:** CHI Pro Low blow-dryer (one of the best for smooth strands)
2. **CURLING IRONS:** Enzo Milano curling stick—one-inch barrel (it's easy to use and delivers the most styling versatility); Sarah Potempa Beachwaver Pro
3. **FLAT IRON:** GHD flat iron (fun to use for a stick straight look and even beachy waves)
4. **PINS:** Choose the color based on your hair, and look for the textured pins, that is, the French hairpins with the balls at the ends.
5. **RUBBER BANDS:** Girl's gotta have 'em! I love the no-mark rubber bands and the Japanese Hook Rubber Bands. They are a little tricky, but the be-all and end-all for thick hair.
6. **ELASTIC HEADBANDS:** For a classic, pulled-back look (great for gym time, too)
7. **ROLLERS:** I love the click 'n curl set for ease and good old-fashioned velcro for volume!

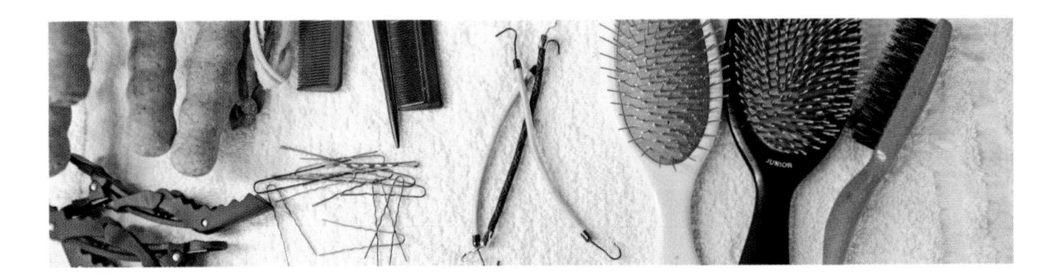

COLOR CORRECT

Getting your hair color right just might be my number one beauty secret it's THAT important. The right color can make your skin appear healthier, your eyes brighter, and you . . . *just better*. And a great color/cut/style combo? Watch out! The three combined take ANYONE from ordinary to *everyday supermodel*. While I'm often some shade of beachy blonde because I think it suits me best, I have tried every color known to man. My first seven years modeling, I had jet-black hair. But I've been platinum, chestnut, dark brown, and I've even had my hair striped like a skunk (which I don't recommend.) My natural color is a medium to dark brown. More recently? I went red for a hair color campaign. Fun fact: Molly Ringwald isn't a natural redhead—she changed it for an acting role and then kept it because she always felt the most like herself. Newsflash: Your natural color doesn't have to be the one you're born with, just the one that makes you feel good! When your hair looks great—you will feel great. And frankly for me, that starts with mastering my color. I will always, always, read-my-lips . . . ALWAYS color my hair until the day I die.

THE QUEEN OF COLOR

God love her, Tracey Cunningham is the best there is. Everyone goes to her. Drew, Gwyneth, J. Lo, Cameron, Kim K . . . I could fill this whole book with her high-profile patrons. Tracey's work is the epitome of what separates the ordinary from the extraordinary. We talked (while she colored, of course), and I got the scoop on how she turns me into Goldilocks and others into Sleeping Beauty, Ariel, and Pocahontas.

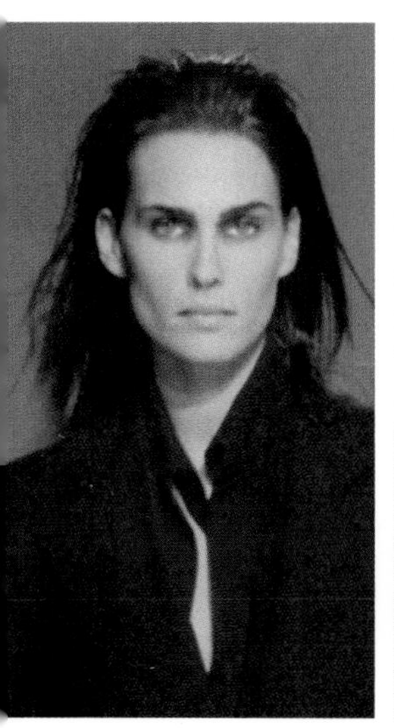
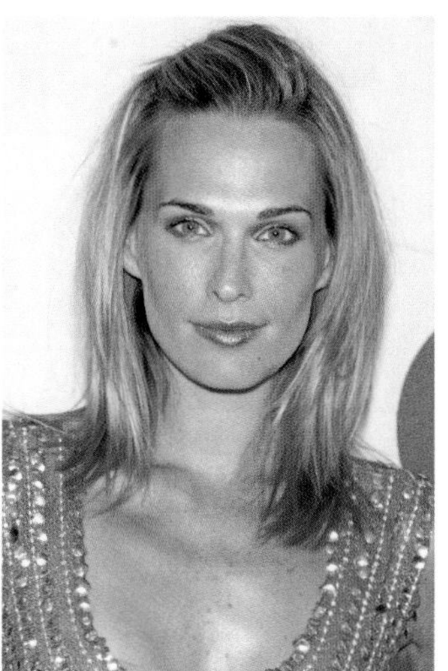
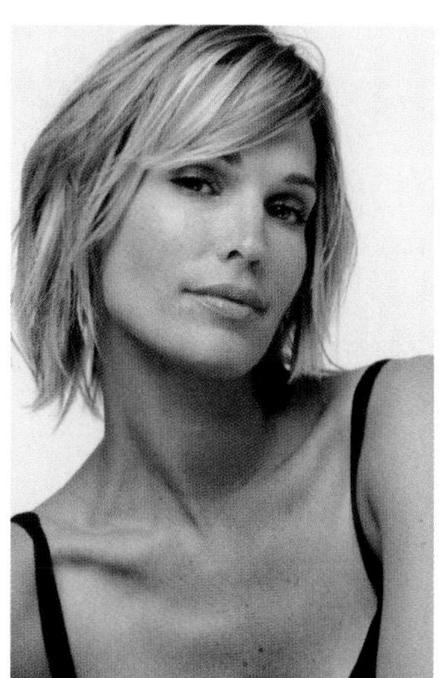
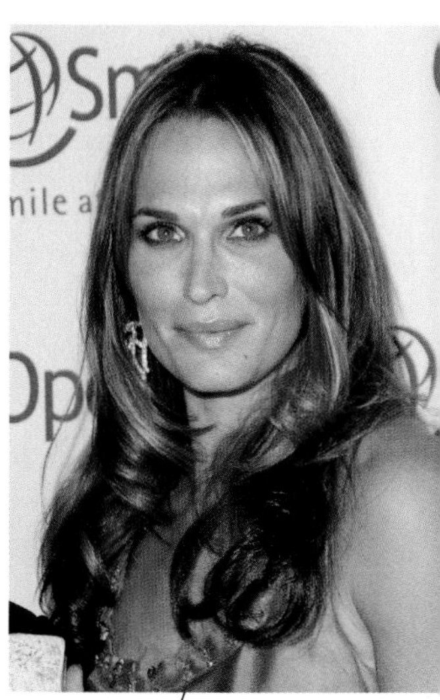

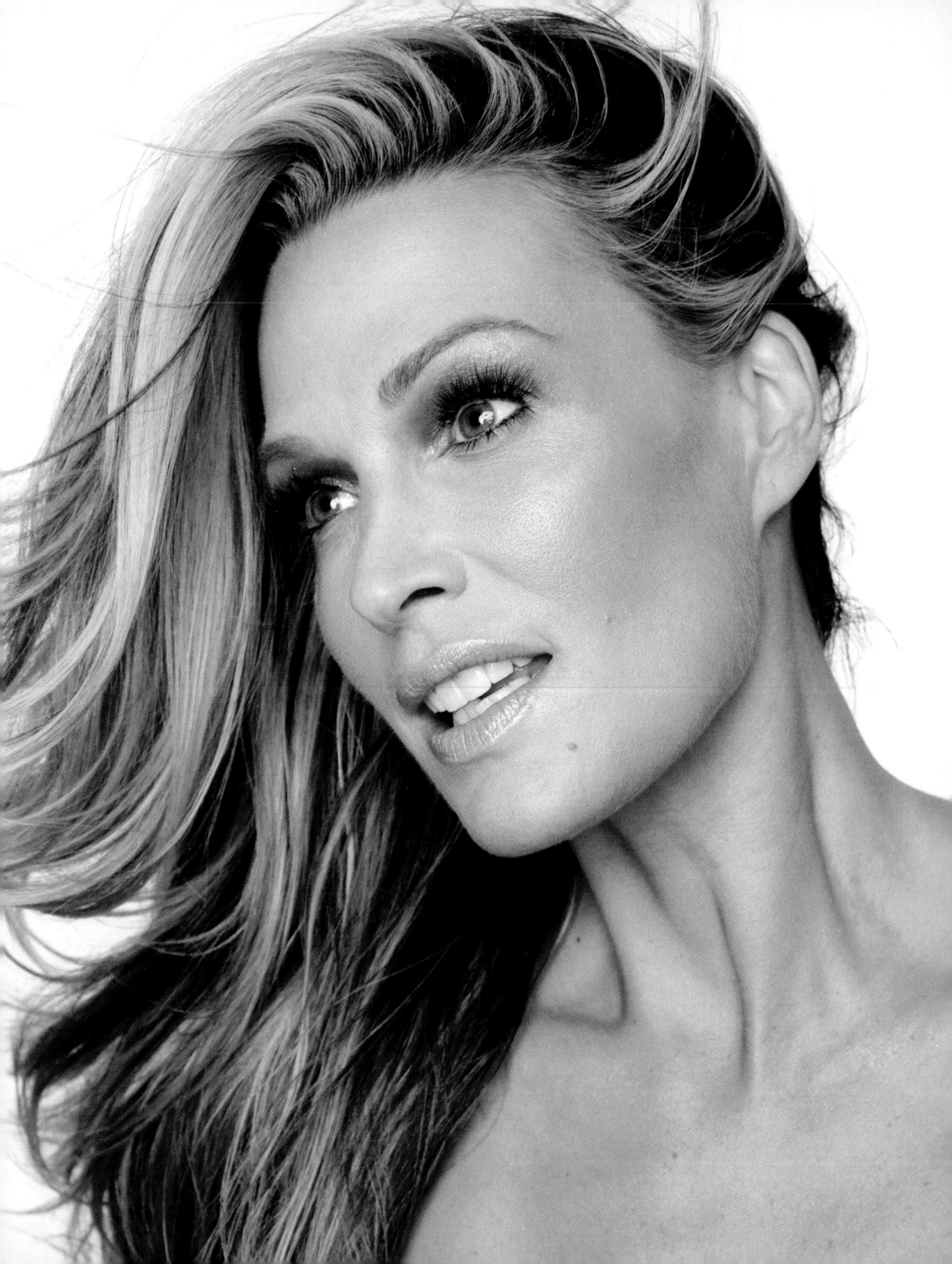

coloring tips Courtesy of Tracey

1. **BE MULTIDIMENSIONAL:** Highlights and lowlights add depth, dimension, and richness. They can also make the hair appear thicker, healthier, and fuller.

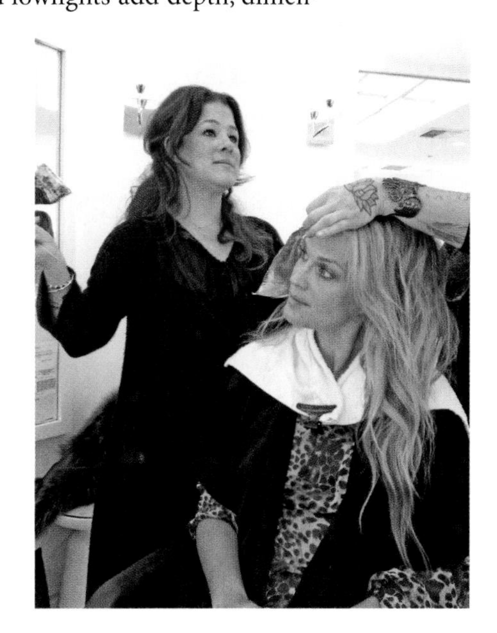

2. **ON MAKING A BIG CHANGE:** This one is tricky—it's good to experiment and get out of a rut, but remember to look at your reasons for changing things up first, or you might regret it.

3. **AVOID OVERPROCESSING:** Be careful not to do too much to your hair. Every day women ask her for things that will really compromise the health of their hair. More blonde! More bleach! Etc. Etc. Be aware, lightening your hair might look amazing, but when you go overboard, you are taking major risks. Listen to your stylist when he or she gives advice.

4. **BEWARE GOING AGAINST YOUR SKIN:** Hair color should enhance your skin tone. Not everyone looks great really dark or really light. Most of us look best a shade or two up or down. And always wear your everyday makeup to the salon. That will help your colorist balance your hair tone with your skin.

5. **GOING TOO HIGH MAINTENANCE:** If you do want to go extreme in one direction, just be prepared. It's a lot of work and can cost you a small fortune. There's nothing worse than high-maintenance color that isn't maintained. It can ruin your whole look.

Your hair is a major investment in every way—time, money, and in yourself. But it's such a worthwhile investment. I've watched women come alive after a change in hair color.

—TRACEY CUNNINGHAM, hair colorist

---

budget Beauty

If you don't have time or money to invest in monthly trips to the salon, consider these options.

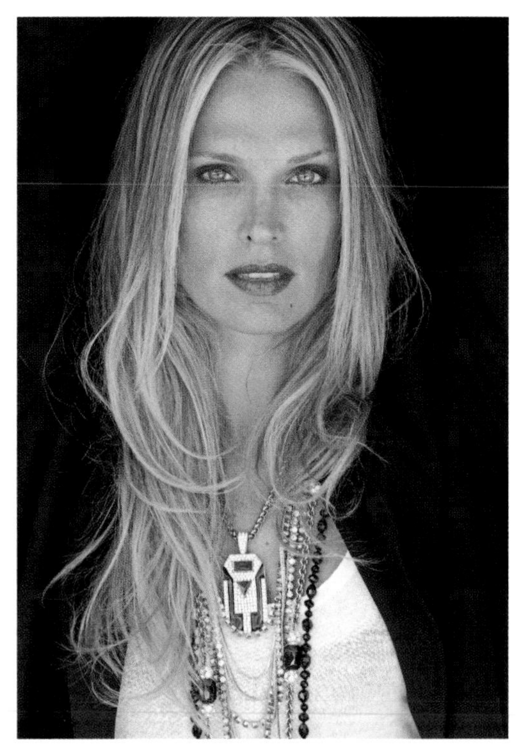

- Subtle highlights are a great way to go. Highlights will enhance your hair and brighten your look. When they are subtle, they grow out and blend in seamlessly.
- Ombré hair is slightly darker at the root and gradually gets lighter, Because there is no hard line at the root, you can go longer in between coloring. And it's beachy, supermodel chic!
- Have products on hand and at home that help to camouflage roots or extend the life of your color. (Think dry shampoos, root touch ups—eyeshadows can work—colorsafe hair products, etc). They will extend the time in between salon visits and save you money.

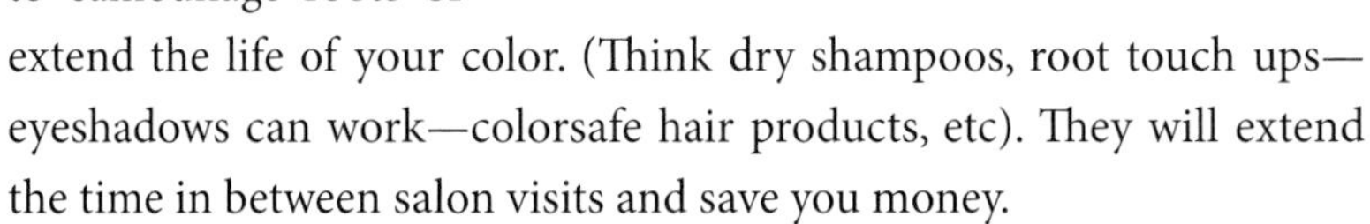

- Michelle Pugh, a colorist also at Meche Salon, recommends your colorist occasionally do a Crystal Treatment on the hair before you color to help extend the life. Also, glossing treatments can be applied after your color; they help protect hair and add luster.
- Just face frame. If you are brunette or dark blonde, placing a few strategic and bright highlights around the face will freshen your look and add a youthful feel—it's quick and affordable.

models **AND THEIR MANES:** Ninety percent of models in the magazines and on runways wear their hair colored in two main styles, ombré (which I mentioned) or in the balayage style. Balayage utilizes the technique where highlights and lowlights are strategically placed throughout the hair—but not in the perfectly uniform way foils and traditional highlighting is done. Balayage highlights are often just painted on in places. It gives hair that sun-kissed look we had as kids. This is my favorite look when it comes to hair color. Techniques like these can be applied to light hair, dark hair, short hair, long hair, and everything in between.

That brings me to my seasonal mantras—as a rule, I usually advise going darker in the winter and brighter in the summer. But every now and again, I'll dramatically switch it up and go superlight in the winter and dark in the summer—just to surprise myself and not get stuck. Just a few tips:

- The point of ombré is to look natural—this black at the root and then superblonde at the bottom should be reserved for rockers.
- Whatever your hair color, ask for the ends of your hair to be lightened. It's youthful. But be aware, bleach does damage. Condition the hair regularly to keep your ends from breaking and splitting!
- Most important tip: Always cut your hair BEFORE you color, otherwise you will cut off the work!

Supermomma Hair Coloring *Tips*

- **BE CAREFUL WITH COLOR IN THE FIRST TRIMESTER:** If you feel you have to, color only subtly and don't touch the root. There's a lot of discussion about what's safe. During my pregnancy, I did subtle highlights but never anything directly to my roots or my scalp. This is a great time to try ombré, because you don't have to touch the roots. For gray, use colored dry shampoos or hair chalks at the roots. Talk to your doctor, do your research—it's really about what feels right for you.
- **DON'T MAKE A BIG CHANGE:** If you have long hair, please don't chop it all off in some hormonally induced rage. You will likely be depressed for eternity. Pregnancy brings on so many bodily changes, the last thing you need is an entirely new hairstyle.
- **THERE ARE NATURAL PRODUCTS OUT THERE:** I've had friends use henna and black tea rinses to freshen up color—they aren't the same but can work in a pinch if you want to avoid chemical dyes.

On Making *the cut*

I've had almost every hair length and style imaginable. Let me tell you, getting the right cut is crucial. Stylist Caile Noble discusses how to get a supermodel-cut.

1. **CONSULT BEFORE YOU CUT:** Have an idea of what you are looking for and talk it through with your stylist. Show him pictures. Ask questions. Have a real conversation. When choosing a cut based on a picture from a magazine, keep in mind the hair is usually *styled* to look like that—not cut to.

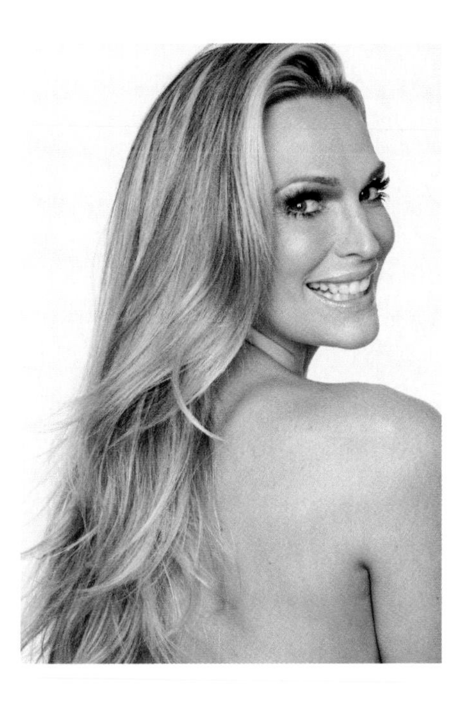

2. **YOU, ONLY BETTER:** Always go with a cut that works well with your texture, your lifestyle, and *your budget*. For example, shorter looks often require more trips to the salon for upkeep, meaning more cash. When it comes to styling, don't be afraid to ask your stylist to teach you how to style your cut too.

3. **TRIM TIME:** Don't be so obsessed with gaining length that you forgo a trim. A little dusting of the ends every few months will help your hair grow longer and faster. When you trim the ends, you prevent the split ends from working their way up the hair shaft and ultimately breaking the hair.

4. **TOO MANY LAYERS:** Do not let someone go all Edward Scissorhands on you. For some reason, a lot of stylists go layer crazy. Although layers can add volume if you have fine hair, you also lose hair when creating layers. With the exception of a very few people, no one looks good with layers cut above the chin.

5. **VERSATILITY:** A great cut is versatile. You may have a favorite way to wear your hair, but the cut should never only look good one way. Long or short, you should have several styling options.

hair looks *I love, love, love!*

While I've had every hairstyle imaginable for editorial shoots, runways, and red carpets—I have my favorites. Whatever the event, one of these styles will almost always fit the bill! I have them down pat, and if I can do them myself—so can you.

Meet my favorites: Polished Pony, Beachy Bombshell, Runway Woman, Sophisticated Bob, Ballerina Bun, Low Chignon, and the Veronica Lake.

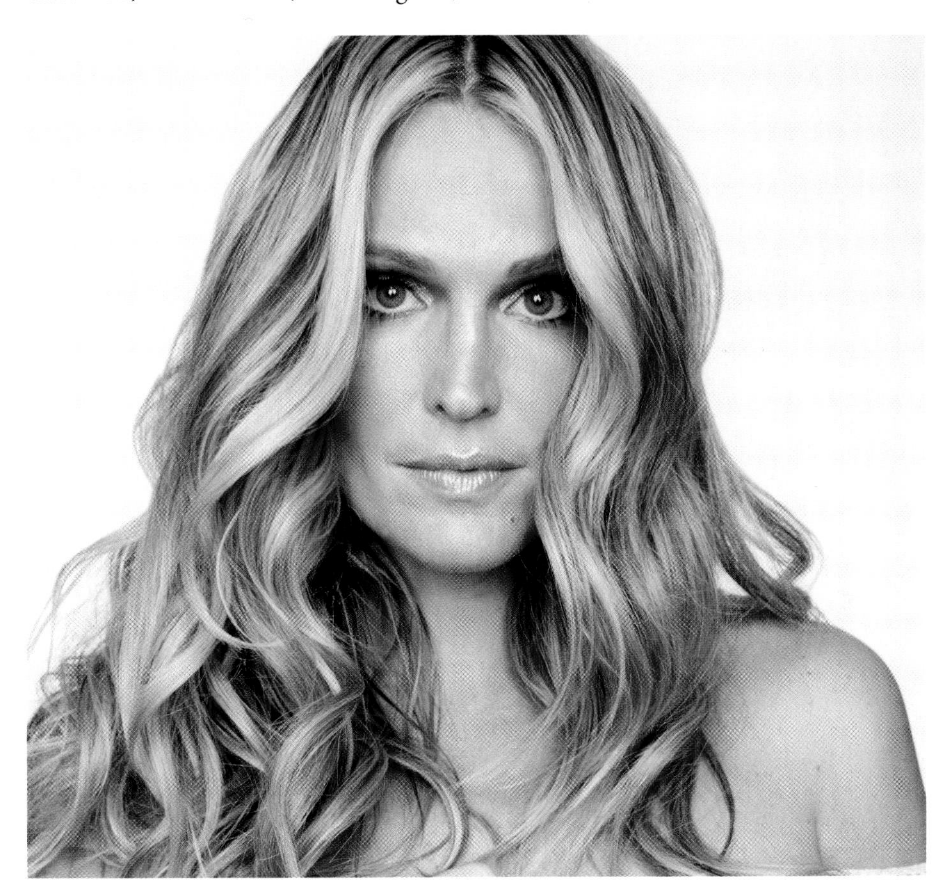

Molly likes to change up her look, but she definitely has her favorites. These looks are in constant rotation. One night it's relaxed and wavy, the next it's in a pony and polished. All these styles are versatile and easy to do at home. Each one is a classic look that can be adapted for any face shape and most hair types.

—DAVY NEWKIRK, hairstylist

---

look one
POLISHED PONY

Confident, fresh, sophisticated, and fun, this look is oh-so-stylish at any age.

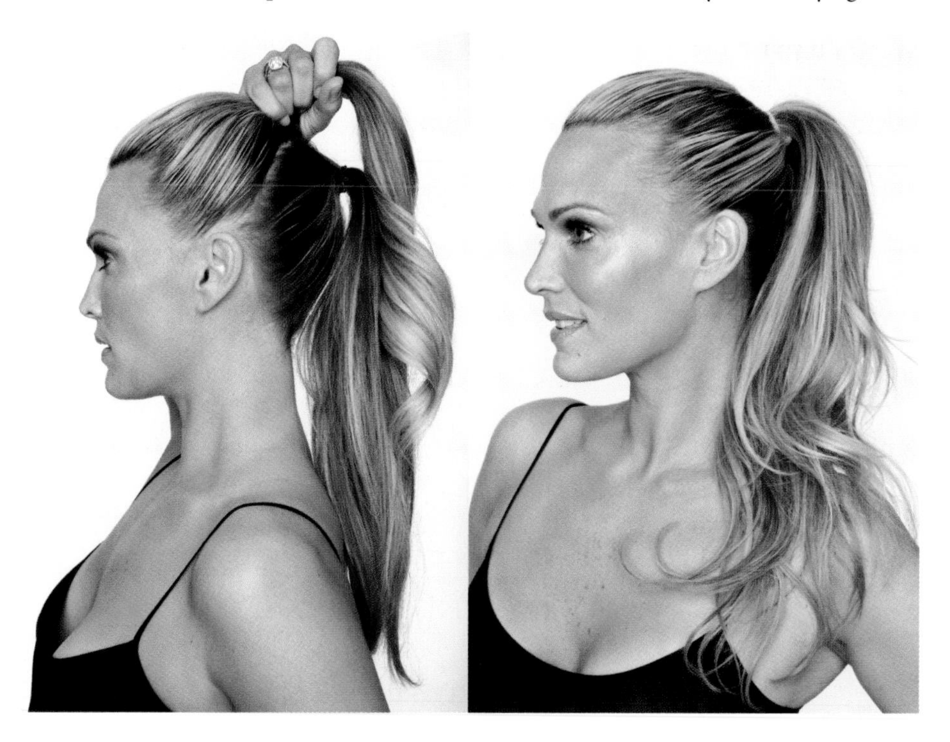

step 1: Blow-dry the hair upside down adding your favorite mousse for volume.

- **ALTERNATE:** If your hair is frizzy or curly, straighten the hair with a flat iron before step 2.

step 2: Section the hair across the back vertically into two parts and pull the top section into a tight pony at the top of the back of the head. Take the bottom section and pull into a tight pony.

step 3: Combine both ponytails at the top center of the head and wrap tightly with a rubber band.

step 4: To add sophistication, take a strand of hair from the inside of the ponytail, wrap it around the ponytail covering the rubber band, and secure it underneath with a bobby pin.

step 5: Finish by using a setting spray to keep flyaways at bay or a finishing wax around the hairline and near the ears to give it extra polish.

Pony *pointers*

- If you have a longer face, you can make a side part first and then pull back into a sleek pony to give the allusion of a wider face.
- If your face is round, part in the middle first and then pull the hair back. That will give it a little dimension and slim the face by adding height.
- If you are going for a more casual look, the pony itself can be slightly wavy or tousled.
- Short hair? You can always add hair clips/extension to pony up!

---

supermodel *secret*

How to swat flyaways. Magic Move is perfect for smoothing breakage and flyaways around the hairline. Y'all know what I'm talking about! Those sneaky strays that drive us all stray-crazy. A small amount works wonders, less than a dime size. It's great around the edges when wearing a pony or a bun, especially if you aren't into that *Planet of the Napes* look. Which *you aren't*. Unless, you are?

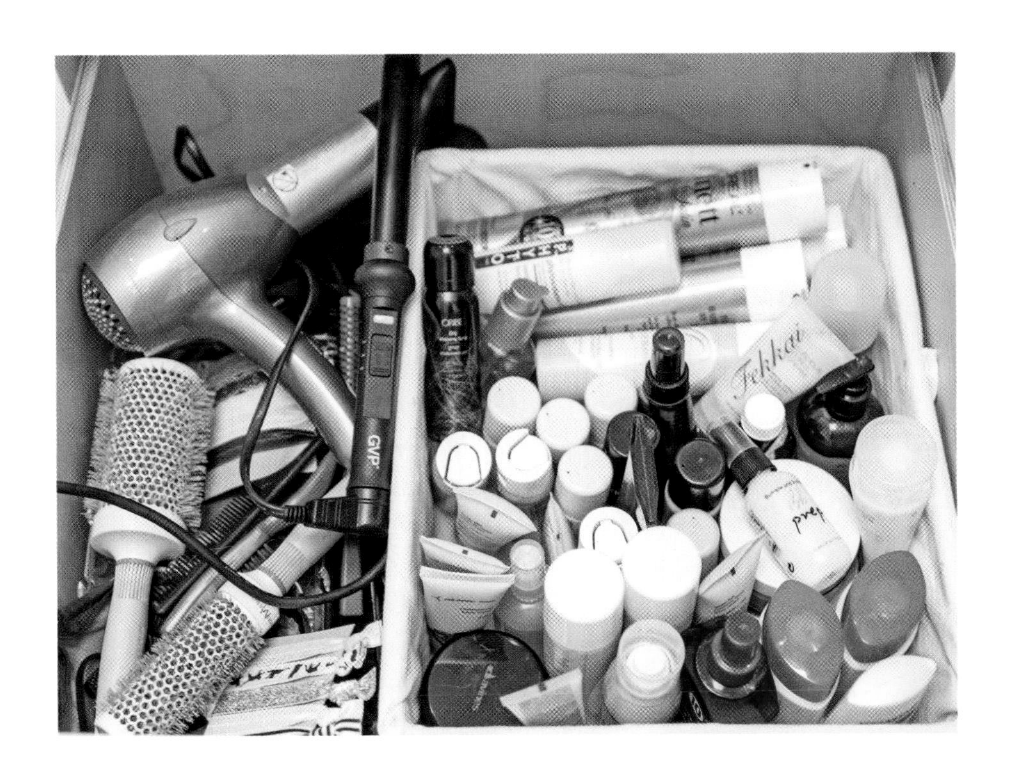

look two
BEACHY BOMBSHELL.

Definitely my day-to-day style. I think these soft, rumpled waves look amazing on all women. It's so feminine and flirty—and sexy—without looking too done.

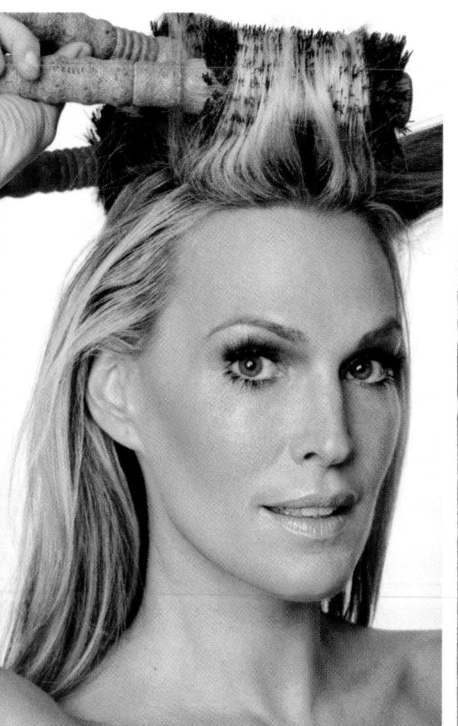

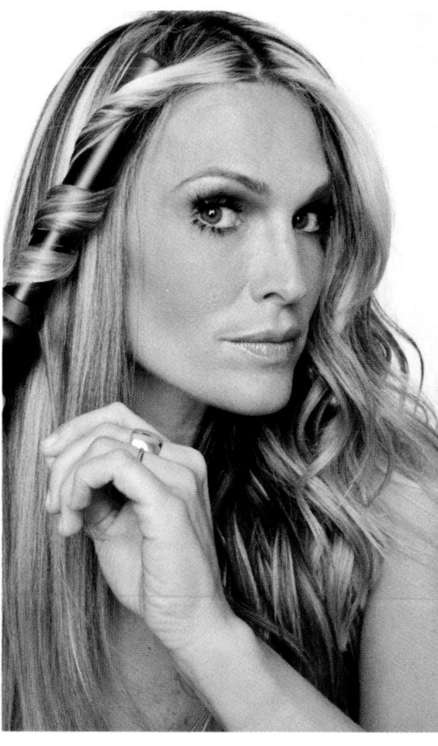

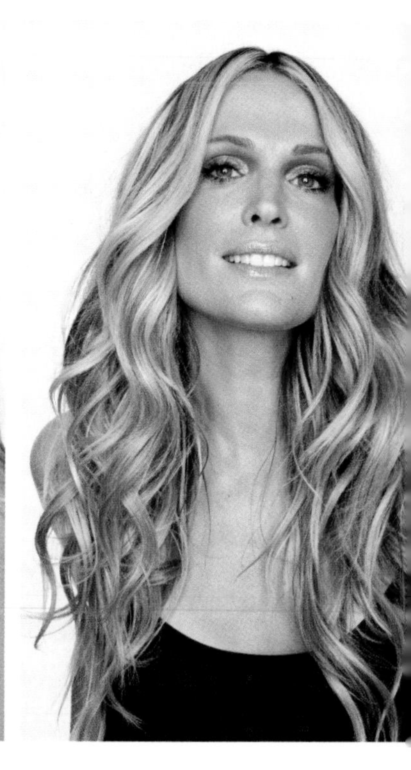

step 1: Start with a great blow-dry using round brushes to add height and volume. If you don't have time for that, spray some texturizing product (Davy loves Frederic Fekkai Beach Spray) into the hair and allow to air dry.

step 2: Using a one-inch curling iron, section the hair into one-inch pieces and curl the hair both forward and backward, alternating directions, from midshaft down. The randomness gives a more natural look. Really important: the front pieces on each side should curl *away* from the face.

step 3: Once finished curling, run your fingers through the hair to pull the curls out a bit.

step 4: Finish with a light dusting of hair spray.

Tousled *Tips*

- For a more modern look, don't take the curl all the way up to the root. Stop at about the eyeline. And leave the very end out of the curl.
- If you like a piecier look, run a little bit of wax through the ends of the hair to define the curls.
- This is a gorgeous style for anyone with hair that is a little longer than chin length and beyond.
- If you use a flat iron instead of the curling iron, the waves will be a slightly tighter
- I DON'T like too much roundness along the forehead. First pull down or blow-dry down height so it's not too much of a circular arch—that just emphasizes and gives the appearance of a modern forehead.

---

supermodel *secret*

DONE/UNDONE

Davy is the king of this look. We mentioned it in fashion, but it can be applied to everything style-wise—your makeup, your hair, etc.—it all works together. Too-styled hair or too much makeup is like too much Botox or extra-large breast implants. That's all you notice! Think soft curls not corkscrew. Loose updos. You hair should move and be touchable. Say no to helmet hair!

---

beachy bombshell ALTERNATE

Feeling lazy? For an even more relaxed version that's a little more beachy and less bombshell, work a small amount of texturizing spray or mousse into wet hair and then sleep in two pigtail braids. In the morning unravel the hair, rake through it with your fingers, and voilà! Gisele is in the house. Or, try using the Beach Waver rotating curling iron. It's quick and easy to use and works well for waves.

look three
RUNWAY WOMAN

This is my favorite look, like, *ever*. Davy has been doing this on me since the beginning of time and—you know what—I'll never get tired of it. It's simple, confident, and chic. When I think of the "model" mane—this is it. You can go to Paris, Milan, Sydney, London, or New York and you will see the it-girls wearing it.

step 1: Condition hair well in the shower, and then apply a heat protectant product. Blow-dry with a round brush. It's important that the hair be shiny and swingy to start.

step 2: Part the hair dead center and then straighten the heck out of it with a straightening iron.

step 3: Finish by working the tiniest amount of shine spray or serum into the hair (rub it onto hands first—don't spray directly onto the hair or apply any to the roots).

step 4: Tuck hair behind the ears and then pull it forward onto each shoulder.

Stick-Straight *suggestions*

* Choose a ceramic flat iron as they are less damaging to the hair.
* Watch out! Be careful not to stop as you work your way down the hair shaft. Stopping midway can create bends or dents in the hair that are tough to get out.

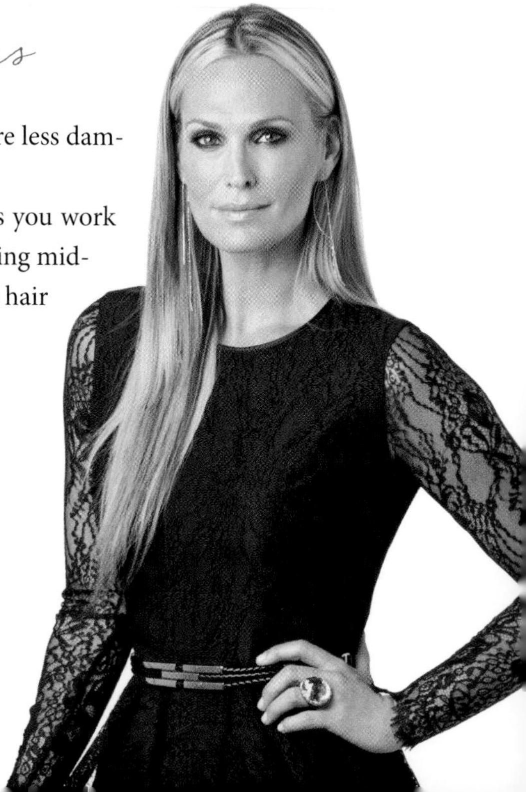

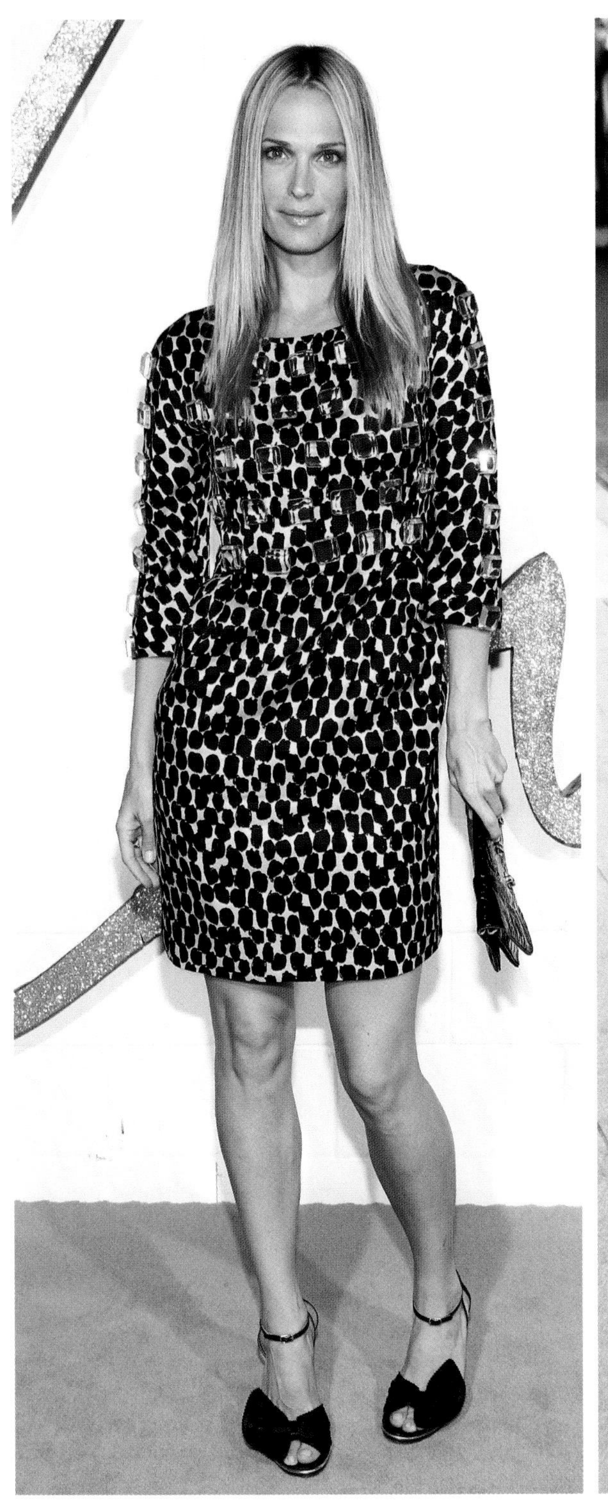

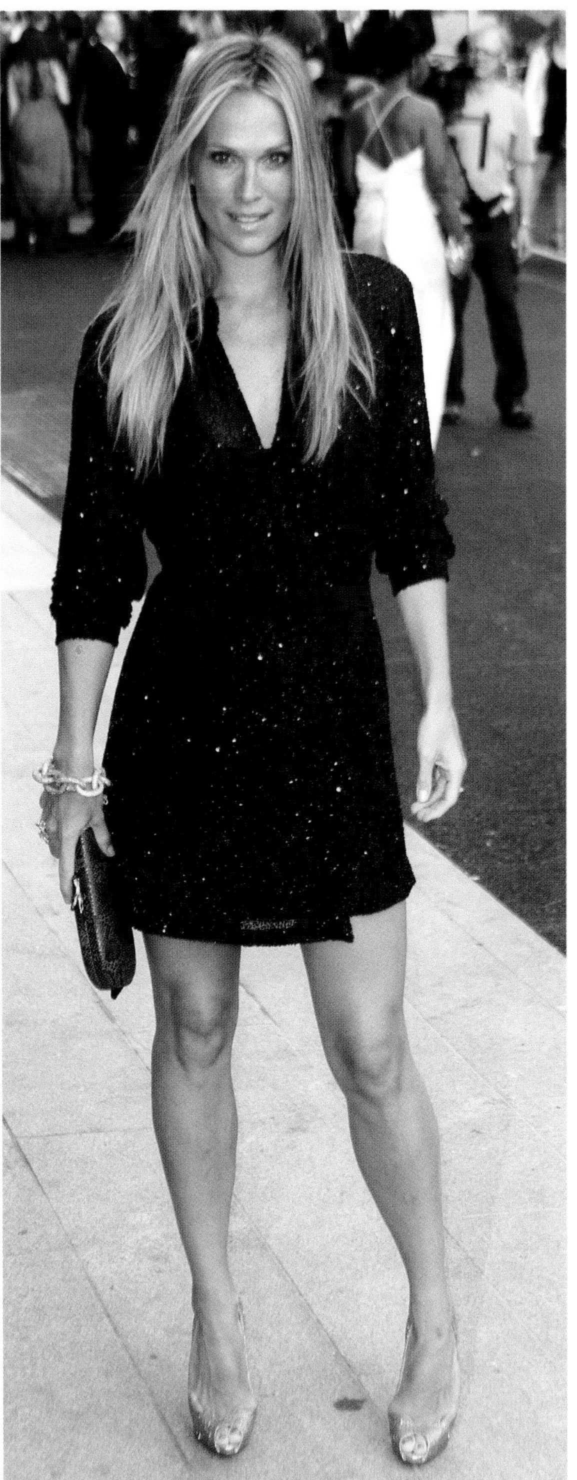

look four
BALLERINA BUN

This look is low on maintenance, but high on style. It's easy-breezy to achieve, especially if your hair is a little sloppy, and slept in already.

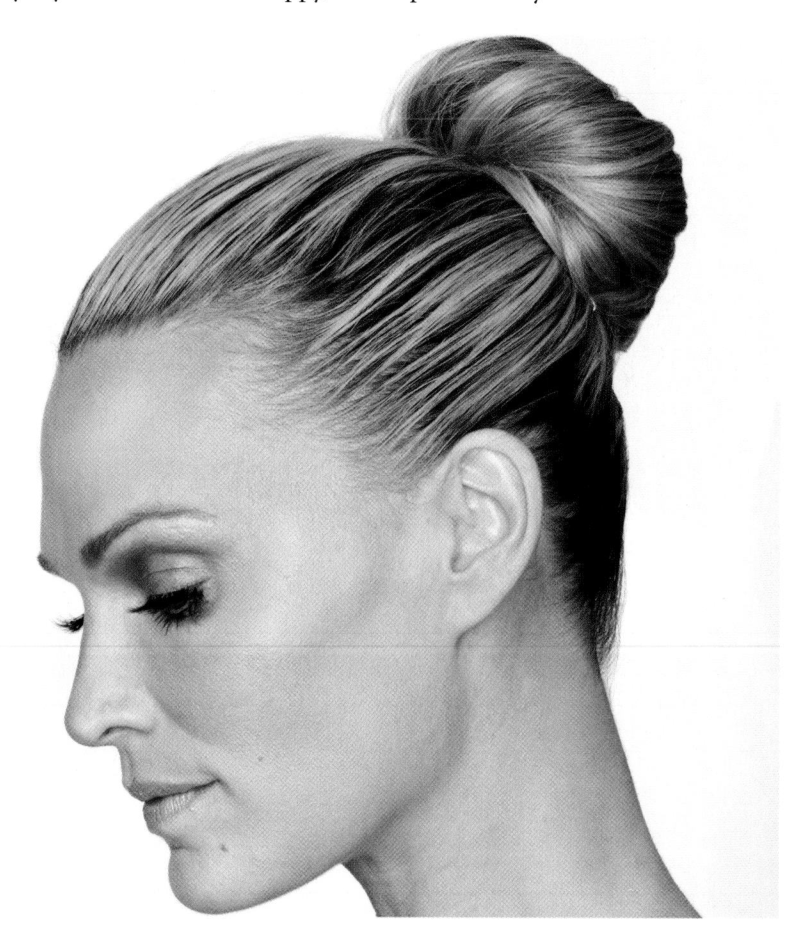

step 1: Gather the hair into a pony high on the back of the head.
step 2: Backcomb the actual ponytail with a large tooth comb by gently teasing the underside of the pony.
step 3: Then gently smooth down the pony, careful to maintain the volume from teasing.
step 4: Twist the ponytail and form into a large bun, securing it with hairpins.
step 5: Set with a touch of finishing spray.

look five
LOW CHIGNON

So pretty and feminine, the chignon is never pretentious—it can go dressy or relaxed and is best worn loose and imperfect.

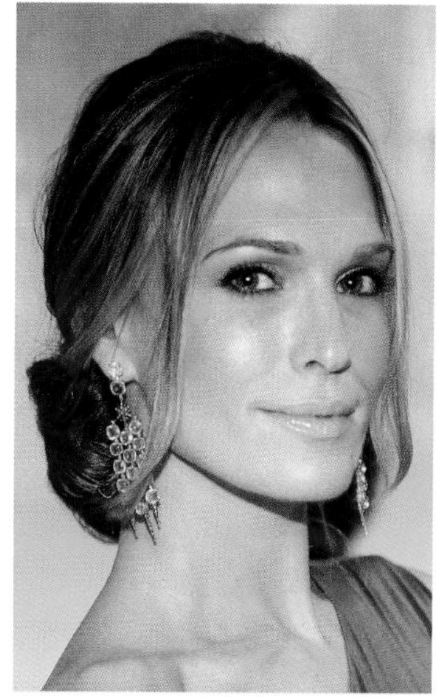

step 1: Blow-dry the hair, then throw in a few curls with a one-inch-barrel curling iron—not all over, just here and there.

step 2: Spray in a bit of texturizing product and run through the hair with your fingers.

step 3: Place a front side part into the hair on either side.

step 4: Secure hair into a low ponytail at the base of the neck (if you prefer, you can position it to the left or right as well so it can be slightly seen from the front).

step 5: Twist and wrap the hair around the rubber band and secure with bobby pins.

Chignon *notes*

* If you have bangs or long layers, pull a few out like wispy tendrils in front for a more relaxed look
* For those with fine hair, tease the ponytail a bit before wrapping into the bun.
* The ponytail can be braided and then wrapped for a more romantic look.

---

supermodel *secret*

PRODUCT OVERLOAD

Don't overdo it with product. Product is easy to add and impossible to take away. You can overmousse. You can overtexturize. You *can* overdo it. Know how much to apply and when to quit. Too much dry shampoo can leave the hair powdery. A mountain of mousse and hair looks/feels heavy. Overdo the beach spray and your strands look like straw. Excess gel or shine serum and, congratulations, you are the next cast member of *The Jersey Shore*!

look SIX
SOPHISTICATED BOB

You can actually have bob-length hair . . . or you can fake it (we faked it!). Either way, it's a flirty look, sweet and sexy all at once. If your hair is long like mine, the style works best, and looks the most natural, if you have a few layers in the front.

step 1: Rough dry the hair, and when it's fully dry, place loose curls (with a round or a flat iron) throughout the hair. Alternate the direction of the curl with each strand.

step 2: Fold and roll the hair under, and then secure to the scalp with small bobby pins.

step 3: If you have layers, pull a few pieces out in the front, and run the curling iron through them again.

step 4: Spray a light layer of setting spray over the whole head.

Bob *beware*

When creating your bob avoid the soccer mom situation—make sure hair isn't too blunt at the bottom. When the hair is slightly shorter in the back and a little longer toward the front, the look is fresher and more modern.

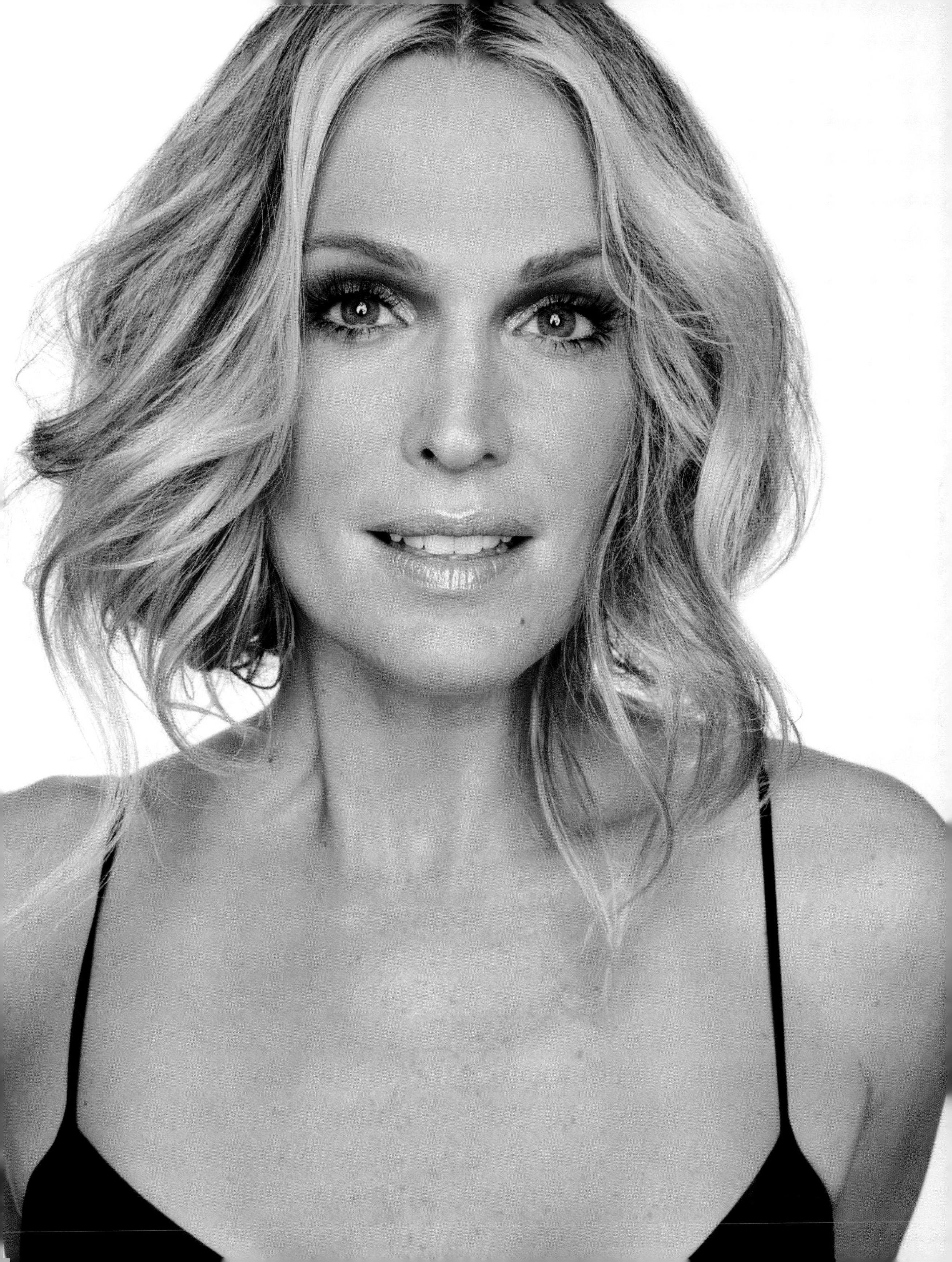

look seven
THE VERONICA LAKE

The Veronica Lake is a classic Hollywood "set." It's one-hundred-percent box-office bombshell . . . and epitomizes glamour. There isn't an actress around who hasn't copied her sultry, signature waves. The key to the look is the S-curve shape.

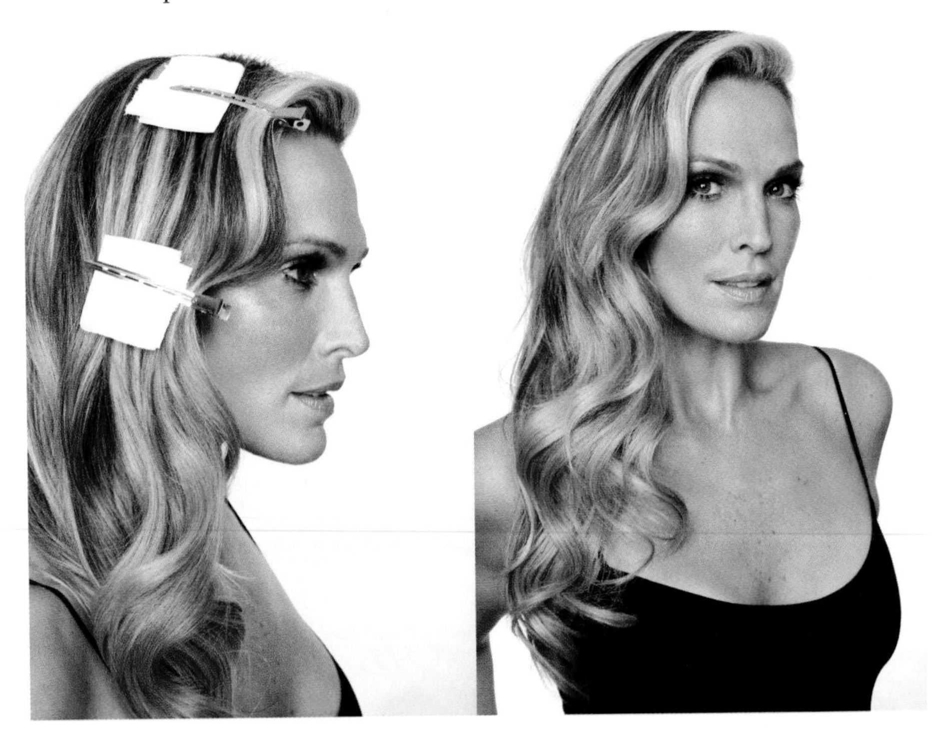

step 1: Start with a beautiful blowout with volume.
step 2: Then, using a one-inch curling iron, curl the hair forward by sections that are small and even. *Tip: Use bobby pins to help set the S shape into place.
step 3: Once all your hair is curled and it has cooled off, brush the hair downward all the way. This allows for the curls to loosen, and lengthen.
step 4: . To keep the curls together, use hair spray on the brush, and keep brushing them down, until you attain the desired look.

the veronica lake
ALTERNATE

For an easier version, place a set of hot rollers all over the head. Let them cool, release and then spray your hair with a brushable/lightweight finishing spray. Gently brush through the curls with a paddle brush for a modern version with Cindy Crawford volume.

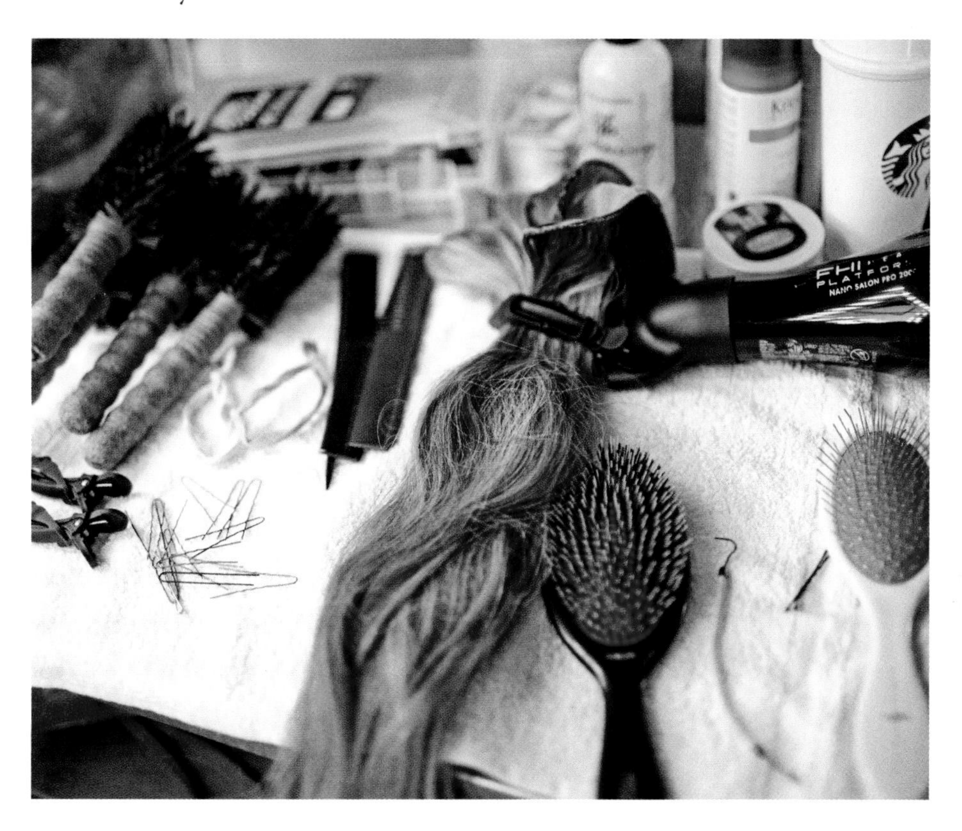

The one-inch curling iron is my personal favorite. It works for all lengths of hair, from short to medium and long. I use it for modern curls, the Veronica Lake look, or period looks, for example. For me, it is the ultimate curling iron for its curl versatility.

—ADRIANA TREVIZO, hairstylist

wild card *look*
THE BOHO BRAID

It's always fun to have a style in your back pocket that's a little different, unconventional perhaps. This braided look is part nymph and part bohemian princess.

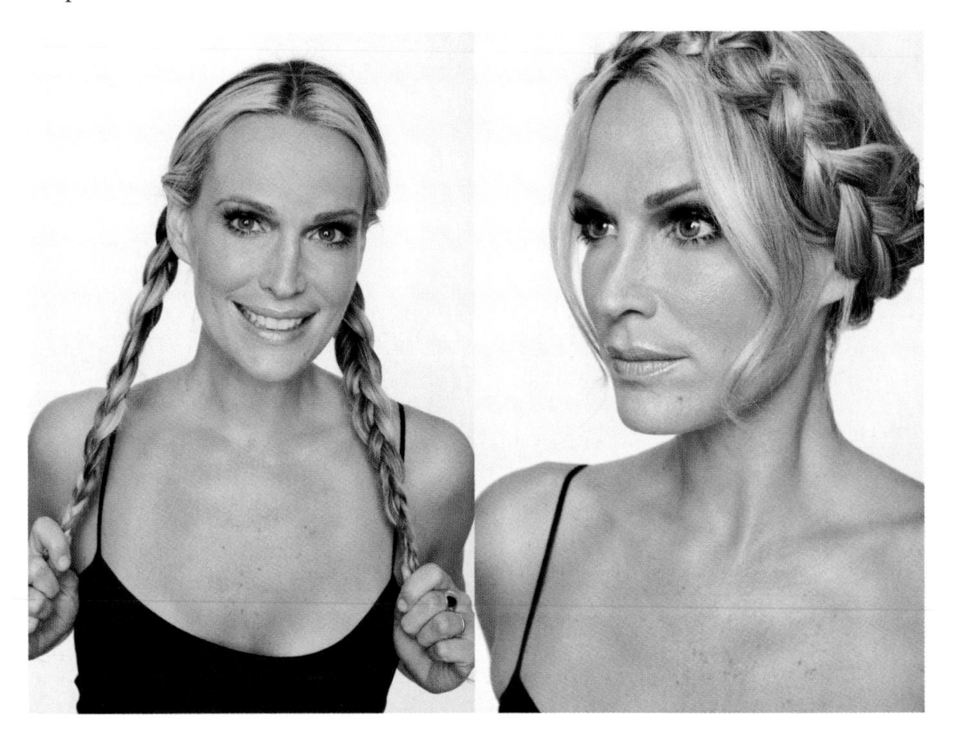

step 1: Split hair down the center and put in two pigtail braids on each side

step 2: Grab the first braid and secure it to the top of the head with small bobby pins in the nearest shade of your hair. Place the pins at both the front and back of the braid. Depending on how thick your hair is, you may use between six and twelve pins for each braid.

step 3: Take the second braid and secure it to the top of the head in the same fashion, creating the "halo" on the head.

step 4: Tuck the ends of each braid underneath the hair and pin to set, creating a halo on the head with the braids.

step 5: To finish, pin any part of the braid that doesn't feel secure and then pull a few strands out around the front to frame the face.

"Halo" *hints*

- For a less polished feel—work the braid a bit and gently pull/stretch it out.
- Have fun with this look! It can be glam and vampy (wear with a merlot lip), or very Coachella (add a flower crown), or romantic and girly (pink cheeks and a rose gloss).

alternate braid *look*

THE FOXY FISHTAIL!

The fishtail braid has been a frenzy on runways and I'm personally obsessed. It makes me think of mermaids—and who doesn't want to channel Daryl Hannah from the *Splash* days?

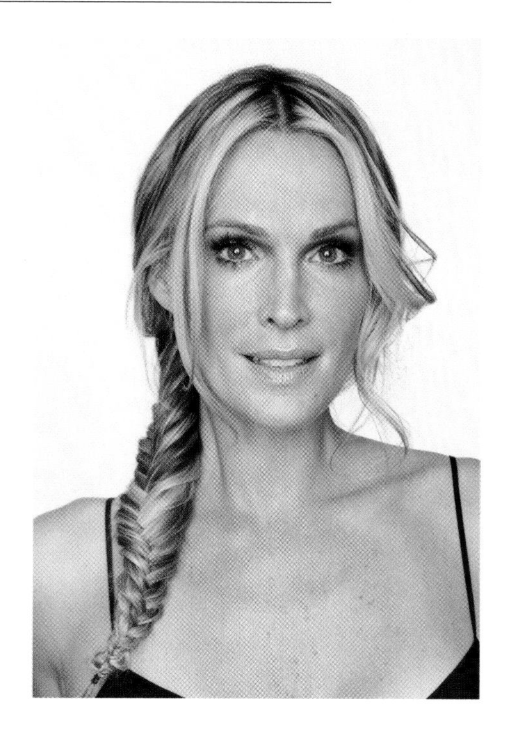

step 1: Pull hair to the side of your head and divide in two sections.
step 2: Grab an outer piece of hair from section one and bring it across to section two. Grab an outer piece of hair from section two and bring it across to section one.
step 3: Repeat all the way down the hair.
step 4: Once at the bottom, grab an elastic or a rubber band and wrap it around the end. You can go back and loosen up the fishtail to give it a loose feel.

Hollywood *hair dos*

There is so much Hollywooding that goes on to get people camera ready. Here are a few simple things that models and actresses do to get red carpet ready that you can do too! I have done every single one of them.

1. **JOIN THE CLIP-IN CLUB:** On television, and in photo shoots, nine times out of ten a model or actress is wearing hair extensions. Glue-in extensions can be a nightmare and screw up your hair. These days, clip-ins are king. The key? *Secure a set that matches your hair color exactly.* Best bet? Find a local hair supply or wig shop so you can clip a set in and take 'em for a test drive. Nothing near you? Look for a good-quality set online, you can always have your hair colorist color them to match if they are made with real hair. The Hair Shop has locations in California and New York and is also a great online resource: www.HairPiece.com.

2. **TEXTURE & TEASE:** This is a one/two punch that really helps to fake flawless hair. Start by spritzing in a texturizing spray and rough-drying your hair. Use your hands to comb through the hair and don't worry about getting it completely dry. Then, gently backcomb and tease the roots under the hair. Finally, smooth over the hair with a paddle brush. It adds volume quickly.

3. **ACCESSORIZE:** Add a little sass to your hair by accessorizing. Try a leather headband, a jeweled hairpin (I did for my wedding), or even a colored clip-in hair extension. You don't have to go all Helena Bonham Carter (she's known to store trinkets in her hair), but these extra details can be a way to have fun without committing to crazy.

---

supermodel *secret*

I've been collecting clip-ins for years, so now I have all the colors I will ever need, even as my hair color changes. Consider building your collection slowly. Start with just a few, or even just one wide strip that can be placed at the base of your hair for added volume. Attention doyennes of dating: Unexpected sleepover? Clip-ins are more discreet than a head full of glued-in hair. You can swiftly snap 'em out and slip 'em into your handbag in no time flat. Your little secret.

I generally don't apply extensions above the earline, because it does't look natural. Hair is all about proportion. You want the volume toward the bottom, not above the ears. For a lot of the Victoria's Secret shoots, I'll just put one broad clip-in extension at the base of the head, just below the earline, that extends all the way across the back of the head. I always slightly tease the hair where I clip it in so it doesn't fall out.

—FRANKIE FOYE, hairstylist

FRINGE *benefits*

Bangs are a great way to experiment with little risk. Michelle Obama made international headlines when her stylist, Johnny Wright, gave her bangs. As he says, "It was a bang heard 'round the world." Similarly, cyberspace went cah-razy when Kate Middleton fringed out. That just goes to show how a small change can make a big impression. If you are thinking of having some fun with fringe, here are a few tips from me and Davy to keep in mind:

- Try it out for size first. Get a clip-in bang and wear it out a few nights.
- Don't forget you have to style bangs every day—do you have the time?
- Bangs can be fun because they offer an immediate change when you cut them, and also they give you different looks as they grow out.
- If you have a larger forehead, blunt bangs are great. If your forehead is smaller, go with a longer, more side-swept bang.
- Fringe is phenomenal as we get older for hiding forehead crinkles and wrinkles!

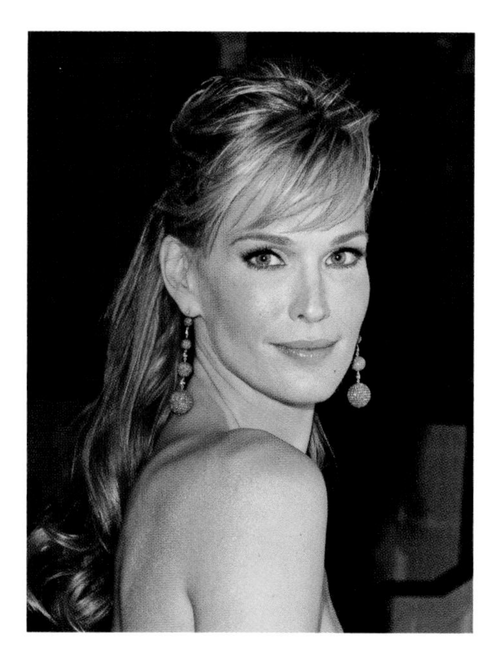

hair-care in a *hurry*

No time? No cash? Still no excuses. Now that you can get an A-list blow-dry for thirty dollars in thirty minutes, there just aren't any reasons for not taking care of yourself every once in a while. Here's a list of treatments that deliver results. They are things you can do on your lunch hour for (almost) less than your lunch money, honey:

- **BLOW-DRY BARS.** Drybar streamlined a service that's been happening in salons everywhere for years. Do you have tempermental hair? A secret: almost no matter how hard up your hair is, these places are affordable and do a bang-up job styling. There are also fun salons that have specialties, like the John Barrett Salon braid bar. So boho chic.
- **HIGHLIGHT TOUCH-UP:** You might not have time for a whole highlight session. And you might need to save a little cash. Did you know that you can cheat your color to extend the time in between? Just ask your colorist for a little touch-up. It will take half the time and will be one-third the cost.
- **AT-HOME HELP:** Rinse your hair with a solution of 1 part apple cider vinegar to 4 parts water. This detoxifies and helps hair get rid of built-up product (can you say Elnet?). After your hair dries, put on a protein mask and let it sit for about fifteen to twenty minutes. You can use a scoop of mayonnaise, an egg or even full-fat milk. Rinse off and hair will shine like a new penny!

A woman's hair is one of the first things that speaks before she even utters a word. It says a lot about you. If the hair isn't moving it has no voice. Your hair is sending a message whether you know it or not, so it's important to consider what message you are sending.

—JOHNNY WRIGHT, hairstylist to First Lady Michelle Obama

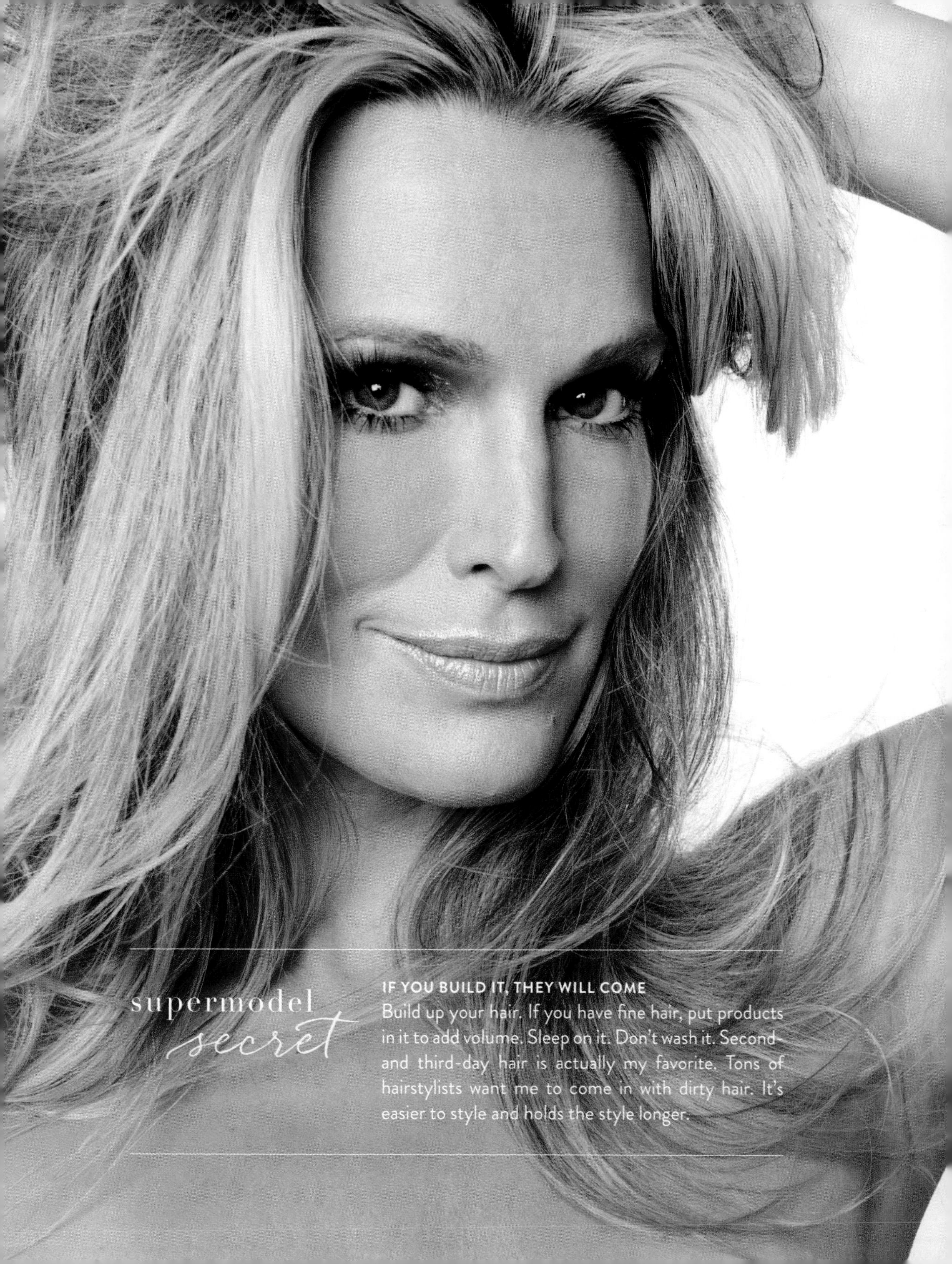

supermodel *secret*

IF YOU BUILD IT, THEY WILL COME

Build up your hair. If you have fine hair, put products in it to add volume. Sleep on it. Don't wash it. Second- and third-day hair is actually my favorite. Tons of hairstylists want me to come in with dirty hair. It's easier to style and holds the style longer.

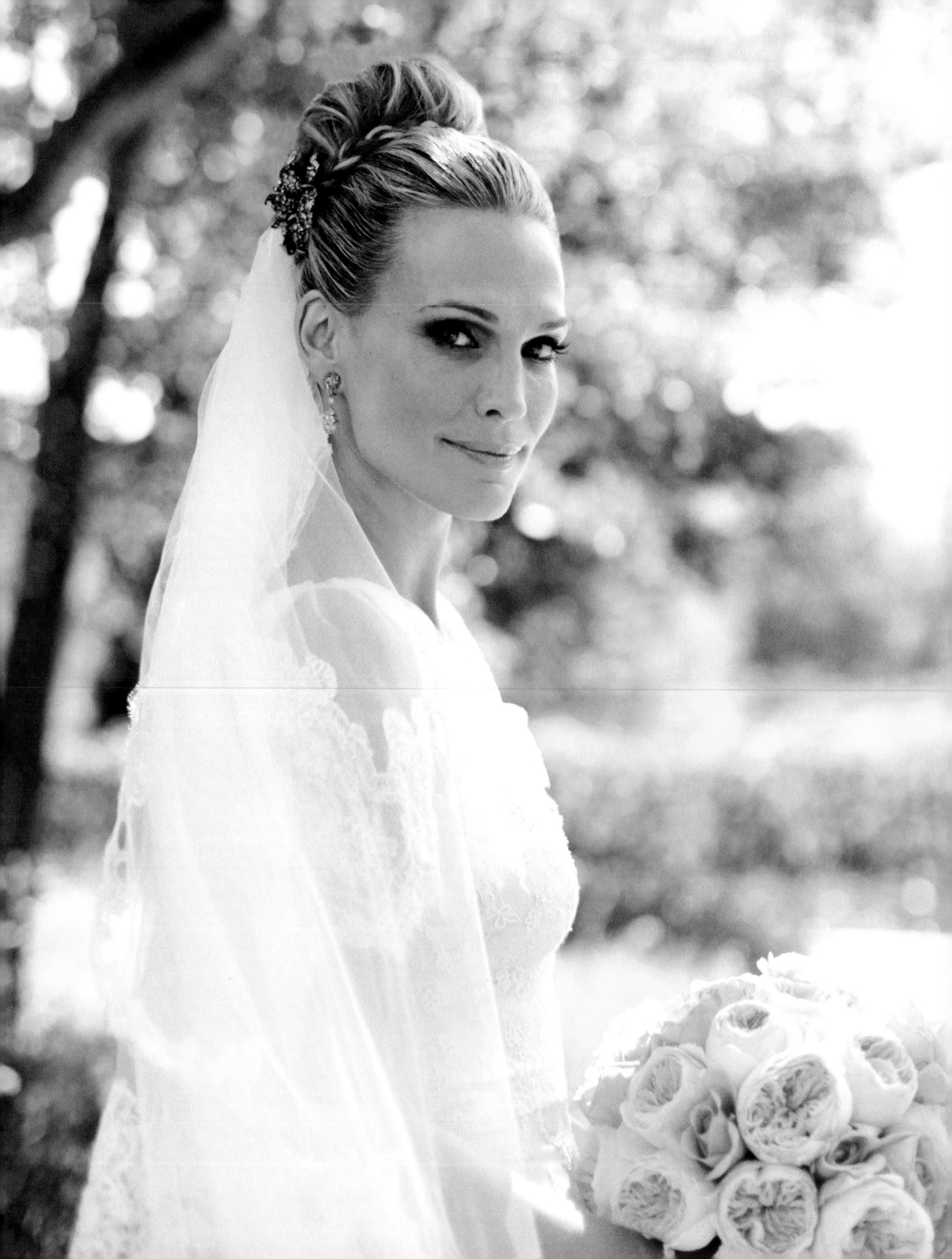

MY *bridal* HAIR AND BEAUTY

SEPTEMBER 24, 2011

Napa Valley, California

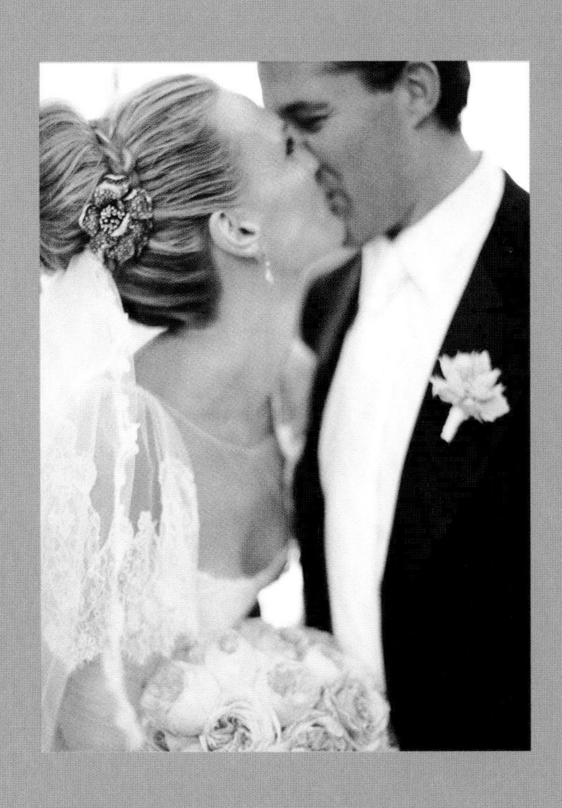

hair BY DAVY NEWKIRK

- We blew out Molly's hair for the rehearsal dinner, so we started with "second-day hair" on the big day.
- I brushed out the knots and then sprayed on a bit of Oribe Thickening Spray. I tousled her hair with my fingers while using a blow-dryer to get a base texture.
- I used a ponytail hairpiece and secured it with bobby pins at the highest point on the back of the head.
- I gathered Molly's hair and secured it around the hairpiece with a bungee as an extremely high ponytail.
- I then backcombed the ponytail with a large-tooth comb, making sure to keep the volume even. I smoothed it out with a boar-bristle brush.
- I then twisted the ponytail and formed it into a large bun, securing it with hairpins.
- TIP: I also roughed my fingers over the hair pulled back to give it a bit of texture and body. Then I applied a small amount of Magic Move (light hold) over the bun and base.
- FOR HOLD: I sprayed the style with the Aveda Control Force firm hold hair spray.
- THE DETAILS: For a something a little extra special, I made a small braid with some extension hair and wrapped that around the base of the bun and then pinned an antique diamond broach at the base of the braid.

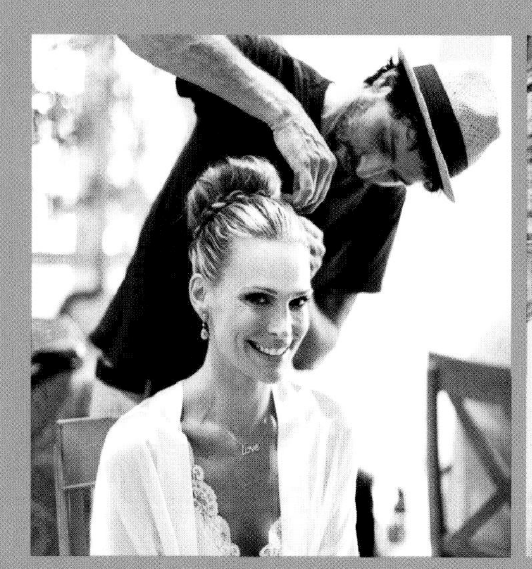

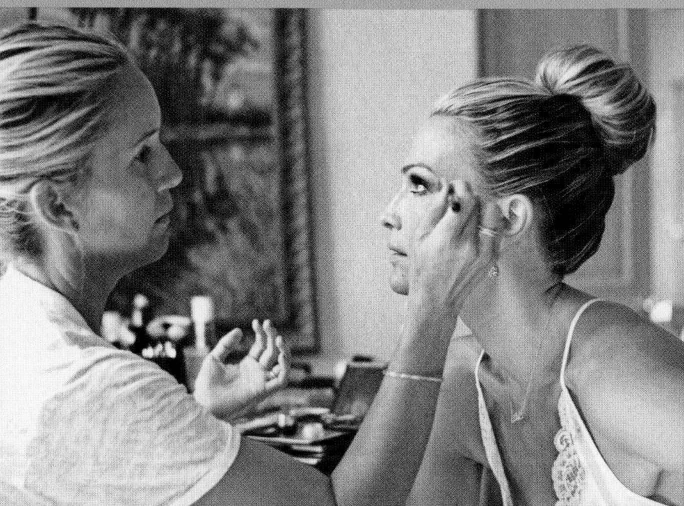

makeup BY MONIKA BLUNDER

- For a flawless foundation we used Armani Luminous in 5.5.
- On Molly's eyes, I lined her upper and lower lashes with a bronze eyeliner pencil by Nars.
- I then used Bobbi Brown gel eyeliner in black on a thin brush and lined in between her upper lashes to give her lashes more intensity.
- I used a shimmer Nars eye shadow in All About Eve on the upper inner corners of her eyes to highlight.
- Then I applied Nars eye shadow in Kalahari, a bronze color, on the outer upper and lower lashes to create depth. I also used a little bit of the bronze color in the crease to create more definition.
- To finish the eyes, I used three coats of Dior Show mascara and applied false, flare eyelashes.
- I contoured Molly's face just a little with the Chanel bronzer.
- I then used both Bobbi Brown Pot Rouge in Pale Pink and Summer Tan on the apple of her cheeks to get the perfect flushed bride effect.
- I also used a little bit of the Mac Hush highlighter just on top of her cheekbones to highlight her face.
- To complete the look I used Chanel Chintz lipstick. This color is my favorite for a bride because it has the perfect light pink color.
- I finished this look by powdering just the T-zone with Laura Mercier loose powder.

molly's *tip*

I love wearing my hair down, but I felt it was too risky for a hot afternoon. I did not want wedding hair-mageddon by midday. I wanted a style that was chic, fresh, and youthful . . . and, most important, would look good all day and for years to come (in the pics). The makeup I wanted a little bit sexy, but still soft.

HAIR *elsewhere*: BROW AND BODY HAIR BASICS

This hair story isn't finished yet. If you are like me, there's more where that came from. Let's move from our scalps to our foreheads . . . and then down below.

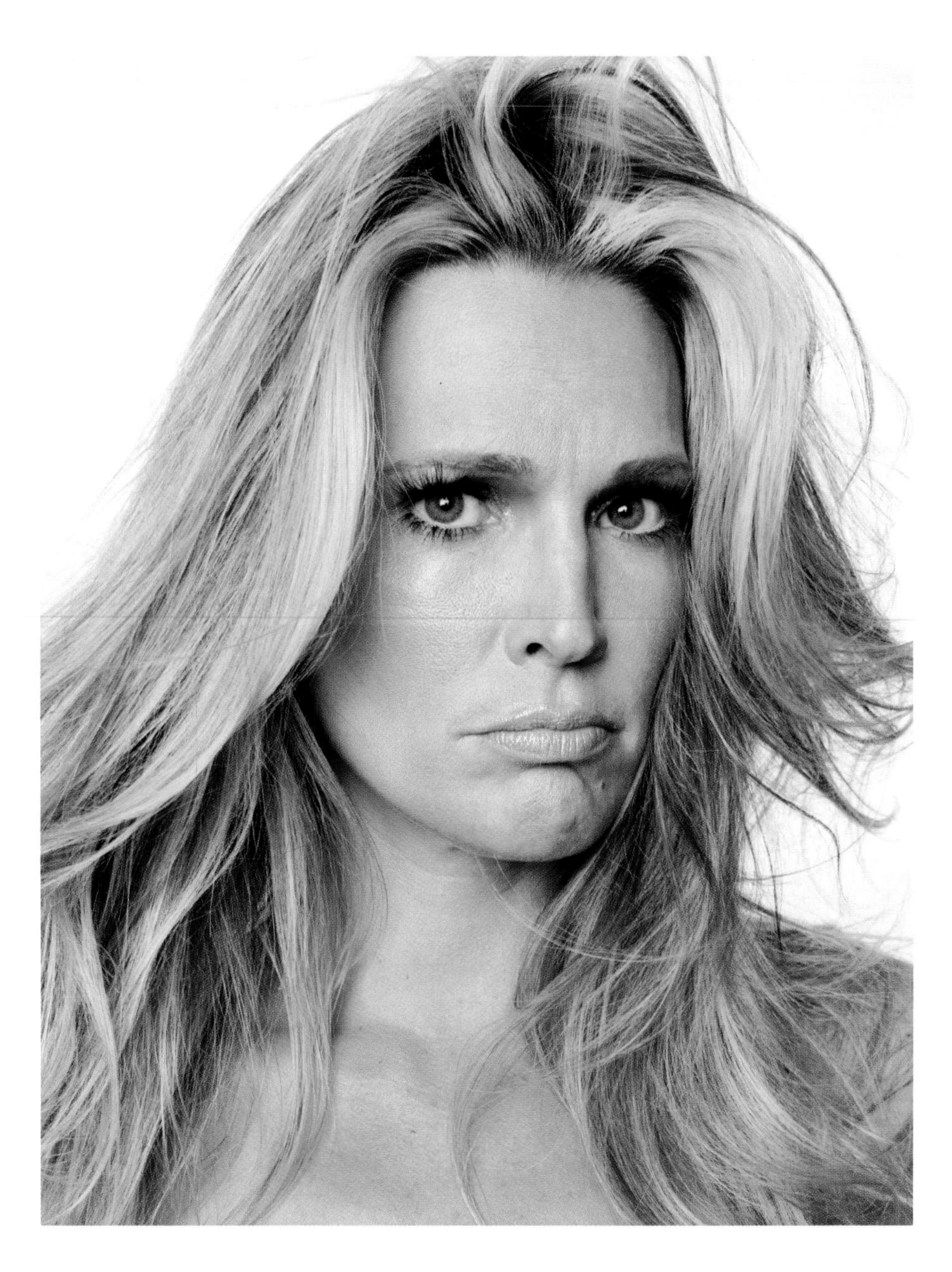

archfrenemy

BECOME BESTIES WITH YOUR BROWS

When I was nineteen, my brows were so intense, Frida Kahlo had nothing on me (refer to my earlier photos). Naturally, mine are as black as night, and to me, they just look harsh and heavy. So I've lightened them considerably for as long as I can remember. Kristie Streicher, makeup artist and bicoastal brow banshee, has brow care down to a science. Here's her advice on how to brow wow:

1. SPACE TO GROW: Overtweezing is a crime. Ladies, put down your weapons/tweezers. Already gone too far? Give your brows three or four weeks to grow in. Assist the efforts with a brow-enhancing growth serum. Once they've grown back—start fresh. See a professional eyebrow artist and have them show you how to shape.

2. STEAM MACHINE: If you are sensitive, tweeze your brows after you wash your face or shower. The steam will ease the release of the hair from the follicle. And always pull in the direction of the hair growth—never against. When tweezing, another tip: tug in a well-lit area and in a regular mirror. Not a big, bad 5x mirror! When you magnify, you can't see both brows at a time, and that is crucial for creating symmetry.

3. FEATHER-FILL: Only fill in where you see there are holes. And never angle your line sharply downward toward the nose or you'll risk looking cranky. Also fill along the top line of the brow rather than the base to lift and broaden the eyes. Make short feathery strokes in the direction of the hair growth and use a color slightly lighter than your natural brow shade.

4. COLOR CONSIDERATION: Dark brows can age you. Consider lightening dark brows or warming them up if they are ashy. This can also enhance eye color. If your brows are superlight, darkening them slightly will help to frame your face. Do this with a professional, please; don't try at home.

HAIR *down there* AND ELSEWHERE?

Let's talk hair horticulture! This ain't the '70s, people, although I guess this "vintage" look is making a comeback. For me personally, I want it all gone. But I understand that's not for everyone. You've got to do what makes you (and, yes, your partner) most comfortable. The point is: *Do something.* Riki B, my below-the-belt beautician, is here to give you the ultimate lowdown on the *down low*. Riki knows more about wax than Madame Tussaud. She's been waxing Hollywood poetic for fifteen years and has made hair removal her personal and professional passion.

WAXING *wisdom* WITH RIKI B

How to Find the *right* Waxer

1. **CREDENTIALS ARE KEY!** In most states, a waxer needs to have a cosmetology license. A lot of nail salons offer waxing, but they are not credentialed, so enter at your own risk. Also, you want someone whose main bread and butter is waxing. For example, if they do 90 percent facials and 10 percent waxing, they just aren't going to have the same light touch as someone who waxes day in and day out.

2. **HYGIENE QUEEN:** Look around! Is the place clean? You should want to eat off the floors. The environment can be cozy, but the operation needs to be clinical.

3. **TRUST IS A MUST:** You don't need to be best friends with the person, but you have to be comfortable with her. You are exposing yourself and your nether regions and may need to ask her a question or two. It's important you are made to feel at ease. Referrals from savvy friends are the best, but websites with personal reviews, like Yelp, are helpful too.

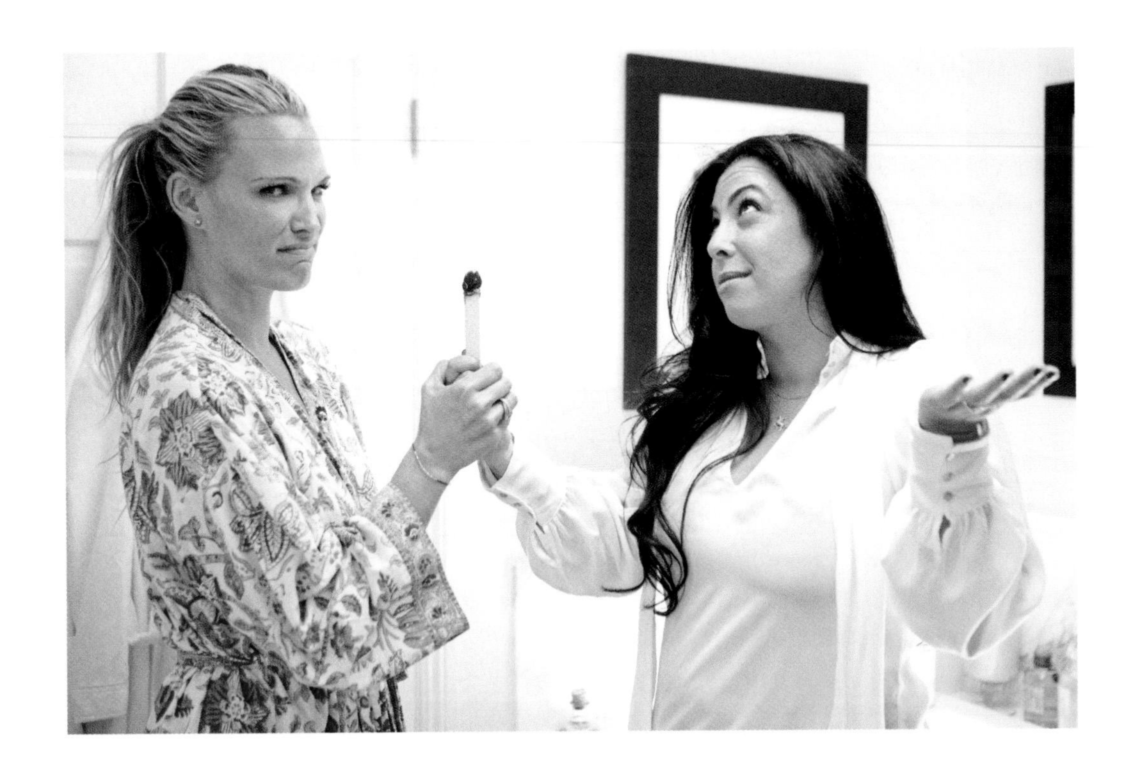

pointers for Posh Pubes

- The best time to wax is the week after your period has finished. NEVER wax during your period (or for that matter, do any laser hair removal). First, for sanitary reasons. Second, you are way more sensitive to pain while on your period. Ouch!
- If you are sensitive, Bare Ease is an over-the-counter numbing cream that you can ask your waxer to use. And for do-it-yourself yanking, Bliss makes a fairly user-friendly Poetic Waxing Kit.
- Hands off! After you wax, leave the area alone. And that also means no steam, sauna, swimming, spinning, or sex. Give it at least a day or two before any of these S's.
- Witch-Hazel Wash: Don't slather on lotion. Lotion can clog the pores and lead to pimples or infection. A splash of witch hazel is perfect to banish bacteria and prevent blemishes from forming.
- Try NOT to shave in between waxes. Instead, use a depilatory. The depilatories out there are very effective and won't create the itching sensation that shaving does.
- And finally, don't forget, there are also safe/effective at-home laser hair removal devices if waxing ain't your thing. Expensive at first, but can save you cash in the long run.

---

supermomma secret

WAXIN' WITH CHILD

I waxed during my entire pregnancy—all the way up to the birth. BUT I'm a baby when it comes to pain—and it's not advised to use numbing cream during pregnancy. My tip: use ice packs to numb the area first. It works like a charm!

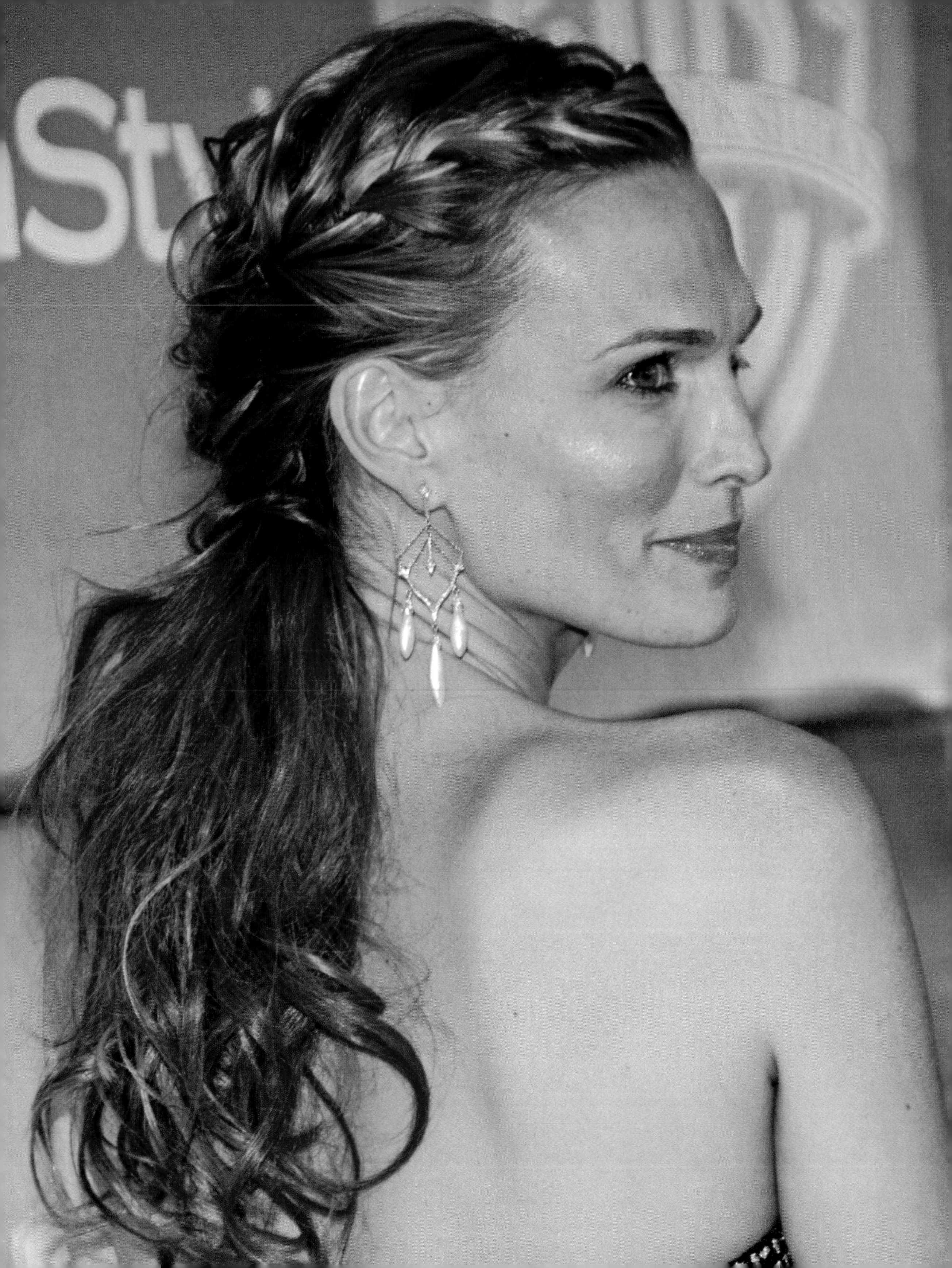

the *everyday* supermodel TOP 10 takeaways

1. Consult with your stylist and get a versatile haircut that suits you, that you can style on your own, and also works for your lifestyle and budget.

2. Be kind to your hair. Beware the chemical cut. Don't overprocess. Watch out for too much heat styling. Every now and again—do an at-home mask or use an intense conditioner. Take supplements to enchance growth, shine, and your hair's general health.

3. Hair color can transform you! Get your color right and you'll thank *you* for it. When your color is right, everything in life is just better.

4. Try out looks like balayage and ombré for the signature supermodel look . . . and don't worry about the upkeep . . . they are looooow maintenance, ladies!

5. Experiment with different hairstyles, play with extensions, try out classic looks (like we feature in here), and get to know your go-tos for common occasions to save you time and stress.

6. Find the one or two products that work for you and learn how to use them. But don't overdo it with product. And always remember, second-day hair always styles best.

7. Use tools like the one-inch curling iron for relaxed looks or more formal. It's the *everyday supermodel*'s secret weapon for a look less ordinary.

8. Master the done/undone look. Create looks that take a little time, that aren't stiff or too structured, but are polished.

9. Do not overpluck. Just stop already! Fuller brows are more youthful at every age—and consider going a little lighter or darker to frame your face.

10. Thou shalt keep your woman parts (and other parts) groomed!

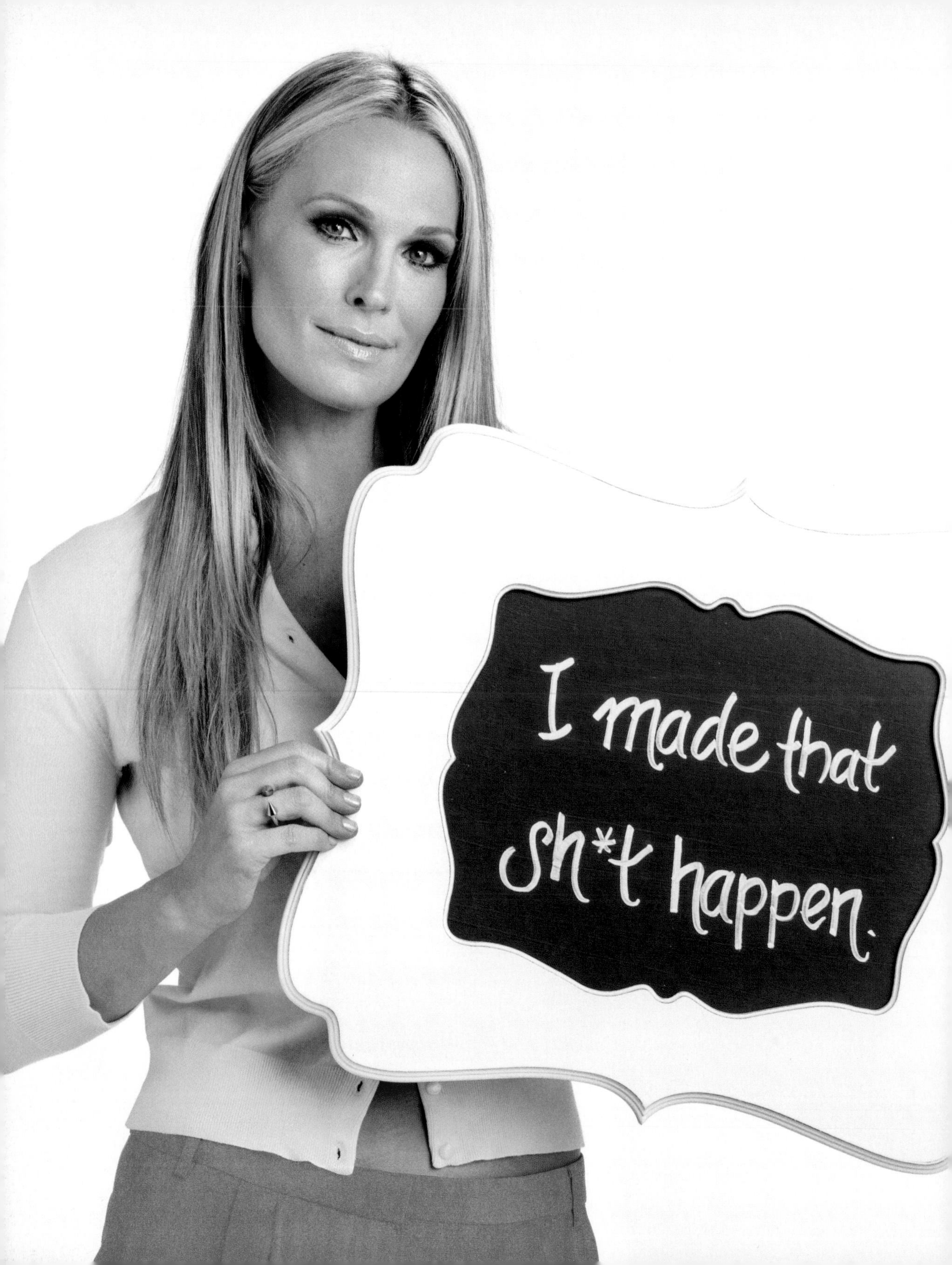
I made that
sh*t happen.

ch/6

i made that sh*t happen

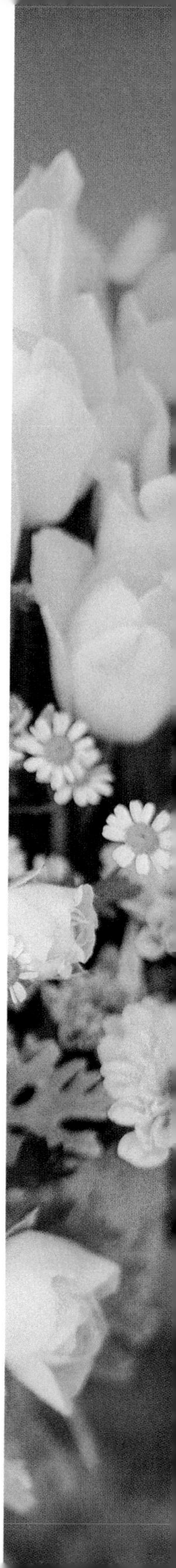

This is the story of how I went from double dumped and depressed to engaged, married, and pregnant in a little over a year, ladies! (Okay, maybe two.) And if that can happen—I'm telling you—*anything* is possible. Of all the chapters in this book, I felt most compelled to write this one—because I'm so blessed to be here. I've come a long way, baby, and it's taken a lot of work, but I made it. The past few years have been a series of milestones (that feel like honest-to-God miracles). I found a life partner I respect, admire, and am crazy about. I got hitched and had a fairy-tale wedding in Napa Valley. And . . . I became a momma for the first time. Oh, and let's not forget, I entered my forties (and am proud of it!). Once you get to this decade, you have a bit to reflect on. Today, I have to pinch myself I'm so happy and grateful. But it's been a loooong, winding, bumpy road to get here. Trust me, just a few years earlier I was swimming in a sea of anxiety, depression, Debbie-Downer-doubt, and despair. My dreams of finding a husband and starting a family seemed light-years away.

Here I was—I had worked a dozen-plus years as a successful model, was wrapping up a dream-come-true television series that had a five-year run, and yet my personal life was in shambles and I was in a downward spiral. Without a daily 5 A.M. call time for *Las Vegas,* I was left to face the facts. I had spent so much time focusing on my career that I had neglected my personal goals. I had applied all kinds of success secrets and strategies at work—but not at play. *And definitely not when it came to love.*

Life is beautiful. We know this because of the Oscar-winning movie, but it's also full of challenges, disappointments, broken hearts, and broken bones. It is all too easy to become weighed down, lose the joy, feel the pain, and not want to push on and fight for what we want, who we are, and who we want to become. It's easy to give up and give in, and to fall asleep at the wheel . . . *of our own lives.* I've done it—specifically when it came to my romantic life. I hadn't just fallen asleep at the wheel, but I was in a full-on coma! I had been in a dead-end relationship for over four years but couldn't make a move. I was scared. Insecure. Codependent. But one day, I woke up and decided that my personal goals weren't just going to materialize without my personal involvement. If you want something, you have to take an active role in it. I decided to wake up, take the wheel, and DRIVE—the next few months would be my version of the *Fast and the Furious.*

This chapter is about *that.* It's about how instead of giving up when I wanted to at times, I *giddy upped* and MADE THAT SH*T HAPPEN. But how? I filled my tank with petrol and stepped on the pedal! With more than a few decades under my belt, I have taken inventory of my life—what's worked/what hasn't—and I have a few ideas about it all. This chapter isn't meant to be a lecture or to air my dirty laundry; it's meant to motivate you and help you to *make that sh*t happen* in your life too. I've learned through trial and lots of error—all outlined here. You can be a passenger in life, or you can get behind the wheel. So let's make sh*t happen together. *Everyday supermodels . . .* Get in, hang on to your hats, and *let's drive!*

DOUBLE DUMPED TO LUCKY IN LOVE

I was on the verge of giving up. I was thirty-six and feeling . . . (gulp) desperate. My life had become one long, cold, clammy sweat. I was dying to meet *the* guy. To start a family. And yet, I was in an unhealthy four-year relationship with someone eight (yes, eight) years younger than me, who was living with me (or rather, off me). A friend told me he was looking at wedding rings and I got physically sick. I desperately wanted to have a life partner, but picturing my life with this person? Check, please! I won't go into all the reasons why it was sad and wrong; just trust me—it was sad and wrong. I woke up and finally said to myself, *Molly, get it together*.

I was terrified to leave because I hated being alone and didn't want to be. The backstory: When I was a young, working model, I was always alone, separated from friends and family and common comforts. I had boyfriends, but I traveled so much and was always on the move. In my twenties, I dated some truly exceptional men, like Stephane Dessant, who helped guide me throughout my career and was my family when I had no one. But in my thirties—for whatever reason—that wasn't the case. I just wasn't in the place in my own life to choose the right partner. So at thirty-six it took this "aha!" moment to see that I was very seriously in the wrong place, with the wrong person, and I needed to get out of both the place and the relationship. The truth is, I had never felt more alone in my life than when I was in that relationship.

When something isn't going right in your life—identify the problem. There's your *make that sh*t happen* Tip #1. Don't ignore it. I did for way too long. I had settled for a fraction of what I wanted and deserved. I worked up the courage and despite my fears, I finally ended the relationship and went to live in New York for three months. I was determined to not make the same mistakes again. I needed to change it up—so I changed my coordinates. No, I don't believe in running away from problems, but I wholeheartedly believe a change of scenery can help you refocus. I tell my single girlfriends all the time to *change it up*! There's Tip #2: **If what you're doing isn't working, try something new.** I took my own advice. Change can deliver newness and freshness. It can introduce new opportunities, people, and perspectives and shift things around when they are stuck in neutral, or even reverse.

I had to dust off, look at myself in the mirror, and face my "home alone" anxiety. So there's Tip #3: **Face your fears and look them in the eye.** Like Abraham Lincoln said, and I semi-quote, if you turn your back on the fire, you'll get burned in the rear—and then have to sit on your blisters! Or something like that. Face the fire, whatever your fire is. It's not going away. My fire was my disastrous love life. I let myself cry, whine, complain, lament, and basically feel sorry for myself. I started seeing a therapist. We talked about all those fears and feelings. Then it was time to stop the sobbing.

So that's quick Tip #4: **Cry. Purge. Mourn. Do all that. And then . . . Stop feeling sorry for yourself.** What was in the past— is in the past. Let's face it: You cannot be in two places at once. You have to choose. I chose and I wanted to be in the future of limitless possibilities—not in the graveyard of past mistakes. That brings us to Tip #5: **Choose the present. Yes, learn from those mistakes. Find the message in the mess. And then get grateful and get going.** Those relationships, jobs, and experiences that disappointed you or didn't work out—all taught you something. They taught you what you want and what you don't. By evaluating past experiences, not only do we learn from them, but we also see our present and future with more clarity and determination.

Once you've learned the lesson, loosen the ties . . . Tip #6: **Let it go**. *Let it alllll go.* Throw your hands up in the air. I've found this to be a necessary, and even redemptive, step that propels us out of neutral into a forward direction. Get quiet, pray, shut yourself in a room, block out any noise from family, friends, anyone, and ask yourself a single question: What do you want? And don't sell yourself short. Tip #7: **Identify what you want and what you don't.** FOCUS. For me, first order of business was to make sh*t happen in my romantic life. For you, it might be time to concentrate on your career, your health, your self-image, or maybe your relationship with your family or your finances. Whatever "it" is, now is the time you put YOU first and take an active role in your own happiness. The *everyday supermodel* does not just sit around and wait. Here's a little example of me finally putting ME first:

What did I want and what didn't I when it came to a relationship? I made a list!

WHAT I *didn't* WANT:

* Someone too young, selfish, or immature
* Someone moody and unpredictable
* Someone I had to mother, someone I had to fix
* Someone wandering through life, without a passion, without a purpose
* Someone who wasn't my emotional, social, moral, or intellectual match

WHAT I *did* WANT: (Aim high. Shoot for the moon—even if you miss—you'll land among stars. Don't make excuses for what you want. Be specific and honest with yourself.)

* A supporter, a participant, and a friend
* Someone balanced, stable, and trustworthy
* Someone independent, responsible, and on his game!
* A lover, a fighter, with a purpose and a passion
* My missing piece or other half: my emotional, social, moral and intellectual match
* To summarize: A modern-day gentleman who respects me, loves me, supports me, keeps me on my toes, but occasionally sweeps me off my feet!
* A TRUE PARTNER

I got specific, I got honest with myself, and I decided to stop selling myself short. I advise you do the same. I was a great girl. I deserved a great guy. I just had to write it down— writing down words makes ideas more concrete. They go from the untouchable, invisible world of thoughts inside your head—to the tangible, visible world of possibility on paper. So when you know what you want, write it down and shout it out. Writing down your goals helps to further clarify them. And shouting them from rooftops lets those around you in on what you want too—that way, maybe . . . *they can even help*! People aren't mind readers.

Tip #8: **NOW GO AFTER IT! Make the first move**. The best defense is a good offense they say in sports and war. So declare war on your sh*t—and your greatest good will appear. Whatever your sh*t is—the sh*tty job, the sh*tty relationship, the sh*tty body image you have—whatever it is, identify it and tell it to go to hell! A little lesson in physics, yep, from the supermodel: Once you make that first move, it's easier to keep on going. An object in motion stays in motion, an object at rest stays at rest. Start moving away from what you don't want and toward what you do!

Relationship-wise I had been at rest for four years, so it was time for me to make a move. There was a guy I'd always thought was attractive, so I asked a mutual friend of ours to set us up. Before I knew it I was on a date. (FYI: Dating scared the crap out of me.) Talk about taking risks—I had been out of the game for a long time and things had changed. I had to learn how to date in my late thirties. I had posed countless times half naked, and yet I was terrified to have dinner with a "friend-of-a-friend." But remember: face your fears. Before long, *oh boy,* I was in love (at least I thought I was). I remember being at a Coldplay concert with this guy, gripping his hand, dreaming how my first name would sound with his last . . . I'm kind of exaggerating, but you know what I mean. I started fantasizing about a life with him. A week later HE DUMPED ME. Fade to black.

I was devastated. I thought I had found *the One*. He, on the other hand, didn't feel the same. Feelings of fear, failure, regret, and past heartbreaks came out of hibernation. If you are single, in your thirties or forties, and yearn to be a momma and have a family, then you might relate to how I was feeling. You've likely watched many of your friends partner up, have children, and transition smoothly into the next chapter of their lives—while you dog-paddle in purgatory. But guess what? I spent a few weeks slaying dragons . . . and then I let it all go. I had tear-filled eyes—but they were still on the prize, people!

Now let's talk time. Most people say you need time to get over heartbreak, to rise above loss. Fine. Take some time and then get moving again. Why? Because the time is now. Remember, the past is the past . . . the present is what it's all about! Tip #9: **Don't wallow. Bounce back. Persist.** The best way to get over something is by exploring something new. The most brilliant book on this subject is called *It's Time,* by my sometimes therapist, Mary Goldenson. Do yourself a favor. Read it. (Later, I give a roundup of some of the best advice she's given to me.) It's an unbeatable guide for getting off your butt and getting over your "buts."

That's exactly what I did. After just a few short weeks in mourning, I got off my but/butt, treated myself to a little pampering (I'd been living in pajamas), called my manager and everyone I knew and made a demand. *Set. Me. Up.* I said what I wanted, asked for help and surprise, surprise—I got it. Friends delivered! I went on a bunch of setups. (*Not-gonna-lie*, it was kind of torture. Think *Groundhog Day* with breadsticks and bad jokes.) Then out of the blue, a gentleman I knew socially (and always had a crush on) became single. So, ladies, like it or not, I made the first move and put fate into my own hands. I mentioned my crushtastic feelings to our mutual friend and mumbled . . . *Set me up?* In a week's time we were swapping better jokes over breadsticks (no, I didn't eat the breadsticks).

There was a spark. He was smart and artsy and masculine. He had his career together, he was independent and fiercely passionate, and he had dreams, goals, and desires. We had two months of dating bliss. And then the Thanksgiving holiday was upon us. Should we spend it together? He freaked out. And then, dumped me, *cold turkey* (sorry, couldn't resist). Who knew poultry, mashed potatoes, and stuffing could not only lead to heartburn, but also *heartbreak*? If you are counting, that's two breakups in twice as many months. I could almost read the imaginary Page Six headline in my head: "Molly Sims: *Sports Illustrated* Supermodel, Star of NBC's *Las Vegas,* and Man Repeller. Dumped Again!" What was wrong with me? Was it ever going to happen? Dating is tricky, but I don't think it's much different from acting or modeling. It's not about the hundred auditions you don't get—it's about the one you do that matters. My acting coach, Leigh Kilton, has a personal mantra for accepting no's and moving on: "Thank you for getting out of the way so I can get where I need to go."

There was a brief moment after the double dumpings that I almost threw in the mating towel. But deep down I've always believed that most people give up just before something really big can happen for them. I refused to be that person. I refused to be TKOed. From that point on, I simply decided that I wasn't going to let anything keep me down. I would be like an inflatable bop bag. Thank Jesus, I didn't give up! The next man I dated became my husband. That reveals Tip #10: **Do not give up on yourself or your goals.** If you want something bad enough, and refuse to give up, I believe you can have it.

Scott and I had known each other for quite a few years through work. One night our fates aligned (because I wasn't at home eating ice cream wallowing in the dumped-ster), and we ran into each other. I sensed a bit of sizzle factor between us . . . and the next day I got an e-mail from him. He was tall, clever, handsome, and best of all—f***ing funny (his friends will say the same!). Not to mention, he has great hair. I was over being single and over settling for less. Scott was so much more. And we both knew what we wanted in a relationship; from the start, we were on the same page. I didn't play any games and neither did he. That brings us back to an earlier tip: in dating, in relationships—and in life—don't be afraid to *say what you want out loud*, clearly and calmly and confidently. You deserve it. Your boyfriend, or your boss, or your friend—whoever you are having that conversation with—will either listen and step up to the plate or won't. Even if you don't get the response you are looking for, they will respect you, but more important, *you will respect yourself* for being your most authentic self.

I was up front with Scott out of the gate about where I was in my life and my personal goals. We had just started dating, but I knew that if my honesty scared him off, then he wouldn't be the right partner for me. The holidays came and went (this time it was Christmas)—*smoothly*. We spent more and more time together and began to merge families and friends. I loved the simple moments we shared as much as the more glamorous ones, and I started to feel like I was part of a team. As I've said before, I am always going a million miles a minute, but Scott made me feel calm. I could relax when I was around him. Within about six months of dating, *I knew*, and I remember the exact moment. I was lying in bed one morning and he was out of town for work—and suddenly in one moment I realized this was it, I didn't want to be with anyone else. It was the best feeling, followed by a moment of panic, because I knew I did not want to lose him. From that moment on, *I couldn't picture my life without him*. I had fallen in love with Scott not only for the man I knew that he was, but also with the man I knew he would be: a great husband, father, and true partner.

Pop the cork, *everyday supermodels,* Molly was gettin' hitched. After a year and a half of dating we got engaged, six months later we married, and the day after that (on our honeymoon) we conceived our boy, Brooks. See what I mean? Things can change almost overnight. Not long before I had been freaking out, settling for less than I deserved, and crying over men that were—I can say this now—*wrong for me.*

During that time, my career took a backseat, because after years of neglecting the personal, I made it top priority. You have got to focus on what you want most and put that at the top of your list. I've never shared this publicly, but I was so afraid that I wouldn't get pregnant, and that I was too old, that even before we were engaged I asked Scott if he would freeze embryos with me. In other words, I asked my *not yet fiancé* to start the process of IVF (in vitro fertilization). I know, you are probably thinking, *whoa*—that's a big ask! And it was. But it was time for me to say what I wanted and not hold back. I knew Scott wanted to have kids, so it didn't scare me. As a side note: I will say this to any of you out there "getting up there"—if you are getting to that age, don't have a partner, but do want to be a mother, look into freezing your eggs. Why not? It's okay! It's worth investigating. It doesn't mean you'll have to use them, but it is an insurance policy I don't think you'll regret.

In my head, the clock was ticking every day, and Scott was a little older as well. So I chose to be fearless, asked, he said yes, and we did it together. Ask for what you want. Ultimately, it turned out that we had no trouble getting pregnant—but I braved that topic and it took pressure off me. Suddenly I wasn't afraid anymore, or alone.

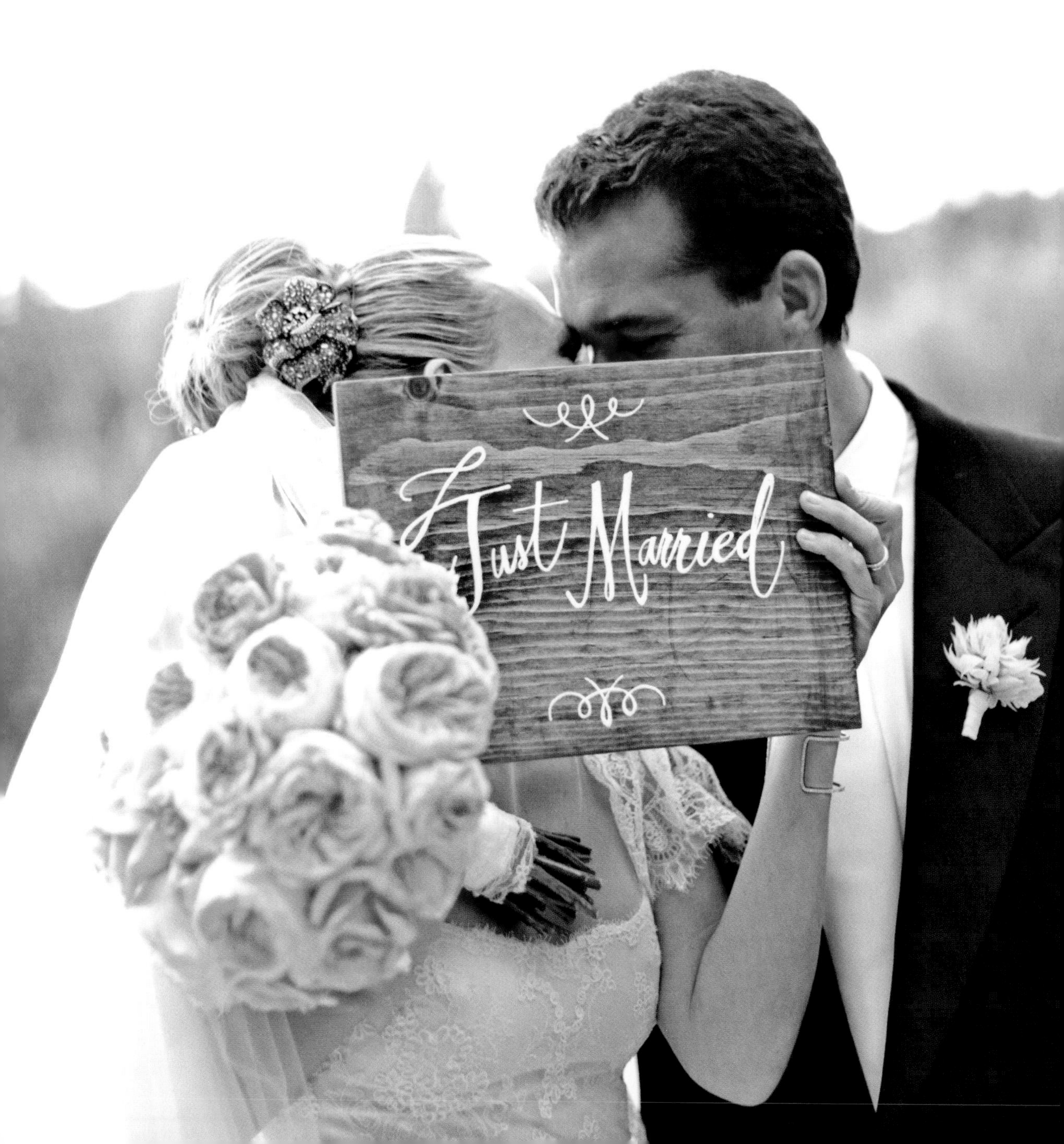
Just Married

Maybe that's one reason conceiving went so smoothly for me—we had that insurance policy (and the fertility smoothie!).

Today, as new parents, we are faced with a whole new world of joys and challenges. As a mother, I continue to apply everything I've learned in life and love to this new adventure. It's not been easy—and there have been times where I've been scared sh*tless. Exhausted. And insecure. But like I've done in work and love, I just face it head-on and do my best. And now I have Scott to do it with me. He truly is the-best-thing-ever, and I absolutely LOVE him. Not to be too dramatic, but where I am in my life is a place I've always dreamed about—but at times—wasn't sure would materialize. And yet, deep down, I knew I was never going to take no for an answer. I said it earlier, and I'll say it again. If there is something in your life that you want, *everyday supermodels,* go after it with your gut and gusto! Make it your number one priority and let yourself loose on it!

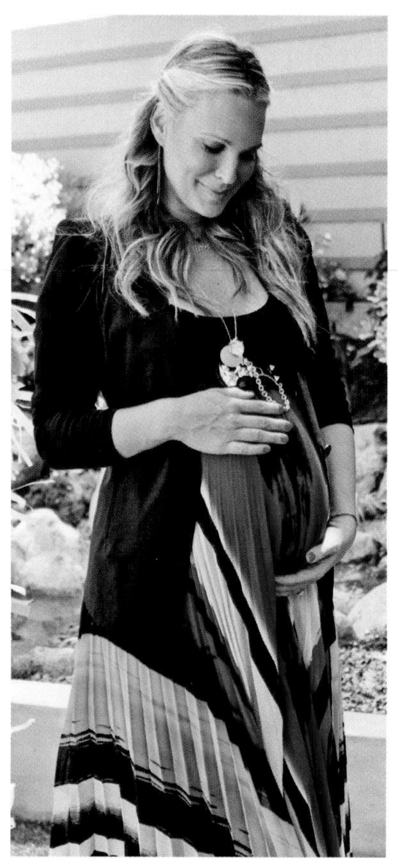

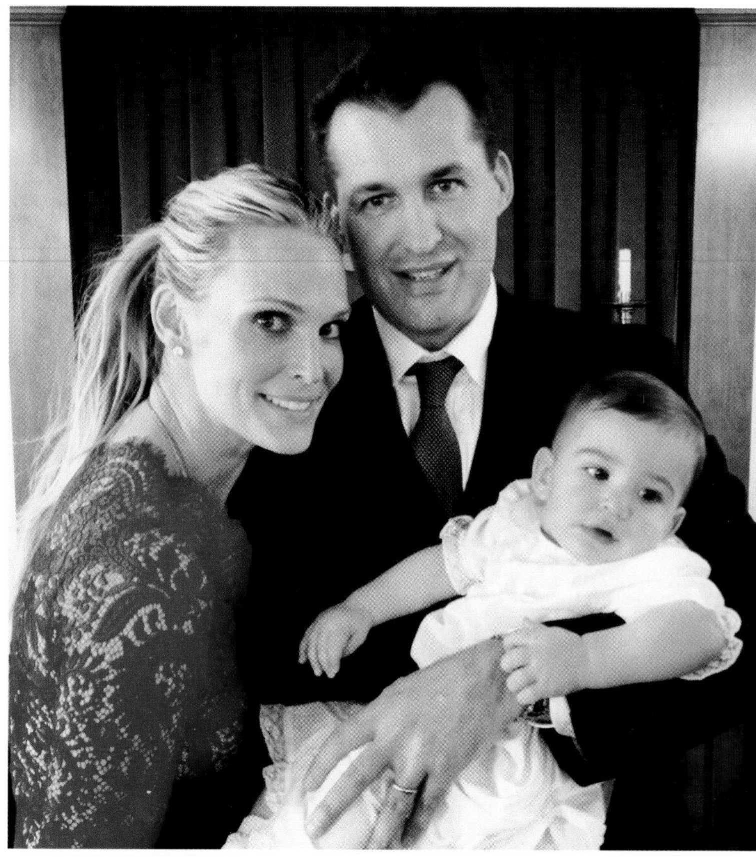

supermodel success *secret*

Do not be a prisoner of your past. Start being in charge of your life now. Everyone who knows me knows that I am a HUGE fan of soaps, and if I've learned anything from them, I've learned: (1) You have only One Life to Live . . . and (2) These Are the Days of Your Lives. So make 'em count!

live a *golden* life

Success Strategies from Mary Goldenson, Ph.D.

- IT'S TIME: Right now, ask yourself, what is it time for me to address in my life? Yes. Now. Why wait? Begin to live with a sense of urgency!
- PRACTICE WHAT YOU WANT: Practice what you want to be good at, because what you practice will improve. Practice complaining and you'll only get better at complaining. On the other hand, practice good communication, trust, and love and *you'll get better at good communication, trust, and love.*
- BE COURAGEOUS: Like Mark Twain said, courage is resistance to fear and mastery of fear—*not absence of fear*. Courage is the key, it's what it takes to begin a great journey.
- ACCEPT LIFE 360°: Open yourself up to all of life. Suffering, joy, success, failure, love, grief, change. The primary cause of most mental anguish is opposition to an acceptance of change.

One trait successful people share is resilience. Molly is successful because she is incredibly resilient. It's not that successful individuals never fall down, quite the opposite, they all do. The difference is they refuse to stay there.

—MARY GOLDENSON, Ph.D.

kick-ass career tips: GO BIG or GO HOME!

Some of the make-sh*t-happen strategies I finally applied to my personal life . . . I had long been applying professionally and didn't know it.

I started modeling when I was nineteen years old, I modeled throughout my twenties and became a television host, and then, I embarked on a full-time acting career in my late twenties and into my thirties. Early on, there was little career/life balance. It was all career, all the time. I was driven and I was focused. But nothing was ever handed to me. I made sh*t happen left and right. I worked so hard for every yes I got, and worked equally as hard for every no. As a model and an actress you hear the word *no* so often you think it's your first name.

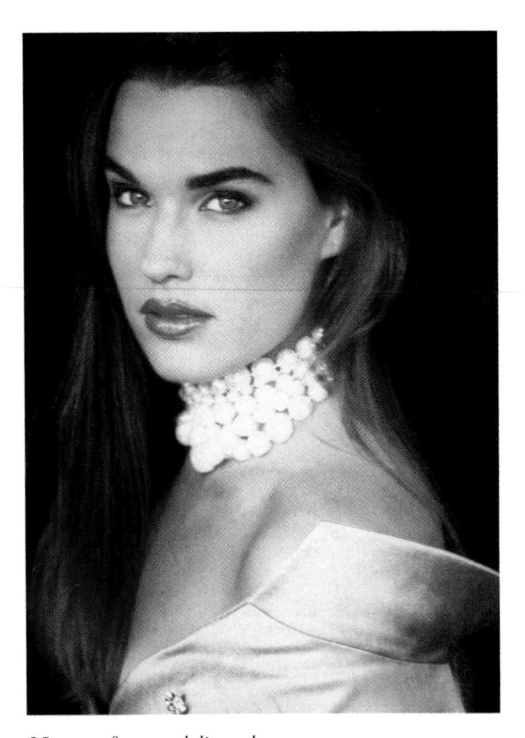

My very first modeling photo.

In 1991, I was enrolled in prelaw at Vanderbilt University, but that was about to change. At the end of my sophomore year, a girlfriend who had done some modeling suggested I take pictures with a fashion photographer she'd worked with in Memphis. It wasn't something I had considered before, but the second she said it, I knew it was something I wanted to try. I drove my butt down to Memphis a few weeks later, took my first-ever modeling shots with the photographer and days later, we sent the pictures to all the New York modeling agencies.

A few agreed to meet with me, so my momma and I flew out to the Big/scary/exciting Apple to take meetings.

Straight out of Murray, Kentucky (population less than 15,000), I walked into my first meeting at Next Model Management wearing pearls, pantyhose, and carrying a leather briefcase. I looked part preacher's wife/part tax attorney—*zero part model.* We had our meeting; I was nervous but remember feeling overwhelmed with excitement. At the time, Next was owned by Jean Luques, Lorenzo Cedrini, Joel Wilkenfeld, and Faith Kates—I met with all of them. Jean Luques and Joel *did not want me*. Literally, when they saw me, they thought "Next!" But not Faith; she saw something in me they didn't see. If it wasn't for Faith's faith in me, I would not have a career. She got her way and Next took me on. She gave me my first ever big break, backed me from day one, and I have been with Next ever since because of that.

All it takes is just ONE—one person to believe in you, and have . . . Faith in you. She did. The irony is not lost on me. Having just one person who believes in you can make all the difference in the world—if you find that person, keep that person close and stay cuddly. Career Tip #1: **When someone believes in you, believe their belief. Don't be humble or dismiss their kindness or encouragement.** Accept that person's belief in you. It's so powerful. It might change your life.

When Molly came into the office for the first time, the guys said, she's never going to work. But I saw it, so I said to them, "We're taking her." A few weeks later we sent Molly to Europe, and she worked almost every single day from the moment she got there. She had that fire within her from day one. Successful people know how to get in touch with that fire and use it as fuel.

—FAITH KATES, co-owner, Next Model Management

I worked in New York for six weeks. In those six weeks I realized that I did not look like the other models. Models did not wear pearls and pantyhose and carry briefcases. After I worked a few weeks in New York, Next sent me to work with an agency in Hamburg, Germany, for six months. It was an ideal market to start my career, because there was a lot of opportunity to work, gain experience, and build my modeling portfolio.

I arrived in Hamburg as innocent as a southern daisy. And within moments of my arrival, it was *Paradise Lost*. I checked in to the German agency and the head booker looked me up and down and said, "Absolutely not. You are too fat." Word. For. Word. He asked me what size I was and how much I weighed, and then he actually made me get a pair of my jeans out of my suitcase to show him I was a size six. He thought I was big, but he didn't believe that I was actually *that big*. A six! Gasp. Not only was I too fat (in his eyes) to work, but I also wasn't *the right look*.

The day I landed was the same day he fired me as a client. Can you imagine? I was nineteen! I had never been on a plane that long in my life. I was away from home and everyone I knew and loved. He said I needed to be on the next plane home to the States. I begged him to let me stay long enough to at least pay off what I owed (the German agency had advanced me the fare for my plane ticket to Germany). I begged him to send me out to castings so I could pay him what I owed him ($872!). In my head, I was NOT going home. Believe me, I was devastated, but there was no way I was getting on that plane with my tail between my legs. I knew if I could just get into those rooms, I would book *something*. I could make something happen. Tip #2. **Believe in yourself, even when no one else does.** If you have to lend yourself a helping hand or be your own cheerleader—get over it and shake those pom-poms!

I was young and naive, but it helped. At each casting I told myself: someone is getting this job—why not me? I wasn't the prettiest, the tallest, or the skinniest. I didn't have the clearest skin or the best body. But what did I have? Determination and more often than not, sometimes faux confidence. Tip #3: **Walk into that room knowing you have the job.** It's an extension of believing in yourself. To this day I continue to do this. Did I always get the job? No! A lot of the times I didn't. But I always moved on and focused on the next opportunity ahead of it. The project I didn't get didn't matter. But the opportunity ahead did.

---

supermodel *secret*

When I was modeling, the top girls were getting paid a lot of money per day. If a client's budget was less than top dollar, they'd walk away from the project, giving up what was still really good money. Because there were fewer top dollar gigs, that meant those models were only working a day or two a month—and earning less than me. I didn't let my ego get in the way. I always chose to work more days at a lower price than only one day a month at a princely sum. Thank you Leigh Crystal, it was the best advice you ever gave me. It paid off. Not to mention, the more jobs I worked, the more relationships I made—which ultimately led to more opportunities for me, and eventually, a few princely sums!

After I begged, the German agent agreed to send me out on a few castings. The very next week, I booked a job. And then another one after that. Within a short time, I had paid my German agency back for my plane ticket and had pocketed a few paychecks! After two years of working out of Munich and Hamburg and building a strong modeling foundation, it was time I further establish myself in Europe. I first moved to London and worked there for a few years, and then Paris. That's how the modeling business works when you are building your career. You often switch markets based on your look, where you can build your portfolio and establish a body of print work. Some markets are also seasonal as well, stronger in the summer for swimsuit or in the fall for high fashion.

A little fun fact! When I was living in Paris, years after those first few days in Munich—I ran into that German agent. I can remember it like it was yesterday. At this point, I had become successful in Europe and looked every part the supermodel . . . leather pants, designer pumps, healthy skin, and swagger. Not to brag, but I looked good! There I was dressed to kill, in the Place des Victoires—and there he was—*kinda short*. It was the best revenge ever. He mumbled something, congratulated me—I flipped my hair, cracked a smile, kept on walking, and never looked back! I got my very own *Pretty Woman* moment. And just imagine, *everyday supermodels,* what if I had listened to him? What if I had let his singular opinion of me keep me down? I would not be where I am today. Tip #4: **Listen to what is within you, and don't be afraid to take your life into your own capable hands.**

After working in Europe, a South African named Leigh Crystal from Next kept leaving me messages on my answering machine in Paris. She said, "I'm going to be the one representing you in New York. I'm going to be in Paris. I'd love to meet up." From that moment on we became a team and she's been my agent ever since. I owe my modeling career to this woman. Good and bad, she is always there for me. I LOVE this woman. Making the leap from Europe to New York for a model is a big deal. But like Faith, Leigh fought for me and believed I would have success in the States, and with her behind me—I was crazy enough to believe I could do it.

When it comes to modeling, New York is another level. The girls I was up against were hard-core competitive. They'd Tonya Harding you to win the job. I've never worked so hard in my life. I did everything it took to give myself a leg up. And I was sweet as pecan pie everywhere I went, to everyone I met, and to everyone I worked with. It sounds simple, but Tip #5: **Always be nice.** It will pay off. People like to work with nice people. And believe me—you will stand out. There are a lot of a-holes out there!

When I was working in Europe, I was known as a "catalog girl." That meant that I would do catalog work, steady work, *not a lot of prestige*. But I wanted to do magazines. Every model does. They are glamorous, you get to dress up in designer clothes, and you shoot with world-class photographers! The flip side? Catalogs pay, and they pay *really well*. Magazines? Not so much. With my catalog money (I had saved and saved like momma taught me), I bought my first house. Boy was I proud of everything I'd accomplished, but it was my dream to do editorial work and ad campaigns for glossy magazines. I just didn't get the opportunities for those jobs, and when I did, I always got a no. It was a constant disappointment.

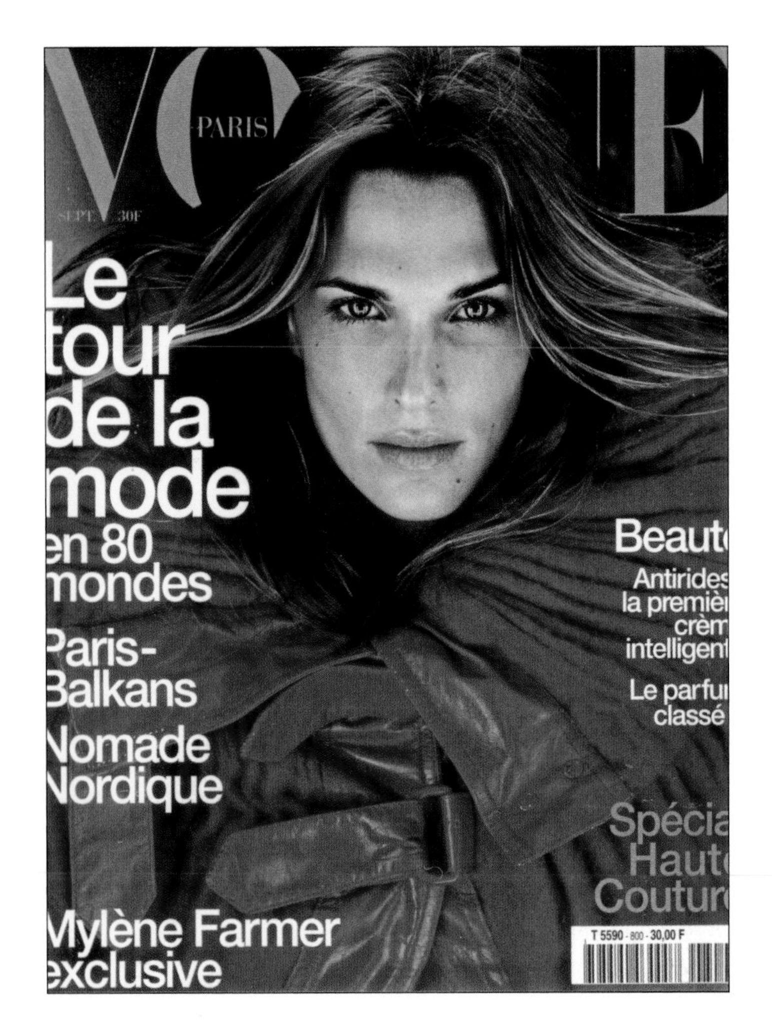

And then one magical day, Leigh let me in on big news at the agency. She called to tell me that Molly Sims had booked the cover of French *Vogue*. THE COVER OF FRENCH *VOGUE*. Did you hear that, people?! In my world, at that time . . . that was BIG. Why did I get the job? I'm not exactly sure. But what I will tell you, Joan Juliet Buck, the editor of French *Vogue* then, gave me a chance. I had done very little editorial work up to this point, but I had put in my dues with her and the magazine, working for next to nothing for an inside spread she did earlier that year.

It was an absolute f***ing miracle that she would put me, *a "catalog girl" from small-town Kentucky* on her cover. It paid close to nothing, but it meant everything. At that moment, I thought, *Oh yeah, Molly, THIS IS IT. You are finally going to do high-fashion.* But guess what? I became even more "commercial." What actually happened after *Vogue*? My *Sports Illustrated* spread. It doesn't get more commercial than that.

As I mentioned in Chapter 1, my *Sports Illustrated* spread did not just come to me on a silver Tiffany platter. I prepped, plotted, prepared, and planned. I did everything I knew I could to give myself the best possible shot.

Tip #6**: Prepare, study, do your homework. And do what you need to do to give yourself a leg up.** Even if there was some luck involved, I'm a big believer in that quote "Luck is what happens when preparation meets opportunity." Bingo. Hard work, perseverance, commitment, and dedication matter. *SI* was a game changer for my career. Doors flung open. Nope, not editorial. But whole new opportunities in an entirely new world . . . a world that both terrified and excited me. Television.

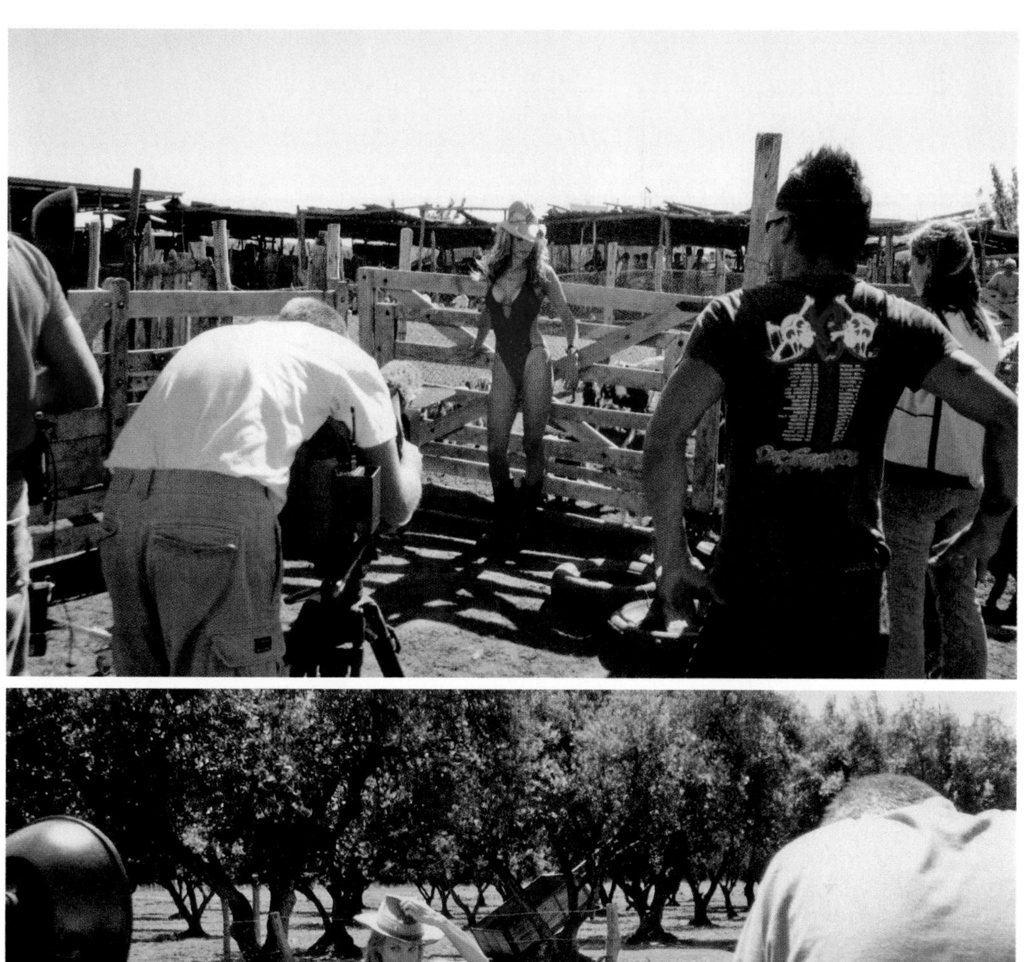

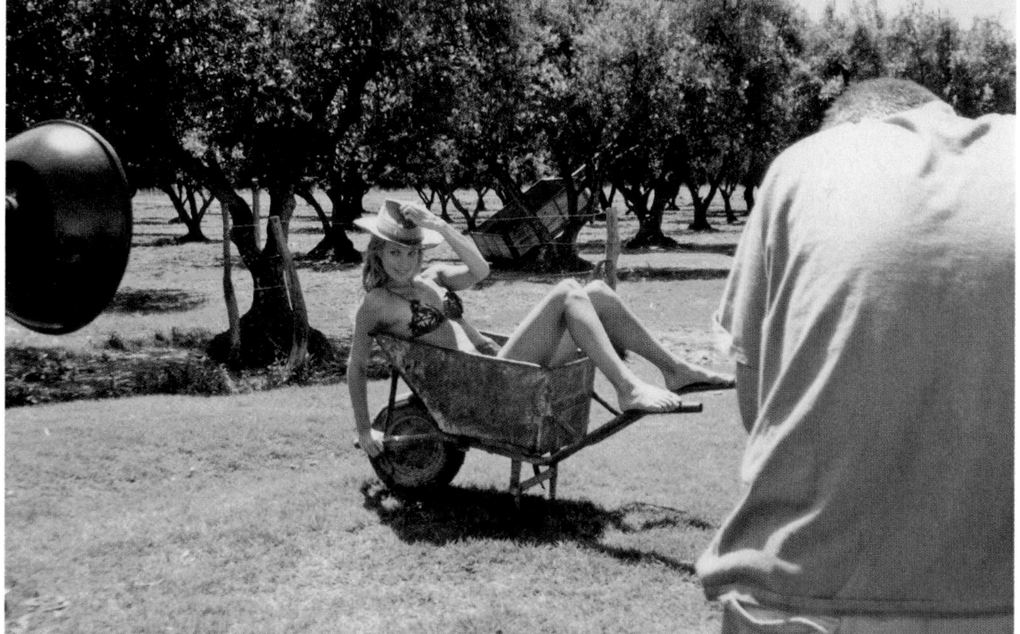

Behind the scenes on my Sports Illustrated *shoot!*

Molly took this work very seriously from the beginning. A lot of girls don't. But she saw it as a business right away. The girls that take their dreams seriously, treat it as a business, and focus on building their careers are the women that succeed.

—MAURY DIMAURO, commercial agent

When I arrived in New York, Next had set me up with Maury DiMauro, a commercial agent who represented models and actresses for film and TV. There's a running theme here, like Faith and Leigh—he also believed in me. He got me the most coveted audition among models at that time: MTV's *House of Style*.

Cindy Crawford was the first host and helped make the series a huge hit. I went through five months of frightening auditions and Maury supported me through it all the way. He sent me to media training because I was NOT *a natural* on camera. There were what felt like a thousand meetings and call-backs. I was a nervous wreck in every single one of them. After a long, hard battle—I got

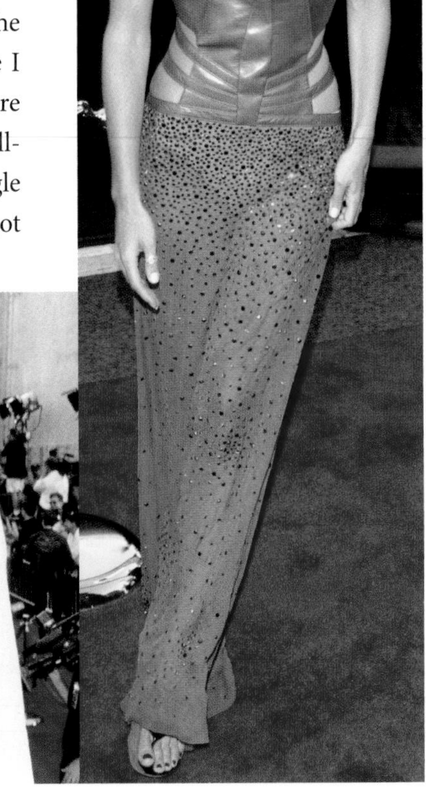

the job—and have producer Chad Hines to thank for taking a chance on me.

I was so inexperienced and greener than spinach in front of the camera. Case in point: one of my first interviews was with the singer Maya. I actually kept dropping the microphone onto the floor. Over and over. And when I wasn't dropping it, I was forgetting to hold it up when she talked. Or when I talked. I'm even embarrassed reliving it now! *God bless.* But think about it. Up until this point in my career I never had to actually talk to model well. The most excruciating part of my new TV gig? I had to watch playbacks of myself in a room with the producers and get "notes" and "feedback." Read: TORTURE.

---

supermodel success *secret*

Do the hustle. The name of this chapter isn't I Made That Sh*t Happen for no good reason. To quote Lincoln again, "Things may come to those who wait, but only the things left by those who hustle." Be one step ahead, not behind. If I were to pin my life's successes on one thing, it might just be this. I'm a hustler, baby.

I had some seriously bad habits. They called me the "bobbing head" because I *never stood still*, but rather would awkwardly swing and bounce side to side. They made me go to voice coaching because my voice was "too high and squeaky." I had to learn to lower the register of my voice and speak more modulated. Despite all the constructive criticism, George McTeague and the other producers were encouraging and made me better. I worked hard. Went to media training. And, little by little, I improved. By the end of the season—*I was seasoned.* One important lesson: I didn't allow the criticism to control me. I took control of it. I worked to make the changes necessary for that show (and me) to be successful. Tip #7: **Use criticism to your advantage.** It sheds a light on areas where you can improve and ultimately excel.

While I was working on *House of Style,* the same producers launched a show called *Mission Makeover* and asked me if I wanted to host it. Compared to what I was making then as a top model, the pay was peanuts. The producers asked me the all-important questions: Do you want to make a name for yourself? Do you want to appear in catalogs or do you want people to *know who you are*? When it came to name recognition as a model, it was few and far between. Name recognition was the exclusive domain of a select few in the modeling world. TV was one of the best ways to do that—to stand out. I remember being overwhelmed by the opportunity and the decision. I was at the height of my modeling career. I finally felt like I had hit my groove and I was making more money than ever. But hosting? I was not the best host, it was such hard work for me, and I had so much to learn. But I believe in doing things that scare you. That's when growth happens. I decided to take the opportunity and dive in headfirst!

I did at least fifty episodes of *Mission Makeover* and had a lot of fun doing it. I cut my TV teeth on that show. I learned how to walk and talk and make it my own. It was impossible not to get good we shot so much. And my hard work paid off—at the end of that period, I ended up hosting the *Radio City Music Awards* with Carson Daly. Who would've thought? By that time, I had caught the bug and I really liked television. There were a few other models making names for themselves in acting—and I decided that's what I wanted to do—dive even deeper into uncharted waters!

Here's how committed I was: during a break from hosting *Mission Makeover*, I moved to Los Angeles to do a month-long intensive acting course and I liked it. But I didn't have a clue what I was doing; all I knew was that *I wanted to keep doing it*. So I bit the bullet and enrolled in the Sanford Meisner two-year acting program with coach Martin Barter, a course that started that fall. In two years, I took seventy-seven red-eyes (basically every weekend) from New York to L.A. for this class. If I was going to act, I wanted to be prepared and to be taken seriously. Exhausting? Yes. However, your *dreams can be your fuel*. As insane as it seemed to travel back and forth across the country, I was so driven, I had to do it. I believed that if I prepared, did my homework, and someone gave me a shot, luck and preparation would collide. Whether you think you can, or you think you can't—*you are always right*. Deep inside, I thought I could. Tip #8: **If you want something, when that bell goes off, and you think you can—that's when you go for it.**

While I was studying acting in L.A., I got an agent with what was the William Morris Agency (now William Morris Endeavor). During my two-year course, they sent me out here and there on auditions, but I wasn't totally ready. I didn't have the acting or auditioning chops. But it was good practice. After I graduated, they started sending me out more and more. Unlike my modeling career, it was slow going at first. Then I got the call to audition for a television pilot called *Las Vegas* for the role of Delinda Deline.

I was so nervous—but like Jimmy Caan says (who became my father on the show), "If you get nervous, that means you are invested. You should always get nervous no matter how good you get or how long you do this." It wasn't a tough audition, but I was still nervous. I did my best. And after a whole lot of acting audition no's, I finally got a big, fat YES! Gary Scott Thompson, the show's creator and director, knew I didn't have much acting experience, but he somehow knew I could do it. I got

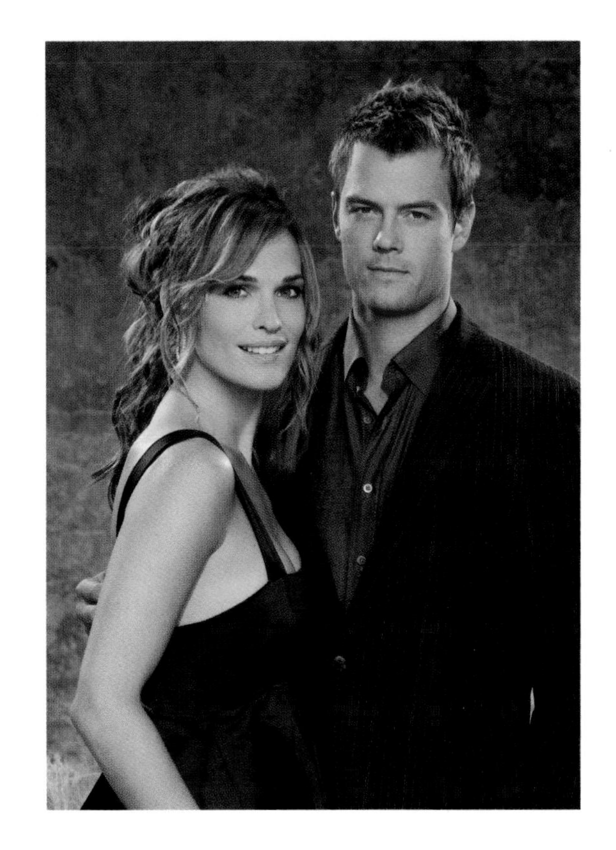

the role of Delinda because I kinda was Delinda and I worked so hard to get there. The role played to my strengths. In a way, everything I had done up to then in my life had prepared me for it.

What's crazy is that role was only supposed to be a one- or two-episode arc. After the pilot got picked up, Delinda was made a series regular. Great news. Amazing news. I had landed a steady acting job; it was the stuff dreams are made of. But it was a huge risk for me. I had to sign a six-year contract. It was all or nothing. That meant I had to leave modeling mostly behind. My bread and butter, the business I knew so well and was really good at. And—I had to physically move from New York to L.A. and actually act, every day. Not model. I was scared sh*tless. Rightfully so! There were scary moments. James Caan, the realest-deal actor you could ever meet—who'd frankly been acting longer than I'd been living—could be SO hard on me and Josh Duhamel, another actor in the cast. We were very inexperienced compared to him. We had to prove ourselves. But that made us better actors. Tip #9: **Surround yourself with people who are better, smarter, or wiser than you are; you learn very quickly:** My manager, Alissa Vradenburg, always says this. Don't hang with turkeys if you want to fly with eagles!

There were other, unexpected situations that were hard. The very first scene I shot was a sex scene with Josh. (Now that might sound exciting to some, but I was petrified.) I was wearing pasties and Josh was wearing—next to nothing—in front of two dozen people. We had to get frisky in front of everyone . . . and we actually fell off the bed. Josh made it fun, but it was still awkward as heck for me, to say the least. *Vegas* had a five-year run, and the cast became like a family to me. I learned to act on that set, and exciting things happened to me during the show's run. It led to a coveted contract with Cover Girl; all of a sudden I was invited to Oscar parties and everything in between, and in an instant, my whole world was different. For the first time in my life, I wasn't living out of a carry-on. *I was rooted in one place.*

I've learned some incredible lessons as I've built my career. One of the most important being: Tip #10: **You have to do things that scare you. All the time.** The second you stop doing things that terrify you is when you stop learning, growing, and expanding. Taking the leap from modeling to acting was one of the biggest risks I've ever taken. Big risks can have big rewards and it did for me.

You have got to take risks in life. Measured risks, calculated risks (to be clear), not idiot ones. You've got to go out on a limb occasionally, because, *everyday supermodels,* that's where the fruit is! So many of us are paralyzed with fear. Fear of failure, of rejection, of screwing up, or of not being good enough, and so on. I know. But like that great quote says, "In the end, we only regret the chances we didn't take, the relationships we're afraid to have, and the decisions we took too long to make." Often, perceived failures open doors to new opportunities. I continue to go out onto those limbs and reach for that fruit! Today, I still model and act, but I've again ventured into new and exciting, and still sometimes scary, professional places. I created and designed a signature jewelry collection, I continue to explore licensing opportunities and brand partnerships, and recently I have focused on building my lifestyle website and social media platforms—balancing this with my newfound motherhood and being a wife.

If it wasn't for the foundation that my family gave me, I don't know that I would have gotten here or had the willpower to get it done. My family still serves as my ultimate inspiration. Both my momma's and my daddy's side have surefire southern grit. Regardless of where you are from, they give good counsel. So let's give the Sims family the soapbox! Here are a few life lessons I've learned from my southern roots.

Fear will say, What if I fail? What if it doesn't work?, which is totally natural, but failure doesn't matter. It's the act of making room for your dream and pursuing it that matters. The act of pursuing it makes room for more dreams and more of your real self to emerge.

—KATE WALSH, actress

---

supermodel KIN success *secrets*

LESSONS FROM MY LOVED ONES

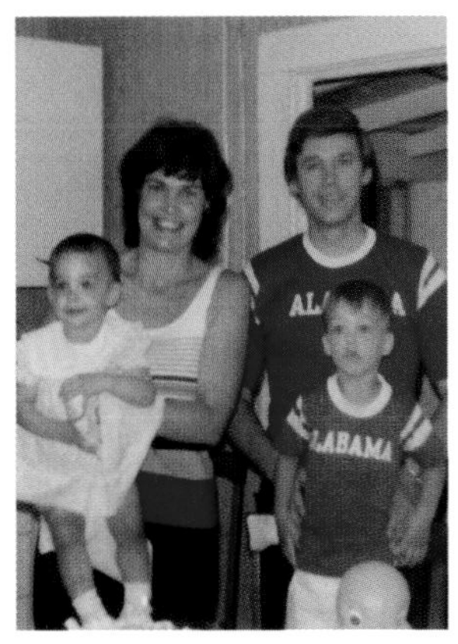

1. GO BIG OR GO HOME: If I got a tattoo (which I won't), it would likely say this. Dream and dream BIG. Fire it up! When it comes to my family's playbook, it's the go-to play. My daddy came from nothing and overcame much adversity. After he came home from the army, he was involved in a car accident that had him left for dead and in a full body cast for six months. He survived and chose to thrive. He taught me to take risks and reach for the stars. I get my guts from my dad.

2. ALWAYS BE NICE (TO EVERYONE): I mentioned it earlier, but it bears repeating. This is straight from my grandmother's mouth. It didn't matter who you were or what you did—she respected everyone. Be nice to assistants. Be nice to flight attendants. Be nice to your boss. Be nice, be nice, be nice. Don't overlook anyone. One day that assistant will be the vice president of the company you aspire to work for. When you are nice, and people like you, they will go out of their way for you.

3. DARE TO BE DIFFERENT: My momma challenged us to not just go with the flow or fly with the flock. There are a lot of rules in the South—but my mother encouraged me to be who I wanted to be. While other moms were encouraging their girls to stay inside the lines, my mom encouraged me to draw my own.

4. GOTTA PICK A LANE: A great piece of advice from my uncle Leslie: You've gotta pick a lane. You cannot drive in the middle of two lanes, or weave in and out of them. Neither can you drive in four lanes at once. Pick one. Choose your direction and drive.

5. DO, HOPE, LOVE: My brother, Todd, always says, "There are three things in life you need: something to do, something to hope for, and someone to love." This is what keeps my head on straight. It's pretty much the definition of sanity and I'd go as far to say, happiness. As long as you can check those three things off your list, you are doing pretty good.

6. FIND YOUR CHURCH: By that I mean, live for and believe in something bigger and greater than you. Maybe it's your community, maybe it's your family—maybe it's your religion. Believe in something.

never FEAR FAILURE

It's quoted a million times, but unbelievable to think: Michael Jordan did not make his high school basketball team. I mean—c'mon! Michael—f***ing—Jordan. I'm writing this section for those who need inspiration, for those who feel knocked down. You might look at successful people and think they've never been knocked down or even out. Trust me we have. But remember, failure is an event, not a person. Some of my biggest failures, or no's in life, are what ultimately led to my biggest successes.

When I was just starting to break into television, there was a model who was getting all kinds of great film and TV roles, and I was envious—I wasn't getting *any*. My agent said to me—let it go. Don't worry about it. You aren't her. You are different. It will happen for you. A few years later, just before I auditioned for *Las Vegas,* there was a role *I really wanted and didn't get*. I was devastated. The next week, I booked *Las Vegas,* became a series regular—and the show lasted five seasons. If I had gotten the other role, it would have prevented me from doing *Vegas*. And that model I mentioned? She has been in and out of rehab and in trouble with the law! The TRUTH IS my whole entire career is failure. I don't get 99% of the jobs I go in for. There have been a lot of things I've *really* wanted and didn't get. But that's okay, because what matters are the jobs I did. I always kept going.

---

supermodel *secret*

SEMPER FI

I've been with Next Model Management since day one—because they took a risk on me and believed in me. I've been with Maury DiMauro, my commercial agent, since we started working together ages ago. Same goes with my manager, Alissa Vradenburg—we've been together almost a decade. I don't have a million friends, but the ones I do have—I would walk across hot coals for. In this career, sometimes you're up, sometimes you're down, and loyalty can swing like a pendulum. I strive, however, to create stability in my relationships, personal and professional—and there's almost nothing more important to me than loyalty. My parents have been married for over thirty years and have given me the best example of that a girl could ask for. *Be loyal.*

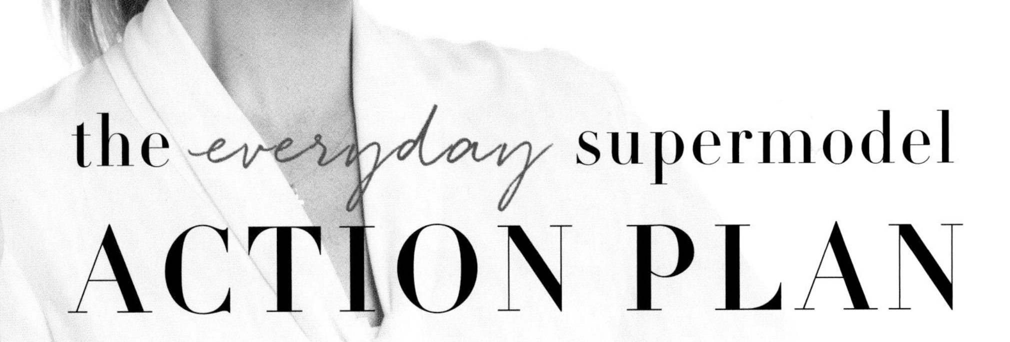

the *everyday* supermodel ACTION PLAN

I have always had a plan. Some of us set goals—as in save money for a vacation, be more organized, or work out more. But what about a life plan? Do you have one? Get one. Where do you want to be two years from now, five years from now, ten years from now? Set goals to go after that give your life direction, meaning, and purpose. Setting and chasing these down leaves a lot less room in your life for shoulda-woulda-couldas later on. As they say, if you don't build your own dreams, someone will hire you to build theirs. So what are you waiting for?

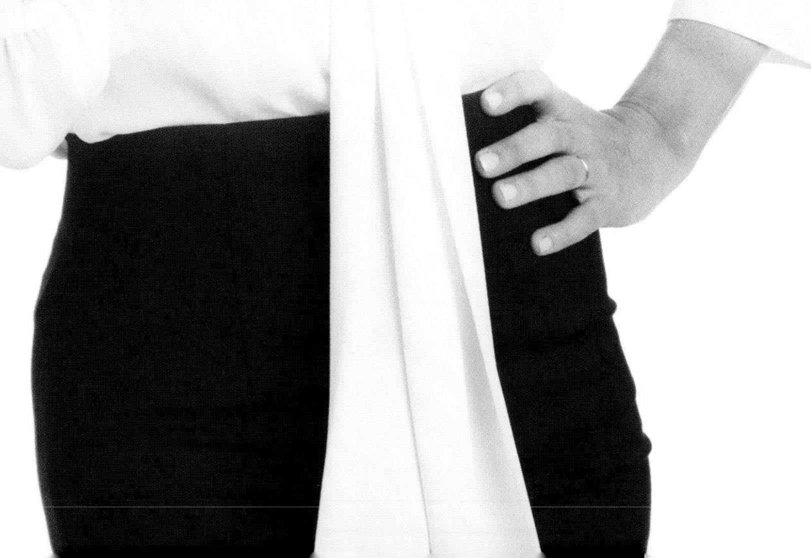

how to *goal* after it

1. **GOALS ARE GORGEOUS:** Make daily goals, monthly goals, yearly goals—and even goals by the decade. If you don't actually take the time to identify them, months and even years can go by—and nothing will have changed. Goal for it!

2. **BE SUPER(MODEL) SPECIFIC:** Be clear and defined about what you want. *I want to be financially stable* should really be =*I want to have XX number of dollars in the bank by XX time and secure a XX raise;* got me? Specific goals can be tracked and measured. Being able to track and measure progress is key to keeping you motivated.

3. **DECIDE AND CONQUER:** Direct energy is much more powerful than energy diffused. I read that Will Smith said there's no reason to have a Plan B because it distracts from Plan A. Focus your energy on the things that you really want and forget the rest.

4. **MAP OUT THE MAGIC:** Print up your plans, type 'em up, scribble them in a journal, send smoke signals. I don't care if you tattoo them on your arm, but say them, write them down, and make them known. Make a list of your dreams, and then create a map to making them happen. Break it down into smaller pieces. Identify people you can contact that can help, classes you can take, and steps you can make toward tackling your target.

5. **SAVE THE DATE:** Set deadlines. Deadlines will hold you accountable. It's all too easy to put things off, suspend action, make excuses . . . and never get around to it. And who doesn't work a little better under the pressure of a deadline? On that same note, prioritize. Don't put your dreams on the back burner. A lot of us do this out of fear. Make them front and center.

6. **SETBACKS = STEP BACKS:** Have specific goals in mind, but be open to them evolving and changing as new opportunities present themselves. Importantly, think of setbacks merely as *step backs*. They give you a chance to recalibrate and renew faith in your cause or redirect if necessary.

7. **GET FIRED UP!:** Get passionate about what you want. And *Rollll Tide!* Goals charged with spirit, soul, and sass have more strength and momentum than your average ho-hum desire. Recruit others as cheerleaders to be excited with you and *for you*. When you are feeling flustered, your fans on the sidelines will empower you forward. And I've said it before, if you have to—*be your own cheer captain!*

8. **CELEBRATE SUCCESSES:** Give yourself credit when credit is due. Take the time to acknowledge the small achievements and the big ones. Celebrate! Feel good about yourself—you did it. Don't just move on to the next goal without recognizing and honoring yourself and the people who got you to this one . . . Review what you did right, what worked to get you there, and congratulate yourself.

9. **HIRE YOURSELF:** If you want to be a writer, start working for yourself and writing. If you want to learn to be great at marketing, read every book and blog you can on the subject. Give yourself a job and just start doing it. Don't wait for someone else to hire you if it isn't happening. You start making it happen on your own—and the rest will begin to fall in line.

10. **GO THE EXTRA MILE:** We really do accomplish more when we push ourselves. Just think about your muscles. It's the same with our minds or our careers. We are often taught to do whatever we can to avoid pain. Sometimes going the extra mile feels good—aka runner's high! And sometimes it's painful—and it hurts. But that's the magic hour. That's when you find out there is *more within you* than meets the eye. You have more strides in you; reserves you didn't think you had. When you push yourself and always do your best—there will never be room for regrets.

---

supermodel *secret*

A NOTE TO YOURSELF

Be the person you *aspire to be*. Get rid of the bullsh*t in your life. Start now. Get to it! If you smoke and you don't like that about yourself: stop smoking. Decide today that you are a nonsmoker, and begin to take the steps toward that status. I did. If you want to start your own business, but don't know anything about running one, start learning. Take a night class. Read some books. Listen to some TED talks. If you want to lose weight . . . stop waiting! Do not do these things for anyone else but you. Get after it and before you know it, you'll have done it.

---

mentor *messages*

Leigh Kilton is my acting coach and mentor. She is a certified Hollywood heavyweight and coaches some of the most well-respected actors on this earth. As if that wasn't enough, she started an orphanage, Friends of El Faro (www.friendsofelfaro.com), and has sheltered, fed, loved, and found homes for hundreds of children. Her coaching is not only relevant to a good scene or a great audition, but it's also relevant to living a full life.

Leigh on Love, Life, and Listening:

1. **Be, be, be, don't do, do do.** "I'm afraid I'm not doing enough—I'm not enough." Does this feel familiar? Take a breath, *take a moment*. We can overact so much in our own lives that all we are doing is *doing* . . . and we aren't *being*. In acting, your performance is as much about *what you don't do* as what you do. *Give applause to the pause.*

2. **Nobody is perfect so stop trying to be.** There is no such thing as perfect. Work hard, try hard—but be real. Authenticity is what is most appreciated and attractive. Be your authentic self and things will start to flow.

3. **Enjoy the process. The struggle is so courageous.** The decision to go after something you want—to be an entrepreneur or an artist or a mom—takes strength. Don't wait to be happy. Don't avoid the struggle or the challenges. The pursuit itself is the point.

4. **Resist the cancer of comparison.** This can destroy a person. Do not compare—when we compare, we instinctively diminish our own light. Trust your own path and follow it all the way. As the saying goes: *Be yourself. Everyone else is already taken.*

5. **Listen with the intent to understand, not respond.** One of my favorite Kilton-isms. We are always in such a rush to tell our story and hear our own selves talk. Are we even listening to what others have to say? Every now and again, shut up and listen!

6. **And finally . . . Don't mistake my kindness for weakness**. Be kind. But be firm. Being kind does not mean being a doormat. Leigh actually made me a T-shirt that says that very thing.

KILTON'S MUST-READS: *The Dude and the Zen Master* by Jeff Bridges, *Spirituality of Imperfection* by Ernest Kurtz and Katherine Ketcham, and *Let the Great World Spin* by Colum McCann.

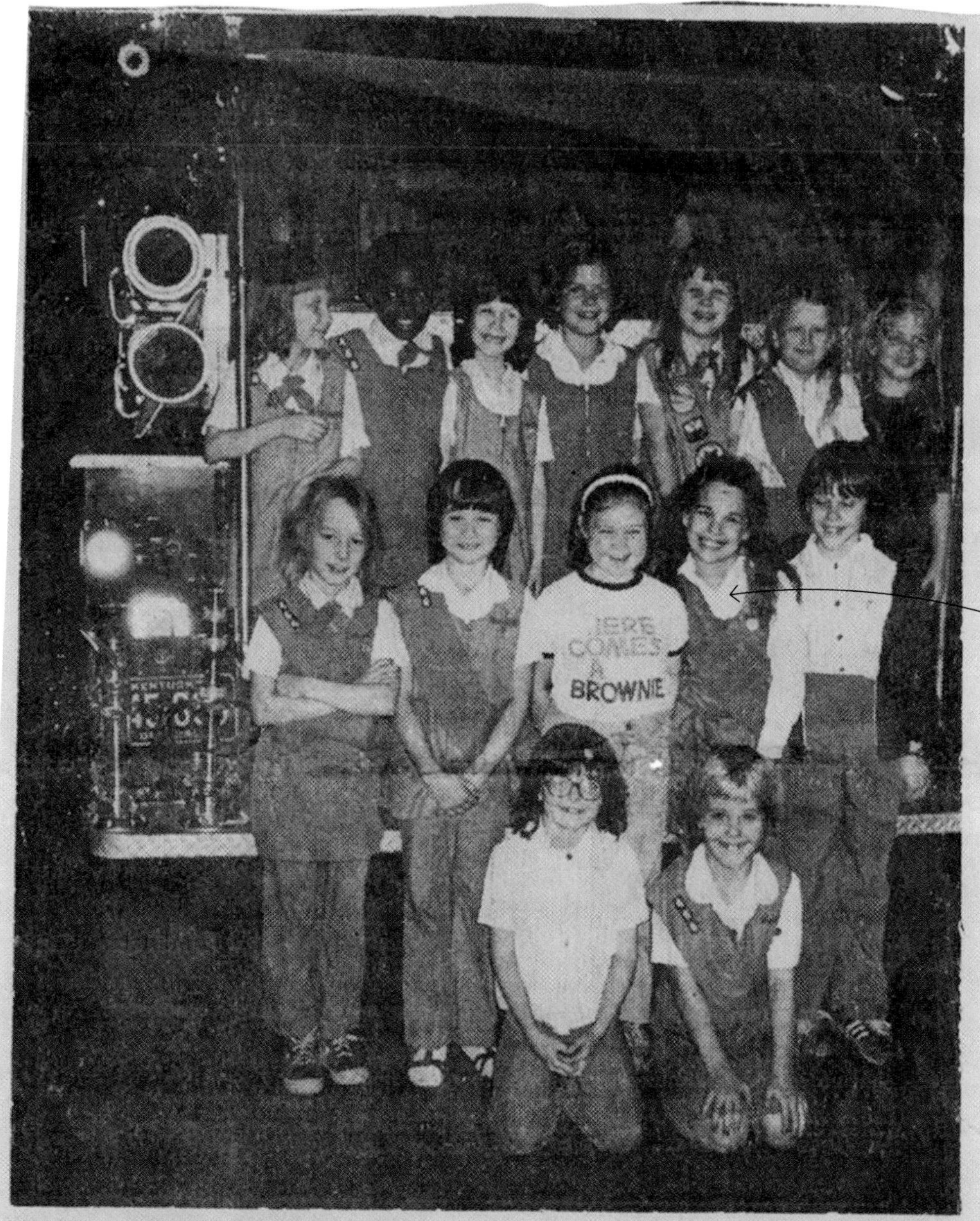

VISIT FIRE STATION — Brownie Scout Troop 466, of East College School are pictured on a recent tour of the fire station on North Sixth Street.

that's me!

Even as a Girl Scout, I knew hard work paid off.

BUILD YOUR *friedship superforce.* Science tells us having a support system is key to a long, healthy life. I wouldn't be where I am without mine (Michelle Lokey Carlson, and the rest, you know who you are). I do believe it takes a village. When it comes to your friends, be good to them. And know their value. Real friends are like family and have proven health benefits that beat Prozac. Know the difference between a real friend and a cyber one. Always support your friend when it's her time to shine. Make her chicken soup when she's sick. Laugh the loudest when she's giving a speech. Know when to offer an opinion—or simply listen.

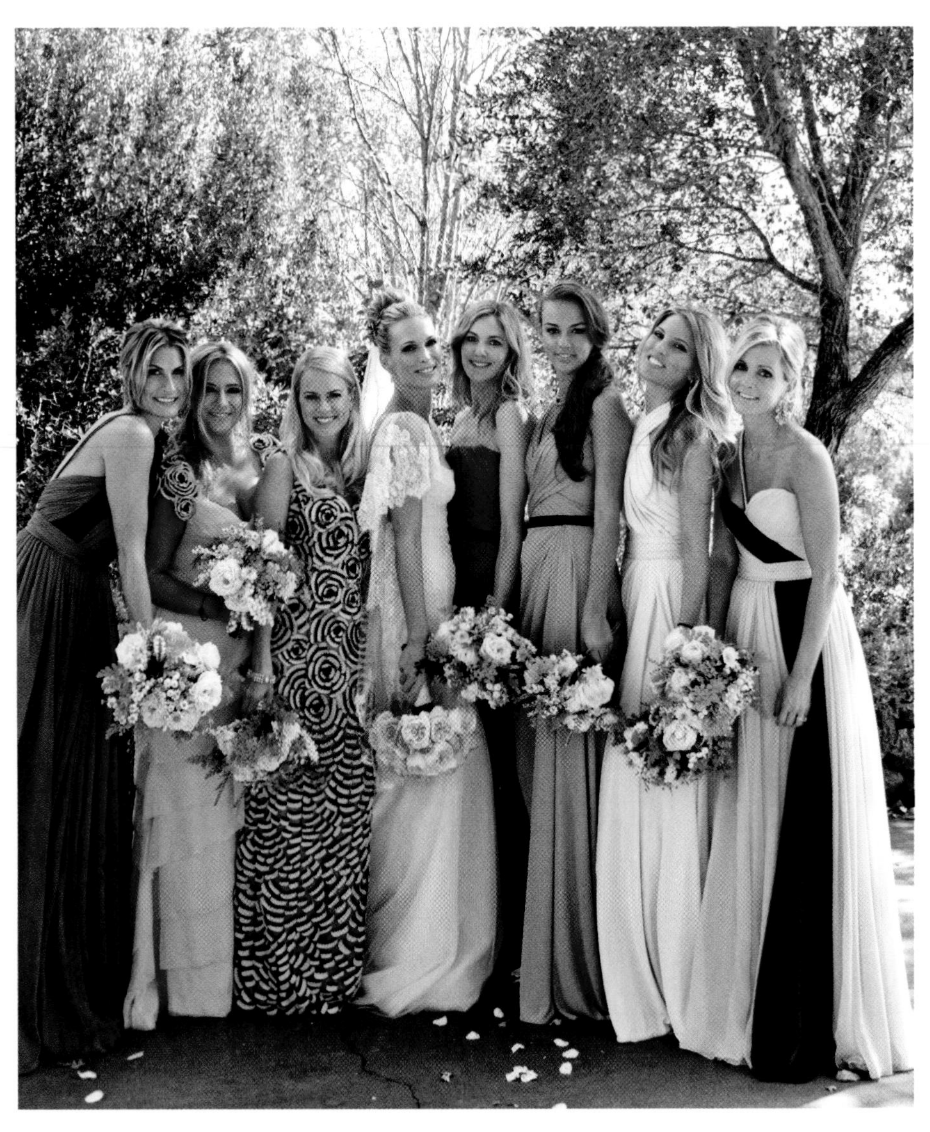

supermomma secret

HELP WANTED.

Becoming a mom for me was something I'd always wanted to do—but it was like learning a new language. So I made mom friends. They were like my Rosetta Stone for parenting. Friend moms told me what stroller was the best, what bottles to use, what supplements to try when my milk wasn't coming in. Psychologically, they helped me too. All these feelings (anxiety, love, fear, exhaustion, elation), were they normal? Without this new community of moms I wouldn't have survived. As much as independence is exalted by the modern woman, we aren't meant to act or survive in isolation. Don't burn yourself out trying to do it all. Rather, build your community.

Road Rules for Being *happy, healthy, & hot*

- **YOU ARE NOT ON SALE:** Listen up! There's a time and a place for free work, trade, and doing things on spec. But *stop* blue-light-specialing yourself. Women are still paid significantly less in the workplace for the same jobs. Many women don't think it's feminine to negotiate and when we do, we often don't know how to negotiate effectively. If you aren't good at negotiating, then find someone to negotiate on your behalf. Know your worth.
- **FOLLOW YOUR GUT:** Studies show that even babies know when *something is off*. Trust your instincts. And, ladies, we are good at this. When someone does something or says something that just doesn't feel right, you may have picked up on something subtle, but that carries a serious message.
- **BLOCK THE DREAM SUCKERS:** There are those who energize and those who suck the energy out of a room. These leechy-von-leechmeisters will bleed you and your dreams dry, leaving you feeling tired and talentless. Choose who you listen to carefully. And be aware. Dream Suckers can be disguised as your friends and even family—so steer clear of these good-vibe vampires at all costs.
- **ASSEMBLE YOUR DREAM TEAM:** Presidents, surgeons, designers, chefs—none of us get where we are without a lot of support. I have an agent, a manager, a lawyer, a nanny—and frankly—the list goes on. As my business and family has grown, so has my team. Your "dream team"

is about support. For each one of us it's going to be different. Find that go-to dry cleaners, the babysitter you can call in a pinch, a financial advisor that cares, a doctor that will actually give you her cell number. Assemble yours.

- **GOTTA GIVE TO GET:** I believe in the Golden Rule, karma, and in paying it forward! For me, philanthropy is more like *Feel-anthropy*. I donate time and resources to several charities. I always feel like I get back so much more than I give! Along with Friends of El Faro, I also work with Baby 2 Baby, an organization that helps mothers in need. By shifting the focus from you to others, you foster a connection to your community and a general feeling of shared goodwill. If you don't feel you have time to volunteer, simple, daily acts of charity count too. A compliment. A helping hand. It all adds up.
- **KNOW WHEN TO FOLD 'EM:** Courtesy of Kenny Rogers. Basically, this is the serenity prayer. When you've tried at something with all your might, and you've given it your best—maybe it's just not in the cards. I had to do this with breast-feeding. I tried absolutely everything, but it just didn't work. Accept and move on. Learn from it. Fuh-get-about-it in a good way.
- **GET GRATEFUL:** Instead of counting sheep, I count my blessings. Gratitude is a lifestyle and it's a way of looking at life consistently. Recognize and give thanks for every achievement and blessed moment in your life. *Watch your mouth and your mind.* Focusing on the negative can expand the negative. Whatever we focus on grows. We can just as easily face the sun rather than turn our back on the light.

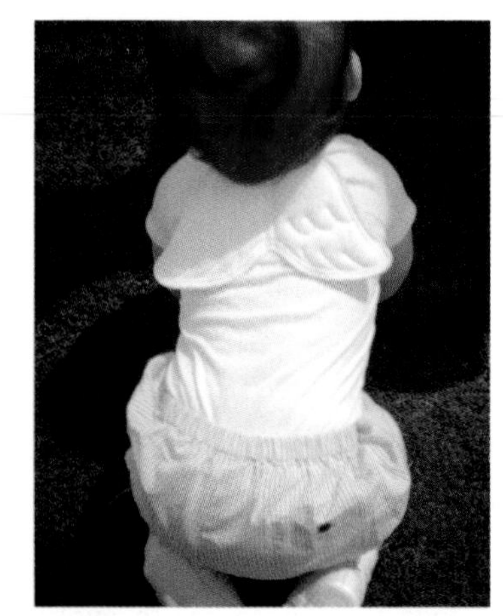

- **HAVE FUN:** Advice courtesy of actress Kate Walsh—and it's so true! "Fun is highly underrated. When I was going through a particularly painful time in my life, a very wise woman asked me every day, 'So what are you doing for fun?' I was, like, 'Fun?! How can I have fun?! I'm being tortured over here!' She made me realize that even in the midst of a sh*tstorm, you can still do something fun."

I still think of this sweet girl from Kentucky. Who wanted something so badly, and she just went for it. She did it, and she did it great. She's a uniquely authentic young woman. Watching her evolve and seeing her become a wife and mother. It just constantly impresses me. She continues to push herself and grow and take on new and different challenges.

—MAURY DIMAURO, commercial agent

SUPERMODEL *secret*: CONFIDENCE IS CHARISMA

You never have to be the smartest, prettiest, tallest, richest, funniest, or whatever-ist to be a success and stand out. Head-turning self-confidence will take you further than any pair of posh pumps ever will. Confidence makes a girl a woman—and it is always gorgeous. There is nothing more powerful and mountain-moving than faith in yourself. It's why I wrote this book. Acceptance, love *for* YOU, and belief *in* YOU are the fundamental elements of confidence. I believe that working to be the *everyday supermodel* version of ourselves does lead to improved confidence, acceptance, and appreciation for the unique individuals that we are. Be the best you, you can be. Be so good that no one will forget you, because they won't be able to! Being an *everyday supermodel* isn't just about looking like one, it's about acting like one.

WHERE I AM *today*

I am now in my forties.

I thought it would feel awful, but it feels f***ing fantastic. What a relief! I am more content now than ever before, and amazingly, at thirty I wasn't. I have a career I love that continues to evolve and challenge me each day. I am constantly being presented new and exciting opportunities—and some crappy ones. But where I am now, I *know that I don't have to take those jobs if I don't want to.* I have worked hard to get where I am today—and will continue to work hard to get where I will be tomorrow. My husband and I love each other, and we have fun

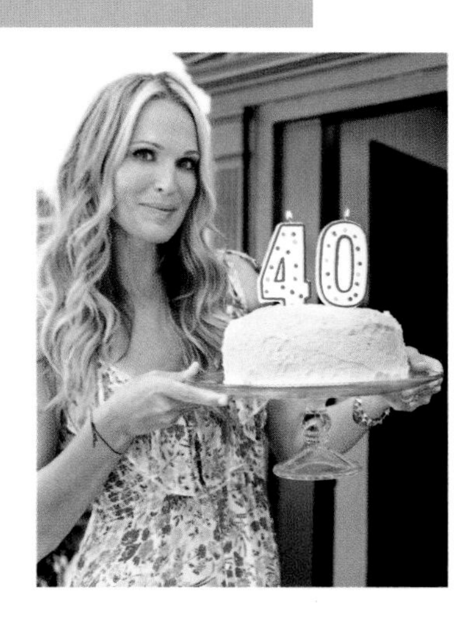

together. We wake up in the mornings and smile because we know we are on this journey together. He is here to support me, and I'm here to do the same for him. It took both of us a while to get here. But let me tell you, it was worth the wait and all the heartbreaks. I wouldn't change anything.

Every choice I've made, good and bad, brought me here. The one thing I do know—I did not get here on my own. It took the love and support of so many people along the way. And this book *clearly shows that*. The movie of my life, up to now—would be named after this chapter, "I Made That Sh*t Happen." The subtitle? "With *a lot* of help along the way!" This super-momma-model did not do this alone. My acting coach and friend, Leigh Kilton, has actors put a Post-it note on the back side of their front door that says: I AM JUST BEGINNING. And I finally believe it. And so are you.

Every day you wake up, you are a given a blank page. It's your time to start fresh. Begin to write what *you want* on it.

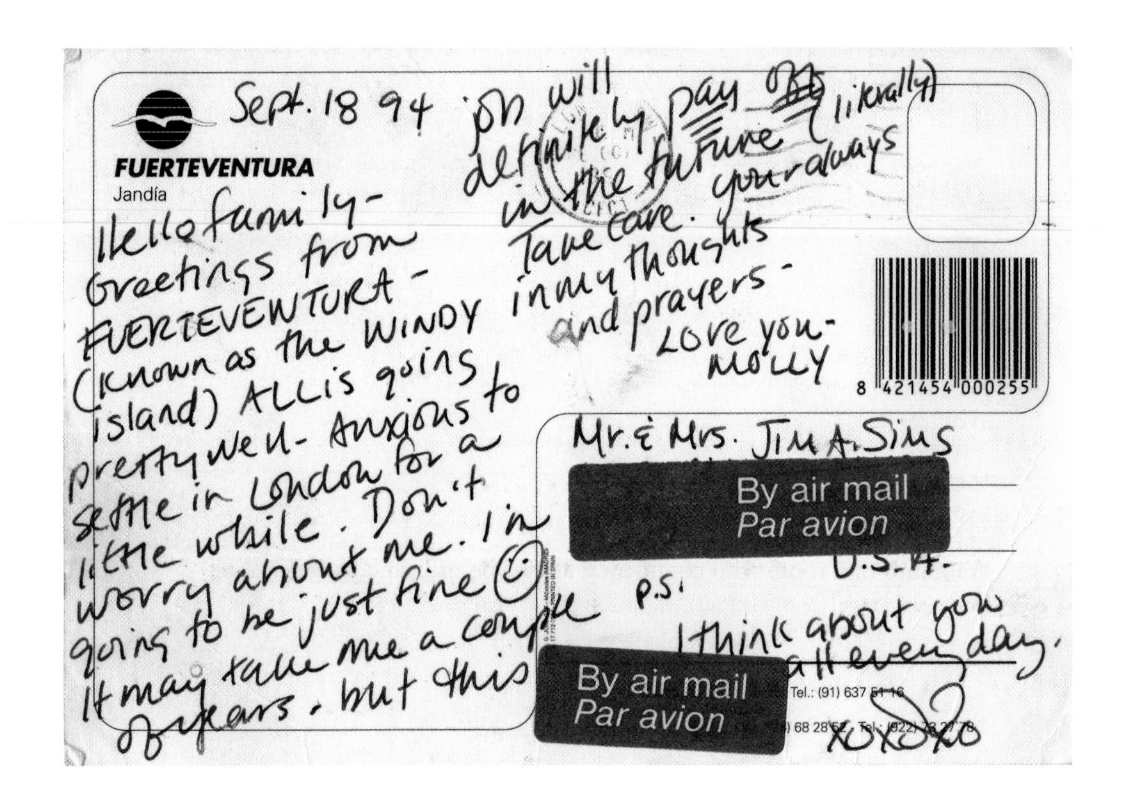

FUERTEVENTURA
Jandía

Sept. 18 94

Hello family-
Greetings from
FUERTEVENTURA -
(known as the WINDY
island) ALL is going
pretty well - Anxious to
settle in London for a
little while. Don't
worry about me. I'm
going to be just fine ☺
It may take me a couple
of years. but this will
definitely pay off (literally)
in the future.
Take care. your always
in my thoughts
and prayers -
LOVE you -
MOLLY

8 421454 000255

Mr. & Mrs. JIM A. SIMS

By air mail
Par avion

U.S.A.

P.S.
I think about you
all every day.
XOXOXO

By air mail
Par avion

the *everyday* supermodel TOP 10 takeaways

1. Start being in charge of your life, right now. There is no reason to wait. You have only one life to live, you might as well live it!

2. Identify what you want and what you don't. If something isn't right, figure out what's wrong so that you can do something about it.

3. Change things up. Doing different things different ways helps you to get unstuck and out of a rut!

4. Face your fears and chase down your dreams. Persist and do not give up. See setbacks as *step backs* and problems as *opportunities* for solutions.

5. Be honest, up front, and open about what you want. Work hard, demand the best for yourself, and don't settle. Expect the best from others.

6. No one is perfect, so don't try to be. Let the past go, embrace the present, and start creating your future.

7. Get a plan. Put it on paper. Write down steps to making it happen. Baby steps and big ones and start crossing things off the list.

8. Recruit your team, friends, family, work associates—your superforce—your village, to help you achieve your goals. You can't do it alone. So don't even try.

9. Know when to fold 'em; let it go and move on.

10. Walk into that room with confidence, always be nice, and leave a lasting impression.

acknowledgments

The Everyday Supermodel was many years in the making!

Special contributors I'd love to thank: Gia Canali and Matt Manus for the beautiful photography. Rebecca Klein and Martina Gordon (The ReStylists), for their styling and timeless fashion contributions. Chef Gavan Murphy for the healthy recipes and Rebecca Baer for nutrition and weight loss strategies. Dr. Karyn Grossman for top-shelf skincare secrets. Joey Maalouf, Davy Newkirk, Monika Blunder Prensena, and Adriana Tesler for hair and makeup tips and styling. Maria Kelling for keeping me toned and Tracey Cunningham and Michelle Pugh for keeping me blonde.

Thank you to all the other mavens of health, beauty, fitness, and fashion who contributed to this book by quote or advice: Cindy Crawford, for her inspiration and wisdom. Tracy Anderson, Alycea Ungaro, Amanda Freeman, Nicole Honnig, and Lori Bregman for health and fitness. Miwa Kobayashi, Kristie Streicher, Riki B., Caile Noble, Gianpaolo Ceciliato, Johnny Wright, Matthew Monzon, Frankie Foye, and Dr. Haleh Bakshandeh for beauty banter. Dr. Shahin Ghadir, and Dr. Michelle Hakakha for pregnancy tips. Dr. Mary Goldenson on success strategies. Rachel Zoe for fierce fashion and Michelle Vick and Erin Bunch for frugal fashion. Stefanie Cove and Yifat Oren for making my world pretty. To the other beauties in my business for sharing secrets: Abbey Lee Kershaw, Ali Larter, Anja Rubik, Brooklyn Decker, Elettra Wiedemann, Fergie, Jessica Alba, and Kate Walsh. Gratitude to companies: SoulCycle, WeCare, Beyond Yoga, and Getty Images.

Thank you Courtney Flynn for your total commitment and make sh*t happen skills. Hugs to my hardworking on-set crew: Todd Parker, Shawn Corrigan, Anthony Francis, Angel Ramos, Clark Perry, Jason Murphy, and Lindsay Groman.

Endless gratitude to my loyal and dedicated team who have been there for me through thick and thin (literally). I would be nowhere without you: to Faith Kates Kogan, Joel Wilkinfeld, Leigh Crystal, Maury DiMauro, James Adams, Leonard Schlangel, and Ekaterina Klimentova. To Adam Sher, the reason I came to LA. To Gary Scott Thompson for believing in me/Delinda. To Alissa Vradenberg: thank you from the bottom of my heart for making my dreams come true. Special thanks to Leigh Crystal for being my mother, friend, and agent for twenty years. Thank you to my website guru, Tracy Reynolds Rice, and my social media guru, Bianca Posterli. Much appreciation to Brooke Slavik Jung and Andy McNicol and my creative and devoted editors: Carrie Thornton and Brittany Hamblin.

To my tribe of girlfriends who support me at all times: Michelle Lokey Carlson, Jessica Berg Prosser, Lauren Kucerak, Leigh Kilton Smith, Emese Gormley, Danielle DeMarne, Mimi Brown, and Robyn Casady. And finally to Tracy O'Connor: Thank you for your vision, making my words sparkle, and bringing this book to life. We did it!

To my beautiful family without whom I am nothing. You taught me to "Go big, or go home!": My parents, Dorothy and Jim Sims, and my brother and sister-in-law, Todd and Alexis Sims. And of course to my baby boy, Brooks Alan Stuber, and my partner and husband, Scott Stuber. I love you more than words can say.

And finally to all my friends and my fans: Thank you for all of your love throughout the years. I sincerely hope this book gives you the tools and encouragement you need to discover the *everyday supermodel* that is within you. It is a pleasure for me to share it with you.

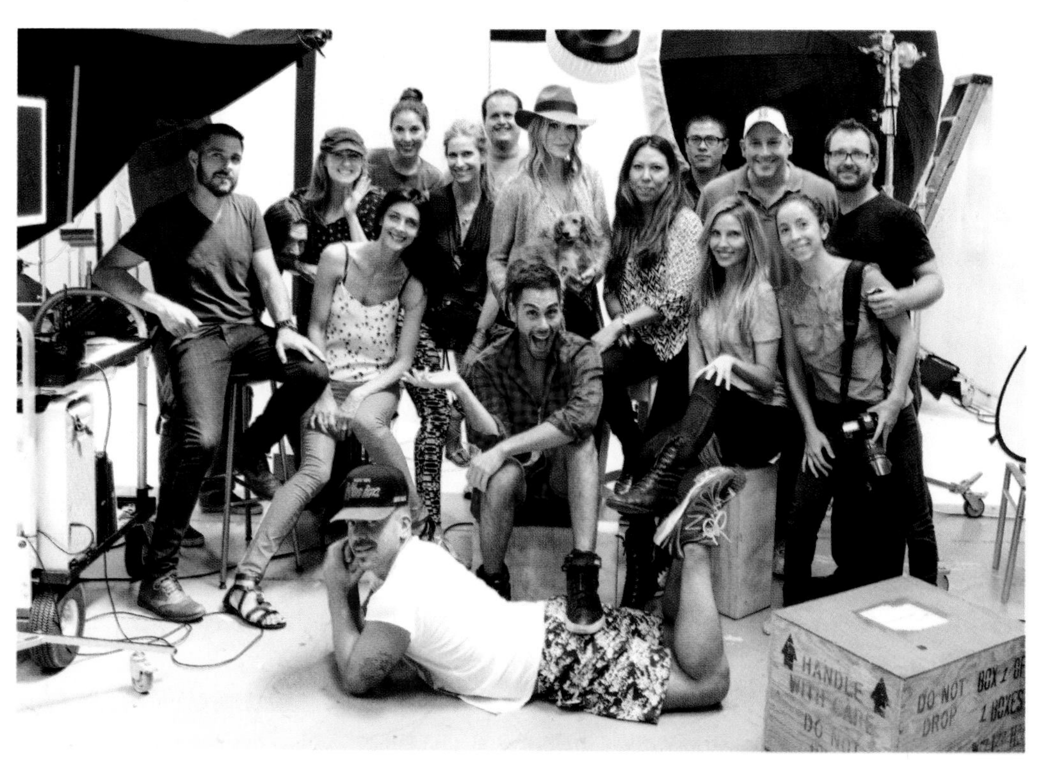

index

NOTE: Page references in *italics* indicate photographs.

---

f

g

h

Photographs on pages: i, xiii, 1, 2, 69, 118, 119, 123 (left), 161 (right), 179, 182, 201, 206 (top), 207, 231 (far left and far right), 242, 243, 251 (left), 251 (middle right), 253, 254, 296 (right), 298, 303, 304 (left), 309, 315, 318, and 320 all courtesy of Molly Sims.

Photographs on pages 3: Justin Lubin/NBC/NBCU Photo Bank via Getty Images; 5: Walter Iooss Jr. /*Sports Illustrated*/Contour by Getty Images; 9 and 112 (left): Jason LaVeris/FilmMagic; 10: Courtesy of *Self* magazine; 27: Creative Crop/Getty Images; 29: Maria Kallin/Getty Images; 35: John Block/Getty Images; 43: Courtesy of Gavin Murphy; 46–47: Tonic Photo Studios, LLC/Getty Images; 49: Walter Iooss Jr. /*Sports Illustrated*/Contour by Getty Images; 77: Courtesy of *Shape* magazine; 112 (right): Kevin Winter/Getty Images; 120: Courtesy of *Lucky* magazine; 121 (top left): Peter Kramer/Getty Images; 121 (top middle): Larry Busacca/Getty Images; 121 (top right) Stephen Lovekin/Getty Images; 121 (bottom left): Jamie McCarthy/WireImage; 121 (bottom middle): Jon Kopaloff/FilmMagic; 121 (bottom right): SGranitz/WireImage; 122: Courtesy of Rebecca Klein and Martina Gordon; 135: Jeff Vespa/WireImage; 144: Courtesy of Rachel Zoe; 161 (left): Evan Agostini/Image-Direct; 169 (left): George Pimentel/WireImage; 169 (right): Stephen Lovekin/Getty Images; 181: Courtesy of *Allure* magazine; 194: Frederick M. Brown/Getty Images; 203: Kevin Winter/Getty Images; 231 (middle): Jeff Vespa/WireImage; 235: KMazur/WireImage; 245: Courtesy of *Cosmopolitan* magazine; 251 (middle left): Jim Spellman/WireImage; 251 (right): Jon Kopaloff/FilmMagic; 263 (left): Alberto E. Rodriguez/WireImage; 263 (right): Marcel Thomas/FilmMagic; 265: Stefanie Keenan/Getty Images for Chopard; 273: SGranitz/Wireimage; 284: Kevin Mazur/WireImage; 302: Courtesy of *Vogue*; 304 (left): D. Kambouris/WireImage; 307: Mitchell Haaseth/NBC/NBCU Photo Bank via Getty Images.

All other photographs by Gia Canali.
